By Mike and Nancy Samuels:

SEEING WITH THE MIND'S EYE:
    The History, Techniques
    and Uses of Visualization
THE WELL BABY BOOK
THE WELL CHILD BOOK
THE WELL CHILD COLORING BOOK

Other books co-authored by Mike Samuels
(with Hal Z. Bennett):

THE WELL BODY BOOK
SPIRIT GUIDES:
    Access to Inner Worlds
BE WELL
WELL BODY, WELL EARTH

MIKE SAMUELS, M.D.
NANCY SAMUELS

illustrated by
WENDY FROST

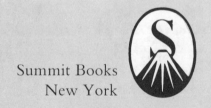

Summit Books
New York

The
WELL
PREGNANCY
BOOK

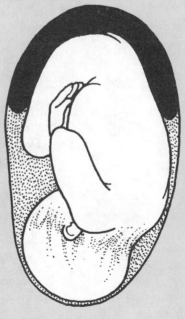

To all pregnant women who look forward to birth with hope and anticipation,
to the people who help them to deliver joyfully,
and to our own mothers, Grayce and Florence

Published by SUMMIT BOOKS
A Division of Simon & Schuster, Inc.
Simon & Schuster Building
1230 Avenue of the Americas
New York, New York 10020
SUMMIT BOOKS and colophon are trademarks of
Simon & Schuster, Inc.
Designed by JENNIE NICHOLS / Levavi & Levavi
Manufactured in the United States of America
3   5   7   9   10   8   6   4   2
First Edition
Library of Congress Cataloging in Publication Data
Samuels, Mike.
The well pregnancy book.
Includes bibliographies and index.
1. Pregnancy.   2. Childbirth.   I. Samuels, Nancy.
II. Title.   [DNLM: 1. Pregnancy—popular works.
WQ 150 S193w]
RG525.S34   1985   618.2   85-9726
ISBN 0-671-55549-9
ISBN 0-671-46080-3 (pbk.)

Contents

Acknowledgments

We would like to thank all the people who contributed to this book—Jim Silberman, our publisher, for conceiving the idea to write a pregnancy book, and Ileene Smith, our editor, for laboring alongside us and helping us deliver the book. Once again we thank our wonderful illustrator, Wendy Frost, for producing the best pregnancy drawings we've ever seen. She continues to draw people's bodies in a way that radiates health and reassurance. We also appreciate the care with which Meryl Levavi designed the book shortly after the birth of her second baby, and the careful way in which Rina Cascone copyedited the manuscript. As always we are indebted to our literary agent, Elaine Markson, and to Geri Toma, for their steady support and good advice.

We especially want to thank two of the people who help women give birth joyfully—Dr. Jon Schwartz, an obstetrician, and Nancy Friedrich, a midwife. Both read the manuscript thoughtfully and commented on it based on their knowledge and skill. Several people generously shared their photographs, and we wish to thank them also—Christi and Joel, Gail, and Regan.

As always, we want to thank our boys, Rudy and Lewis, the babies we joyfully gave birth to, for their patience and understanding during the many times their parents were laboring over this book. Thanks too to the relatives and friends who gave freely of their time to help us or look after the boys: Florence and Iggy; Hope, Owen, Wen, Laurie, and Greg; Linda; Elizabeth, Sean, Liam, and Miss Kate.

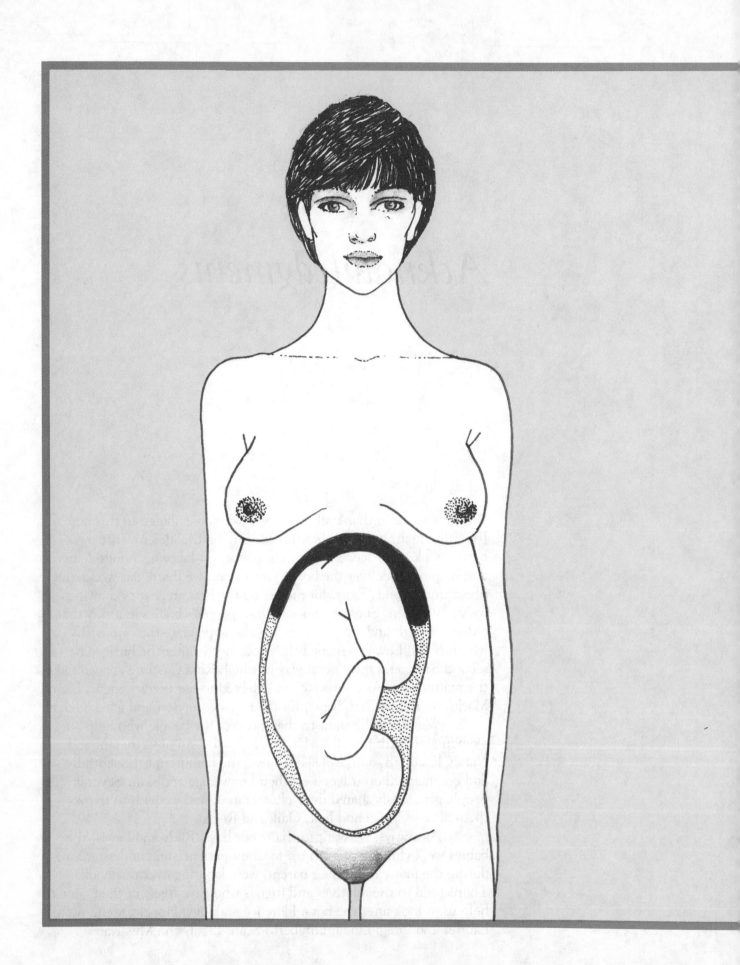

SECTION
I

An
Overview

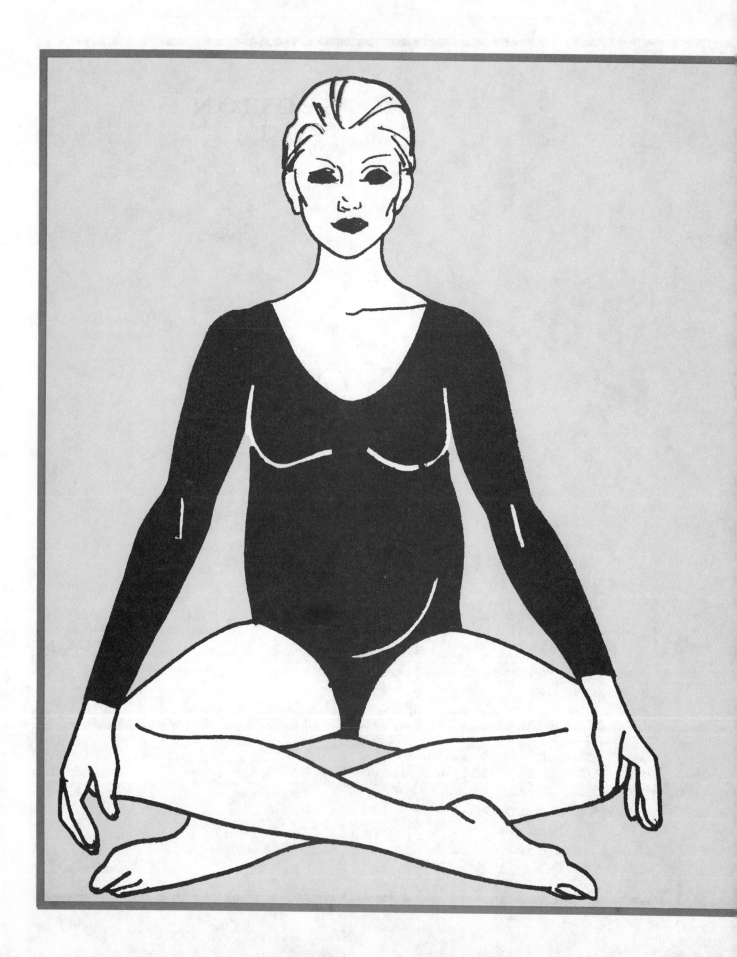

Introduction

How We Came to Write This Book

This is the first book in a series. The second and third books have already been written. In 1976 we wrote a self-help medical book called *The Well Baby Book*, which we began just before the birth of our second child. The book was specifically written for new parents, and its goal was to help create happy, healthy babies. We did not give parents any dogmatic solutions or advice, but tried to provide them with a broad understanding of growth and development, of health and disease, so that they could make their own choices about patterns that would contribute to their baby's lifelong health. Our next book, *The Well Child Book*, was written as our children started to grow up. It also pursued the objectives of wellness and preventive medicine, but for the age group of four to twelve.

We began the present book because we realized that the same concerns needed to be addressed in terms of pregnancy. There was a lot of information that still was not readily available to the lay person, and much that needed to be demystified. We wanted to give expectant mothers and fathers information on the normal processes of pregnancy and childbirth, so that they would develop confidence in the mother's body and a profound respect for the natural changes her body would undergo during the course of gestation. We believe such information helps because it replaces fear of the unknown with understanding, enables parents to avoid those things that might have negative effects on the baby, and gives parents a realistic basis for positive images of labor and delivery. Our goal in *The Well Pregnancy Book* is to help foster happy, healthy pregnancies with good deliveries and healthy babies. In this book we try not to give rigid answers or advice, but to make parents aware of the way pregnancy is currently managed so they will be able to make their own choices and feel comfortable and satisfied with the outcome.

Birth is a natural process that women and babies have evolved over millions of years. Both mother and baby are eminently suited to play out their parts in the processes of fertilization, conception, gestation, labor, and delivery. If a mother were asked to "design" a baby, "grow" it, and bring it forth from her body, she could not do it. Yet her body has the wisdom to do just that in a manner that never ceases to be miraculous. So an expectant mother's learning doesn't have to do with how to grow a baby but with helping her body do what it instinctively knows how to, without getting in its way.

Basically there are two major ways in which expectant mothers hinder their own bodies—one is physical, the other is mental. In terms of the mother's physical environment, her diet, exercise, exposure to chemicals, and general health are all important variables. Doc-

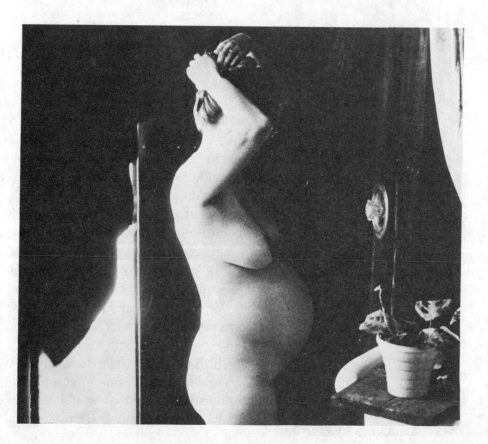

Our goal is to help foster healthy pregnancies, healthy deliveries, and healthy babies. Photo by Michael Samuels.

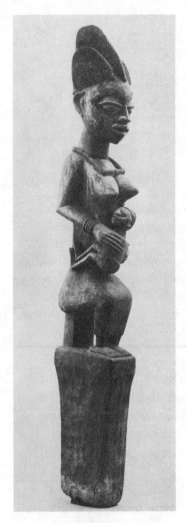

Birth is a natural process that women and babies have evolved over millions of years. Mother and Child, Yoruba. The Metropolitan Museum of Art. The Michael C. Rockefeller Memorial Collection, The Diana Woolman Memorial Collection, 1973.

tors are beginning to learn that certain things in these categories will help the mother's body work at its best, while others may impede it. For example, a baby is much more likely to be healthy if its mother has an optimal diet than if her diet is deficient in calories or protein. In terms of the mother's mental environment, her experiences and her perceptions of them are the important variables. The less fear, stress, and anxiety the mother experiences, the less complicated her pregnancy and delivery are likely to be. Blood flow to the uterus, which controls the delivery of food and oxygen and the removal of waste products, is governed by the *autonomic nervous system,* the unconscious branch of the nervous system. When a mother can relax and visualize positive images, blood flow to the uterus is maximized; her body tends to nurture the baby in an optimum way during pregnancy and to promote the most effective contractions during labor and delivery. A relaxed, reassured mother who is knowledgeable and feels loved and supported is able to keep out of her body's way by releasing tension and fear, and allowing her body to take over with the inborn skills it has evolved over the centuries. In *The Well Body Book,* Michael referred to this kind of inborn body wisdom as the *three-million-year-old healer.* In this book, in a similar way, we visualize that each pregnant woman has inside her a *three-million-year-old mother.* When a woman lets go of fear and tension, her three-million-year-old mother is free to work at her best.

Having a Baby Today

Having a baby at this time in our culture not only requires a mother to let her three-million-year-old mother work at its best, it requires her to be able to understand and deal with technical medical knowledge when necessary. Modern medicine has tools that have helped to optimize the chances of a healthy pregnancy and delivery in certain situations. But these tools and techniques are too new to have become part of any mother's age-old bioprograms or cultural patterns. Mothers may find certain medical techniques to be anxiety producing and in conflict with their instinctual feelings. Thus some midwives, childbirth educators, and doctors believe that medical intervention can be counterproductive in some instances, working against the natural processes involved in pregnancy and birth. This is the dilemma of modern obstetrics, and it has led to a split between those who feel they want as natural a pregnancy and delivery as possible and those who feel that medical intervention during pregnancy and delivery maximizes the health of the mother and, particularly, the health of the baby.

Most women having a baby in the United States today—and an increasing number of expectant mothers throughout the world—will experience some degree of medical intervention during their preg-

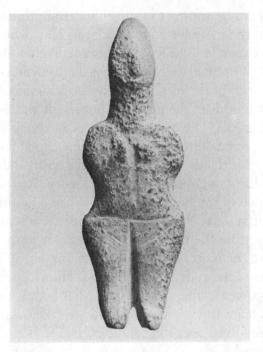

Every woman's body has inborn wisdom about pregnancy and childbirth. We visualize this wisdom as a three-million-year-old mother. Cycladic stone sculpture, 3000–2500 B.C. The Metropolitan Museum of Art. Rogers Fund, 1945.

nancy or delivery. Thus we feel that it is important to include information on the most commonly used procedures and laboratory tests, as well as on cesarean birth. We believe that the more a mother understands about such medical practices, about their rationale and the choices open to her, the less frightened or upset she will be in dealing with them.

Every mother and father hope for a magical delivery, and this is true of many births, but it is unfortunately not the reality of every one. We hope to help *all* mothers achieve as positive a childbirth experience as possible among a realistic range of possibilities. We acknowledge that not every woman will have an uneventful, joyful birth, although our wish is to facilitate just that outcome. For this reason we have not chosen to deal exclusively with home deliveries, technical deliveries, or prepared childbirth. We have attempted to make the book useful for as diverse a group of mothers and fathers as possible. This was a complex task because of the great divergence that presently exists between natural and technical obstetrics, and because of the wide scope in the guidelines for managing certain obstetrical situations. We've tried to make the material in the book as applicable for a mother having a home delivery as for a high-risk mother having a cesarean birth, by concentrating on the fundamental events and feelings as well as on the various ways of handling different situations. We have focused on anatomy and physiology to see how the three-million-year-old mother normally works. And we have shown through numerous studies how different factors affect fetal development and birth. We have emphasized how relaxation and support help *any* mother have a more positive pregnancy and birth experience. All this information enables parents to make educated choices and to take more responsibility throughout gestation and delivery. Studies have shown that the single most important factor in helping to ensure a mother's satisfaction with her delivery is her feeling that she was an active participant and had a measure of control over the situation. To make choices and have control, a mother needs to understand the alternatives and the reasons for them.

We see *The Well Pregnancy Book* as an adjunct for childbirth preparation classes, not a substitute for them. Not only can the birth educator answer parents' individual questions and respond to their specific needs, but the class members generally become a support group for each other. Also we do not focus on one method of childbirth preparation or one labor-management technique, because they vary widely from doctor to doctor and from one geographical area or hospital to another. Each doctor or midwife tends to handle particular medical situations in one of several prescribed ways, depending on their obstetrical philosophy and the specifics of the situation; thus only they, and not a book, can say how they will deal with a particular situation. We have tried to give mothers enough information so that they will be able to question and confer knowledgeably with their doctor. It is our desire that this book help mothers and fathers to increase the health and enjoyment of the birth of their baby. We hope that whatever type of birth experience parents have, they will emerge from it with a sense of satisfaction and completion that will send them into the coming years of parenting with boundless love and energy.

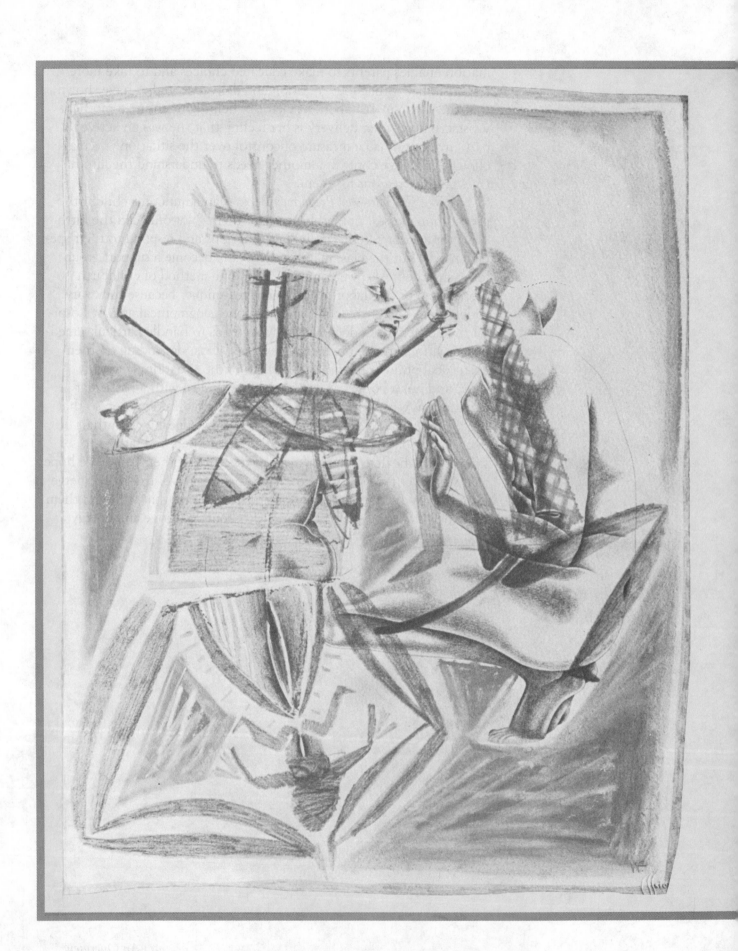

Birth in Different Cultures

Cultural Patterning of Childbirth

Since the beginning of time all cultures have placed great importance on birth. Not only has birth been considered a transforming personal experience for the mother, it has always had broad social and spiritual implications for the rest of the family and the society to which it belonged. People of all cultures have seen the birth of a baby as a special, magical event, one that by its very nature transforms their everyday reality and brings them into contact with forces beyond their control. From the beginning, birth has been linked to the basic spiritual concepts of creation, life, and death. Thus birth had an integral part in religious belief and was at the center of many religious rituals.

Because of its importance to society, birth has also always been the subject of significant cultural patterning. Each culture has evolved many rituals and techniques that relate to the various aspects of conception, pregnancy, childbirth, and the newborn period. For instance, traditional practices in tribal cultures have developed over thousands of years, while the technological aspects of modern obstetrics have grown up over a relatively short period of time. Such practices are symbolic of each culture's world view, of the way they solve problems, and of whether they view childbirth as an illness or a natural process.

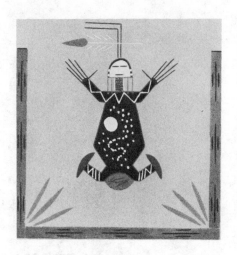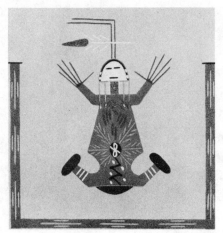

Many cultures depict the creation of the first child as a union between the sky, which is the male principal, and the earth, which is the female principal. Father Sky, and Mother Earth, by John Lee Begay. Museum of the American Indian, Heye Foundation.

To a great extent, the tone of a mother's birth experience is set by her society's practices and attitudes toward birth.

Considering how different cultures look at birth imparts a sense of the diversity of the experience. Not all cultures have a uniform view of birth. At present within our own culture there are many different types of birth experience, some of which vary as much as experiences in different cultures. Knowledge of the variety of cultural practices worldwide, combined with a historical sense of how rapidly birth practices have changed in our culture over the last several hundred years, conveys a sense of the relativity of a culture's birth practices. No *one* practice is necessarily "right" or will remain fixed over time.

Ours is a culture that attempts to solve its problems scientifically and that views childbirth as a medical event that can sometimes be perilous for the baby or the mother. Strangely enough, in spite of our scientific foundation, many of the medical solutions used in our culture have not been subjected to serious double-blind studies that dealt with enough mothers and babies to be statistically significant. Thus many of the current Western procedures have not been scientifically proven any more than have those in primitive cultures. In part, this is because some studies would be difficult or impossible to do, either because of complexity, ethics, liability, or expense. So Western practices often fall into the category of *scientific myth,* which, like traditional practices, are based on a culture's world view, as opposed to scientific fact.

Spiritual Views of Birth

Mircea Eliade, an eminent history-of-religions scholar, has traced birth images back to the earliest myths. Many cultures depict the creation of the first child as a marriage between heaven and earth. Similar myths hold that the sky or heaven, which is male, showers rain on the female earth, bringing new life. This ancient formula is at the heart of

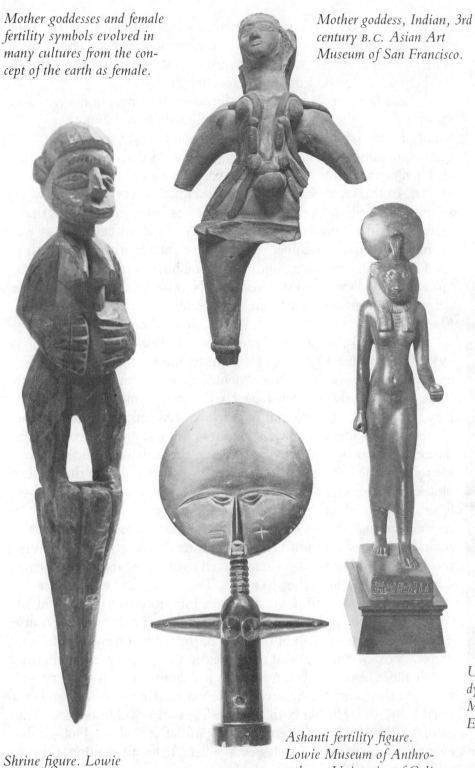

Mother goddesses and female fertility symbols evolved in many cultures from the concept of the earth as female.

Mother goddess, Indian, 3rd century B.C. Asian Art Museum of San Francisco.

Aphrodite, Greek, 4th century B.C. The Metropolitan Museum of Art. Fletcher Fund, 1952.

Uto, Egyptian, 22nd–26th dynasty. The Metropolitan Museum of Art. Gift of Edward S. Harkness, 1935.

Shrine figure. Lowie Museum of Anthropology, University of California, Berkeley.

Ashanti fertility figure. Lowie Museum of Anthropology, University of California, Berkeley.

the world view of both hunter-gatherer and agricultural societies. It is the source of the concept of *sacred places*, particular geographical locations where life springs forth, and for the existence of hunter-gatherer mother goddesses and agricultural fertility goddesses.

Eliade observes that before the causes of conception were known, people thought a baby was put directly into the mother's womb. Prior to that event a child's *spirit* was thought to reside in natural formations. Thus early humans believed that they were truly children of the earth, arising from a particular rock, water hole, or animal. In this creation scheme the father had no early role and was simply thought to adopt the baby after it was born. Eliade states that many present-day practices spring from these ancient beliefs. For example, in Africa a number of tribes have their mothers give birth in the forest sitting on the ground, while in China women lie on the ground during labor, and the Maoris of New Zealand have the mother deliver on the ground near a stream. It is interesting to note that the Maori word *whenna* means both "earth" and "placenta."

A remarkable and beautiful version of this early myth is still alive in the birth philosophy of the Australian aborigines, a hunter-gatherer people who live a nonagricultural, wandering life and use few tools. Although their beliefs have changed with time, many of them may be hundreds of thousands of years old. One of the legends of the Oenpelli aborigines acknowledges that fertilization results from insemination by the male, but they believe that the actual entrance of the life force of the baby is spiritual. At the beginning of time the ancient mother put on earth the spirits of all the people, leaving them for future generations. These spirits are believed by the aborigines to reside in animals or around sacred water holes and rocks in the Outback, where they wait until they can attract prospective fathers. When the spirits see a hunter, they may attach themselves and make themselves known to him if they like him. The hunter and future father, recognizing that a spirit has come inside him, returns to camp and "gives" the spirit to the mother at some future time during intercourse. According to one version of the legend, the spirit travels into the uterus, "breaks" the egg, and then goes on to live between the mother's shoulder blades, only returning to her uterus when it starts to grow. At this point the father tells the mother that he has given her a spirit baby, and tells her both the baby's sex and its clan lineage. Thus among the aborigines conception is a spiritual as well as a biological event, and the parents are viewed as a vehicle for an existing spirit child of the earth to become manifest.

Almost all cultures have views on the moment when the spirit or life force enters the baby. For example, the Canadian Eskimos believe that the spirit enters the baby in the early part of pregnancy, and therefore the mother talks to it and teaches it during pregnancy. The Bambara of Africa believe that the father's clan's spirit enters the

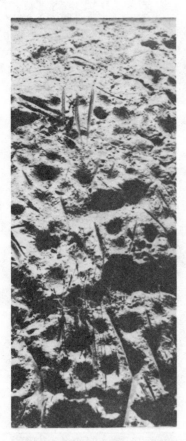

Among some cultures, babies' spirits are believed to live around or to be able to be called forth near particular physical landmarks. Ceremonial Rocks, Baby Rocks, Pomo, California. Lowie Museum of Anthropology, University of California, Berkeley.

The Australian aborigines place great importance on when the baby's spirit enters the mother's body. They believe that baby spirits live around waterholes and other natural formations. Spirit Babies, *Wendy Frost, 1984. Pastel/graphite on lithograph, 18" x 24". Collection, Mike and Nancy Samuels.*

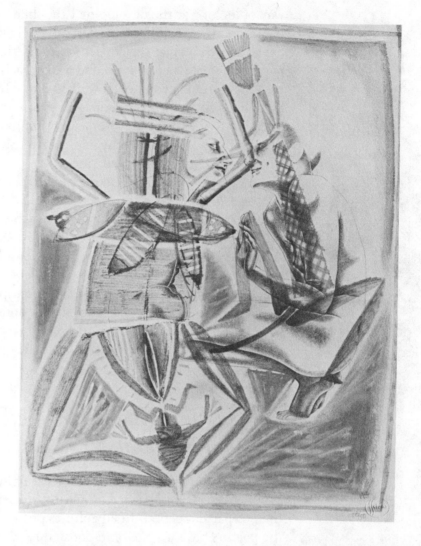

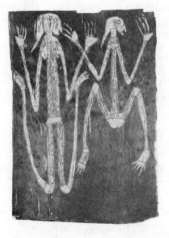

The Oenpelli aborigines of Australia believe that ancient spirit figures left all the baby spirits for generations to come. Oenpelli bark painting. Lowie Museum of Anthropology, University of California, Berkeley.

baby early in pregnancy, the mother's, not until the naming ceremony after the baby's birth. Many other African tribes do not believe that the spirit enters the baby until several months *after* birth, when the baby is named. Childbirth researcher Niles Newton points out that in Western culture the view of when the spirit enters the baby has varied throughout history. The Catholic Church believes the spirit enters with conception; English common law holds that it enters when "quickening" takes place, that is, when the mother first feels the baby move. The question of when the spirit enters is at the heart of the present abortion issue and is becoming an important medical-ethical question for doctors to address as they become able to keep premature babies alive after less and less time in the uterus.

Throughout history most cultures have had religious views about the nature of the baby's spirit. In many cultures the beliefs involve concepts of ancestors, the hereafter, everlasting life, and reincarnation. Obviously such ideas strongly influence how people relate to and treat the baby in utero, because they provide a very different way of looking at the developing baby than does the biological view of parenthood. One of the most pervasive religious beliefs about the baby's spirit involves the concept of reincarnation, which holds that a particular spirit is born again and again, each time in a different body, until its spiritual evolution is worked out. This belief is acknowledged by Hindus, Buddhists, and some sects of Jews and Christians, as well as by many tribal cultures. Reincarnation has been a major topic of debate in modern philosophy and is currently being studied by scientific parapsychology and medicine.

Perhaps the most striking picture of reincarnation is provided by *The Tibetan Book of the Dead,* an ancient Buddhist treatise that is read to people as they are dying in order to guide them through the illusions they will encounter after death. Tibetan Buddhists believe that when they can see through the various illusions without becoming ensnared, they will escape from the wheel of continual death and rebirth. Should the dying person fail to escape, as most do, the book goes on to give an intricate set of instructions for deciding on a womb to enter for the next incarnation. First the person is urged to choose a continent where religion prevails, then he or she is urged to pick the womb of a holy person.

How Cultures Handle Different Aspects of Childbirth

Cultural patterns dealing with childbearing relate to all aspects of the experience, including behavior during pregnancy, labor, delivery, and the postpartum period. In all cultures pregnancy is taken seriously, and the parents have a sense of responsibility about their roles. The Chagga of Africa have a saying: "Pay attention to the pregnant woman! There is no one more important than she." In general, the way of life of the mother and father is thought to directly affect the baby and its delivery. These beliefs have led to long lists of both prescribed and proscribed acts for parents in every culture, the most prevalent of which are dietary guidelines for the mother.

Yale University maintains a Human Relations Area File on 222 different cultures. This file has been a valuable source for anthropologists and shows the variety of ways that people handle childbirth and related issues. All but four out of sixty-four cultures studied by Yale anthropologist Clellan Ford had dietary regulations. Depriving a mother of certain foods, rather than adding foods, is the most common pattern. It is strange from a Western nutritional point of view that the foods most often denied a mother are protein sources such as meat and fish. The reason given for these particular foods being prohibited is that the baby, labor, or delivery may take on animallike characteristics. For example, one Philippino tribe believes that eating a bird may

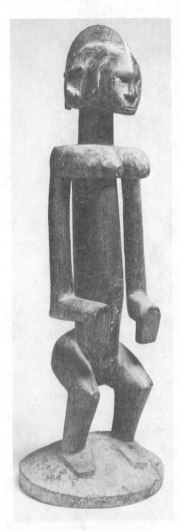

In some cultures ancestors are believed to be able to influence the spirit of the unborn baby. Female ancestor figure, Mali. The Fine Arts Museum of San Francisco. Memorial gift from Dr. T Edward and Mrs. Tullah Hanley.

keep the baby small, and that eating octopus may make the fetus stick inside the mother.

Many cultures also have guidelines for a woman's activity during pregnancy. The most common advice is for the mother to be very active so the baby doesn't become too big. Such advice is given by the Hopi, who admonish mothers to rise early and not sit around, and by the Sanpoil Indians, who have a whole regimen of walking and swimming activities for expectant mothers. Most tropical peoples have the mother continue working throughout pregnancy.

Sexual intercourse is an activity that is discouraged for pregnant women in some cultures and encouraged in others. Ford charted sixty cultures in this regard and found that 70 percent permitted intercourse in the second month, dropping off as pregnancy progressed to only 30 percent approving of intercourse by the ninth month.

Many cultures have descriptions of the way in which violent emotions, stress, or possible supernatural events can affect the baby. For that reason the pregnant woman is often advised to keep a calm emotional tenor to her life, and her husband and the people around her are urged to support and protect her. For example, the Luzon Philippinos say that anger in a pregnant woman will cause her baby to have an angry face, and if the mother quarrels with her own mother or mother-in-law, she will have a difficult delivery. Most West African tribes believe that because the fetus is so close to the spirit world, both the baby and the mother are unusually vulnerable to malevolent spirits. For this reason the expectant mother is told to wear special amulets to protect herself and to avoid doing things that attract such spirits.

Cultures vary widely in terms of whether they think of pregnancy and childbirth as an illness or as a natural, healthy event. They also vary in terms of how seriously or casually they treat it. Niles Newton observes that among the Cuna Indians of Panama the expectant mother goes to the medicine man for medication every day during pregnancy and is also medicated throughout labor and delivery. At the other end of this spectrum are the Jarara of South America, among whom birth is considered such a normal event that it takes place in a passageway in full view of everyone. Brigitte Jordan, a medical anthropologist, notes that even Western countries vary greatly in terms of how they conceptualize birth. Based on her studies, she feels that birth is viewed as a medical procedure in the United States, as a natural process in Holland, as a fulfilling personal achievement in Sweden, and as a stressful but normal part of family life among the Indians in the Yucatán.

Another interesting birth variable is the kind of help the mother receives during labor and delivery. In the great majority of cultures—58 out of the 60 that anthropologist Ford studied—older women are the ones who assist the mother during childbirth. Generally these women are sisters, mothers, mothers-in-law, co-wives, relatives, or friends. Usually men are not allowed to be in the room with the mother, though in some tribes male healers help with labor and delivery. Among the Lepcha of the Himalayas, there is no sex preference for helpers and any knowledgeable person can assist the mother. Marshall Klaus, a well-known American pediatrician and bonding expert, cites a study that shows that not only are helpers generally women, but that in all but one of 150 cultures studied, at least one helper remained with the woman *continuously* throughout labor and delivery. Klaus notes that among the Santa Maria Indians in Guatemala the standard practice was for the native midwife, both grandmothers, the husband, and occasionally the father-in-law to be present for the birth.

Details of labor management also vary widely from one culture to another, for instance, in regard to eating. The African Hottentots feed soup to women in labor to keep them strong, while the Pawnee Indians of America do not allow food or water after the first labor pain. Niles Newton points out that in many cultures what she calls "sensory stimulation" plays a significant part in the management of labor. Among the Navahos of the Southwest and other groups music is played for the mother.

The amount a mother moves around during labor varies widely from culture to culture. Among the Taureg of the Sahara, women walk up and down small hills while they are in labor, returning to their hut only to deliver the baby; whereas among the Hottentots, who are also from Africa, the mother is packed into a small hut with a number of other women and can barely move.

Conversation among the helpers is used either to relax and reassure the mother or to encourage her. Among the Mayans conversation is tailored to the particular stage of labor and to how the mother is doing. As labor progresses, the midwife talks to the mother and demonstrates pushing techniques. Finally, as the contractions become very strong, idle conversation ceases and talk focuses on the mother's labor or on the helper's own birth experiences. If necessary, the helpers repeatedly voice a litany that urges the mother on. A number of cultures have practices in which the mother is kept quite warm or even has heat applied to her back or stomach. Cultures such as the Yahgan of Tierra del Fuego and the Punjab of India massage the mother's back or abdomen with oil during labor.

One of the most widespread labor practices is having the mother held or supported in a particular position by her helpers. For example, among the Mayan Indians of the Yucatán, the mother is supported by the arms and body of a woman who sits behind her. This woman, who is called a "head helper," not only supports the mother's weight, she parallels the mother's action in pushing and breathing during each contraction. Often the two women are in skin-to-skin

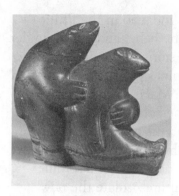

In many cultures a woman assists the laboring mother, sitting behind her and supporting her weight. Two bears, Eskimo. The Metropolitan Museum of Art. Harris Brisbane Dick Fund and Houghton Foundation, Inc. Gift.

contact, which apparently is of great significance because it seems to increase the effectiveness of the helper's reassurance. Ford lists twenty-five cultures in which the woman is supported from behind.

Cultures also vary greatly in whether they attempt to speed labor and delivery or adopt a waiting course. Niles Newton distinguishes these attitudes as the "faster the better" versus "let nature take its course." The Siriono of Bolivia exhibit the ultimate laissez-faire attitude, having the mother give birth in the midst of a crowd of other women in a large hut. Apart from providing conversation and a rope to pull on during contractions, no move is made to help the laboring woman, who gives birth in a hammock that is slung very low to the ground. The baby is actually allowed to slip out of the hammock onto the ground, the shock of which seems to be enough to start it breathing.

In many cultures a number of techniques are used to assist the mother and speed delivery. Applying external pressure to the abdomen is the most common of these. Some cultures simply squeeze the mother during contractions; others apply a belt or binder throughout labor. Among the Arunta of Australia the woman who supports the mother from behind pushes firmly down on the top of the mother's abdomen and utters encouraging words at the same time. Many cultures, nontechnical as well as technical, have medicines that speed the mother's labor much as the drug oxytocin does. Several tribes stimulate the mother's natural mechanisms for making oxytocin, either by stimulating her breasts or by instructing the father to have intercourse with the mother. Among a number of tribes smooth saps or oils may be used to lubricate the vagina.

There are great cultural differences as to what position the mother should be in when she gives birth. Out of seventy-six cultures in the Yale Human Relations Area File, sixty-two have the mother give birth in a vertical rather than a horizontal position. Of those, twenty-one had mothers upright on their knees, nineteen were sitting, fifteen were squatting, and five were standing. In all but the standing position, the mother's back naturally curves forward. As mentioned, many cultures specifically provide the mother with pulling devices such as ropes, poles, or stakes to help her increase the force of her efforts to expel the baby.

Cultures also have their own rituals for cutting the umbilical cord. In the Philippines the cord is traditionally cut with a piece of sharp bamboo and then dusted with powder. In another Philippino tribe the cord is left long enough to touch the baby's forehead, so it will be wise. Midwives in Sumatra cut the cord with a wooden flute in order to ensure that the baby has a good voice.

Much emphasis is placed on the disposal of the placenta and cord, especially in nonindustrialized countries. Many cultures believe that the placenta has to be treated in a special way because it embodies part of the baby's soul. The Bukinon of Mindanao in the Philippines look at the placenta as the brother of the baby, and bury it under the house. They believe that after burial the spirit in the placenta returns to the sky. The Tolong of the Philippines put the placenta in a clay pot, smoke it, and then bury the pot. In Malaysia the placenta is placed in a coconut and put at the back of the cooking stove for two months before being buried. Occasionally parents put a note in the coconut in the hope that it will make the baby more intelligent.

Postpartum methods of caring for the new mother also differ greatly from one people to another. Many cultures isolate the new mother and baby in a small hut, where they remain in bed to rest and recuperate for a period of time. In sixty-four cultures the mother just rests, in a few instances for up to two months. Among the Goajiro Indians of Colombia, a well-to-do mother will remain in bed and out of the sunlight for one month after her first delivery. But in some tribes, such as the Yahgan of Tierra del Fuego, the mother is back to gathering shellfish with the rest of the tribe less than a day after she has given birth.

Different cultures employ a wide variety of physical therapy and sensory stimulation techniques for the new mother. By far the most common is heat. Often, especially in Southeast Asia, a fire is lit in the hut to "smoke" or "roast" the mother. Such heat is believed to relieve postpartum soreness and prevent the uterus from falling. New mothers in Mexico are given steam baths. Massage is another common postpartum treatment. The Punjab in India have elaborate massages for the abdomen and the area around the vagina. Among the Maya, the midwife gives the mother a special massage twenty days after the birth, which marks the end of the postpartum period.

Cultures vary greatly in their patterns of early breast-feeding. Many societies feed the baby right after birth, but others delay the first feeding for as long as two or three days, in some cases because they believe that colostrum, the initial milk, is dangerous. In such cases the baby is given herbal teas or even soft foods until nursing begins.

Among the major differences of various cultures are the patterns of closeness between mother and baby after the birth. Anthropologists refer to the period during which the baby is physiologically dependent on the mother and remains in close contact with her as the *transition period.* Generally, weaning signals the end of the transition period. The time at which weaning takes place ranges from birth, in a baby who isn't nursed at all by its mother, to about three years. Among the sixty-four cultures that Ford studied, one weaned at six months, thirteen at eighteen months, sixteen at two years, fifteen at three years, and nineteen were unclear. In a few cultures breast-feeding continues for up to six years.

Tribal cultures tend to have a fairly long transition period in which the baby is nursed and carried about by the mother, sleeps with

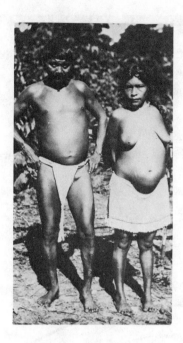

There is now much interest in cross-cultural birth customs. Man and woman, Patamona Indians, British Guiana. Museum of the American Indian, Heye Foundation.

her, and is attended to quickly by her if it cries. As societies become industrialized, there has been a tendency toward a "muted" transition period in which the baby is weaned early, spends most of its time away from the mother in a crib, and doesn't sleep with the mother. Generally in cultures with lengthy transition periods there is fairly wide spacing between babies. This is thought to be due, at least in part, to the contraceptive effects of intense nursing and, in some cases, to taboos against intercourse during the lactation period. The Yoruba prohibit coitus entirely during lactation, whereas the Arapesh prohibit coitus until the baby takes its first steps.

Among the Aymara of Brazil mothers take their babies everywhere with them and the babies sleep with them until two years of age. Among the Tsinghai of China mothers carry their babies with them and nurse them on demand up to the age of five years. Within tribal cultures there are a few definite exceptions to this long period of closeness, generally in cultures in which the women are an important part of the economic structure. For example, among the Alor of Indonesia the mother returns to work in the fields ten days after the baby is born and leaves the baby in the care of a relative, but she does sleep with the baby and breast-feeds it as soon as she comes in from the fields.

There are as many food prohibitions and prescriptions for the mother after birth as there are during pregnancy. In Malaysia the mother's food is severly limited, whereas in Tanganyika her diet is enriched with meat, milk, blood, and fat. Among the Arapesh of New Guinea fresh coconuts are reserved for lactating women and for feasts. In Burma there is a soup made of plants, fish, and fruit that is traditionally fed to new mothers. Among the Philippinos the mother is given a special meal of boiled chicken, corn porridge, and a small amount of cooked placenta. In another Philippino tribe, the Tarong, the mother is given a tea made with charred placenta and root that is eaten to eliminate "bad air." The mother is also given a cigar to smoke.

Medical anthropologist Brigitte Jordan speculates that the reason there is now so much interest in cross-cultural birth customs is that both Western and tribal birth practices are in rapid transition all over the world. Ironically, the traditional methods are tending to become more technical, while the technical methods are being questioned by many birth educators. In Guatemala a number of women are being delivered in Western-style hospitals after being left to labor alone. On the other hand, in the state hospital at Pithiviers, France, under the direction of Michel Odent, women are being encouraged to deliver completely naturally in a supported squatting position. We believe that studying various cultural alternatives helps people to view their own system with a more open mind and make a more informed decision about the kind of birth situation that will be best for them.

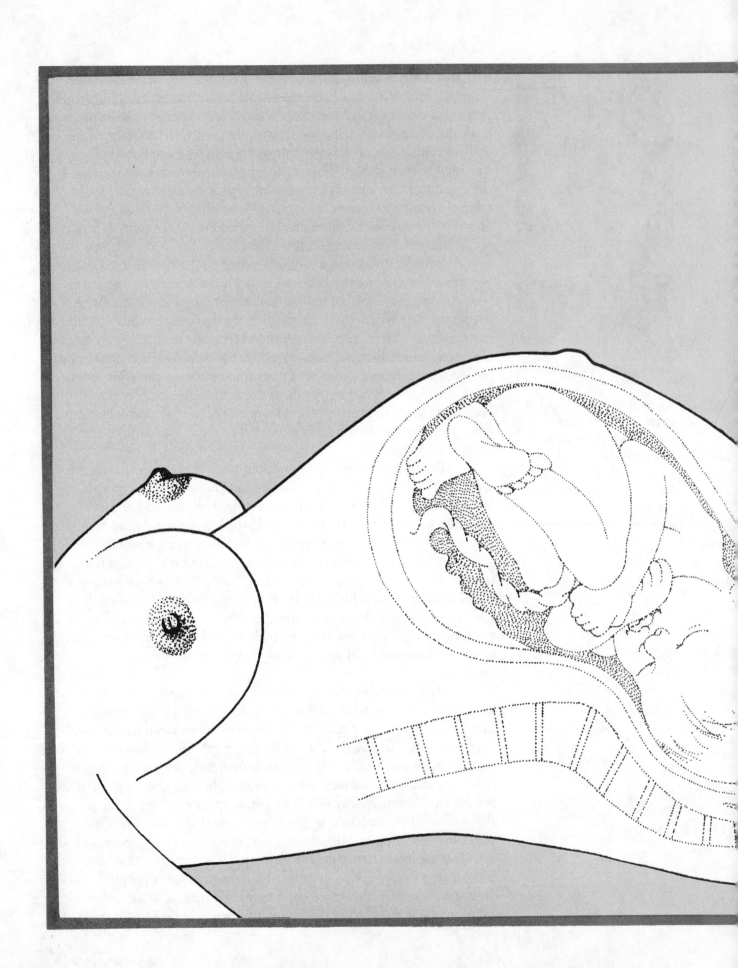

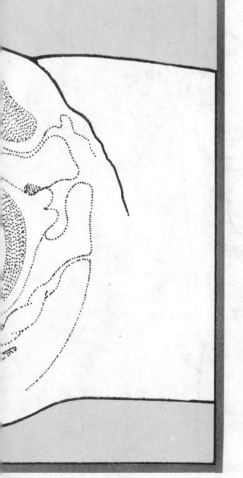

SECTION
II

Pregnancy

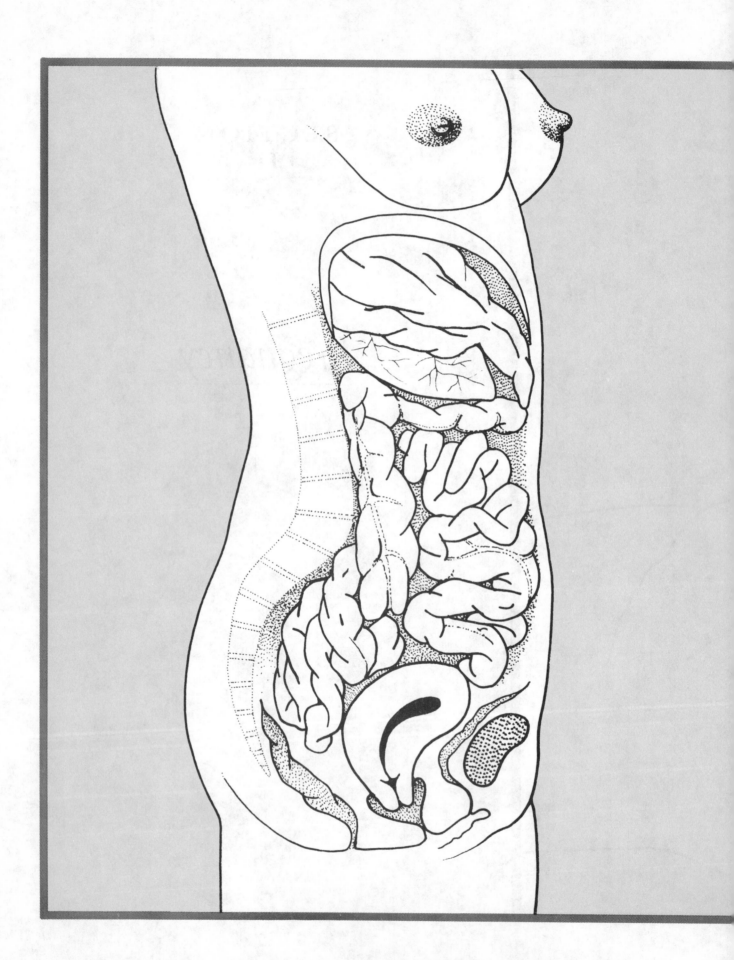

Anatomy
and Physiology
of the Mother

Understanding the Sensations
of Pregnancy

Much of what expectant mothers feel and are concerned about relates to the anatomy and physiology of their bodies. Just as most people are taught little about how a baby grows and develops after birth, they often know little about the anatomy and physiology of reproduction and pregnancy. What this means is that when a nurse, midwife, or obstetrician gives a brief explanation in response to a query, an expectant mother may end up feeling confused or unsatisfied. If a woman does not really understand the answer she is given, her concerns may not be allayed and new questions may arise to trouble her.

When a woman understands what is happening within her body, she is better able to accept and deal with the sensations and changes she is experiencing and to see them as normal occurrences rather than as strange feelings that may be precursors of illness. When pregnancy and birth are seen as natural events, they take place without unnecessary fear or apprehension. The result of such understanding is fewer problems and illnesses during pregnancy, labor, and delivery. This is the goal of prepared childbirth.

In the following pages we will present information on female anatomy, physiology, and endocrinology as they relate to the average pregnancy. Our aim is to make expectant mothers aware of the normal range of sensations and the anatomical and physiological reasons for them. In addition, the material will acquaint expectant parents with terms and concepts that they will hear from childbirth educators and doctors throughout pregnancy.

Female Anatomy

INTERNAL REPRODUCTIVE ORGANS

The female reproductive system consists of a number of internal and external structures that serve to facilitate intercourse, conception, the development and birth of a baby, and the nurturance of the baby after birth. The uterus, which is an organ shaped like an upside-down pear, sits between the bladder in the front and the rectum in the back. Most of the uterus actually tilts forward and lies on top of the bladder. The nonpregnant uterus is about 2½ inches (6–8 centimeters) long in a woman who has never been pregnant, and 3½ inches (9–10 centimeters) long in a woman who has previously been pregnant. It is largely made up of muscle tissue so thick that the front and back walls almost touch, leaving only a narrow slit in the interior. Like the digestive

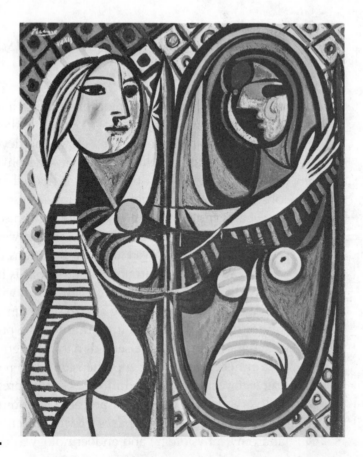

The female reproductive system consists of a complex set of internal and external structures which facilitate the growth of a baby. Girl Before A Mirror, *Pablo Picasso, 1932. Oil on canvas, 64" x 51¼". Collection, The Museum of Modern Art, New York. Gift of Mrs. Simon Guggenheim.*

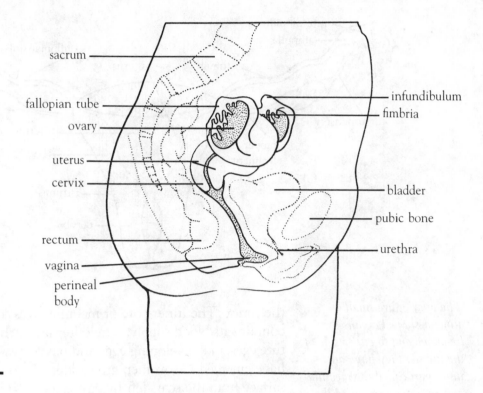

sacrum

fallopian tube

ovary

uterus

cervix

rectum

vagina

perineal
body

infundibulum

fimbria

bladder

pubic bone

urethra

*The uterus is a muscular,
pear-shaped organ that lies
between the bladder in the
front and the rectum in the
back.*

tract, the uterus is made of a special kind of muscle whose contractions
are involuntary. And like the digestive tract, the nerves that innervate
the uterus are not motor nerves that can be consciously directed but
autonomic nerves that are largely under automatic control.

The inside of the uterus is lined with *endometrium,* a pink,
velvety glandular tissue that undergoes cyclical monthly changes due
to the influence of hormones. After menstruation the endometrium is
thin; it becomes thicker and thicker until one week after ovulation
takes place, and later it is sloughed off during the next menstrual
period—provided conception has not occurred.

On either side of the uterus, near the top, are three tough
bands called *ligaments,* which attach to the sides of the pelvis and
support and position the uterus over the bladder. Slightly above the
ligaments, near the top corners of the uterus, are the *fallopian tubes* or
oviducts, which lead from the uterus to the ovaries. These tubes are
2¾ to 6 inches (7–14 centimeters) long and are ⅛ to ⅜ inch (2–8
millimeters) thick. The tubes curve around the ovaries, ending in a
funnel-shape opening called the *infundibulum,* which does not actually
join the ovary but is open to the abdominal cavity. During ovulation
feathery appendages on the funnel called *fimbriae* help to guide the egg
from the ovary into the fallopian tube.

The *ovaries* are a pair of small, almond-shape organs that are 1
to 2 inches (2.5–5 centimeters) long and ½ to ¾ inch (.7–1.5 centimeters) wide. They are located at the top of the pelvic cavity, above
the uterus. Each ovary has an inner and outer part, the *medulla* and

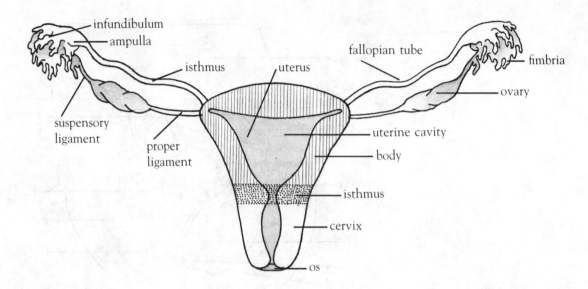

infundibulum
ampulla
isthmus
uterus
fallopian tube
fimbria
ovary
suspensory ligament
proper ligament
uterine cavity
body
isthmus
cervix
os

The ovaries are small, almond-shaped organs that lie above and to either side of the uterus; they have an inner part called the medulla and an outer part called the cortex.

the *cortex*. The inner core or medulla gives the ovary its shape and contains its blood supply. The outer layer, the cortex, contains immature eggs and developing eggs and has scars where previous ripe eggs have emerged. As women grow older, the ovaries develop a bumpy surface from the scars left by past eggs.

The bottom of the uterus narrows into a stubby round cylinder about ¾ inch wide that is called the *cervix.* It projects into the top of the vagina at an angle that varies from 45 to 90 degrees. The *os* or opening of the cervix can also vary tremendously in appearance. First,

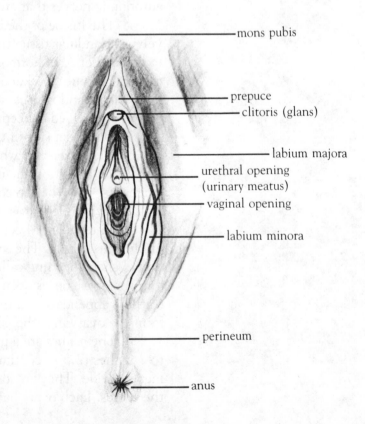

mons pubis
prepuce
clitoris (glans)
labium majora
urethral opening (urinary meatus)
vaginal opening
labium minora
perineum
anus

The vaginal opening is surrounded by inner and outer labia. The clitoris and urethral opening are situated above the vagina, with the anus below.

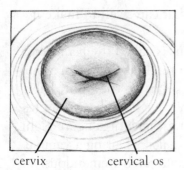

cervix   cervical os

before vaginal delivery

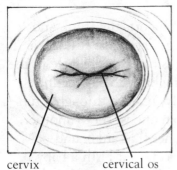

cervix   cervical os

after vaginal delivery

The shape of the cervical opening changes from an oval to a slit once it has dilated for a vaginal delivery.

The pelvic floor consists of several layers of muscle that form a figure eight around the vaginal and anal openings, supporting the organs of the pelvis.

the lining of the os alters at different points during the menstrual cycle due to hormones. Second, childbirth changes the shape of the os: before birth it is a small, oval opening; after a vaginal birth the opening assumes a slitlike appearance. Unlike the body of the uterus, the cervix is only partly muscle; the rest is connective and elastic tissue. Protein molecules in these tissues actually dissociate or loosen during labor, allowing the cervix to stretch around the baby's head and irrevocably changing the way it looks.

The *vagina* is a muscular canal or tube that connects the bottom of the uterus with the outside of the body. The vagina averages 3½ to 4 inches (7–10 centimeters) in length. Before a vaginal birth the canal is about 2½ inches (4 centimeters) wide; after vaginal births it gradually widens and the walls smooth out. Normally the vagina is kept moist by an acidic mucosal secretion from the uterus. The acidity and the slipperiness of the secretion vary throughout the menstrual cycle.

THE EXTERNAL GENITALIA

The opening of the vagina lies between the *anus* and the *mons pubis*, a fatty cushion that covers the pubic bone. On either side of the vagina are fatty folds called the *labia majora*. Within the labia majora are a set of skinlike folds called the *labia minora*. Both the labia majora and the labia minora contain abundant nerve endings. The outer folds become less prominent after childbirth, while the inner folds become more prominent and extend below the labia majora.

At the top of the vaginal opening lies the *urinary meatus*, the opening to the *urethra*, which connects the *bladder* with the outside of the body. Above the urinary meatus, where the labia minora meet, lies the *clitoris*, a small erectile structure that is less than ¾ inch (2 centimeters) long. It is similar in structure and developmental history to the penis: the tip or *glans* is covered with sensitive nerve endings,

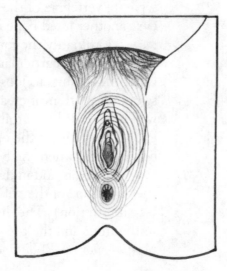

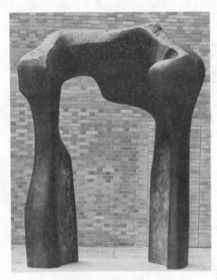

Passing through a hole or tunnel, as the baby does in a vaginal birth, is a primal image of transformation.

Large Torso: Arch., Henry Moore, 1962–63. Bronze, 66⅛" x 59⅛" x 51¼". Collection, The Museum of Modern Art, New York. Mrs. Simon Guggenheim Fund.

and the main body contains blood caverns that can swell to make it erect during sexual arousal.

The area between the vagina and anus is called the *perineum*. The perineum includes layers of muscles and tendons that form a muscular sling that attaches to the bones of the pelvis on the front, back, and sides and supports the organs in the pelvic cavity. These muscles actually encircle the vaginal and anal openings, making a figure eight. Birth educators often refer to this as the *pelvic floor*. During a vaginal delivery the skin and muscles of the perineum stretch tremendously.

THE PELVIS

The pelvis is a bony, bottomless basket that supports the trunk and upper body and is in turn supported by the legs. This basket holds and protects the organs of the lower abdomen. It is through the hole in the bottom of this basket that a baby passes during birth to emerge into the world as a separate being. Not surprisingly, passage through a tunnel or hole is a primal image of transition from one world to another.

The pelvis itself is made up of four bones that are bound together: the *hipbones*, the *sacrum*, and the *coccyx*. At birth a baby's pelvis is a combination of bone and cartilage. The cartilage does not ossify, or turn to bone completely, until somewhere between puberty and twenty-five years of age.

The hipbones lie to either side of the body, curving around to meet in the front at a joint called the *pubic symphysis*, which is held together by four ligaments. The hipbones actually consist of three bones that are fused together: the *ilium* on top, the *ischium* below, and the *pubic bone* to the front. In the rear the hipbones form two joints with the sacrum, a shield-shape bone that sits at the base of the spinal cord. Like the pubic symphysis, these sacroiliac joints are tightly bound by several ligaments. The sacrum itself is pierced by eight holes and is made up of five fused sacral vertebrae. Above the sacrum are the separate vertebrae of the spinal column. Below the sacrum is the coccyx, another fused bone that consists of the last four vertebrae.

Ordinarily the joints of the pelvis have little mobility. But during pregnancy, particularly in the last trimester, hormonal changes cause these joints to loosen and become more movable. The pubic symphysis in front increases in width and moves up and down with walking. And the sacroiliac joints in back can glide up and down enough to increase the opening of the pelvis by as much as ¾ inch (2 centimeters) when the baby is delivered.

Doctors and midwives use several measurements to describe the size and shape of the pelvic opening that the baby will pass through (see illustration). The distance between the top of the pubic symphysis in the front and the top of the sacrum at the back is called the *anterior-posterior (A-P) distance* across the *inlet*. It marks the beginning of

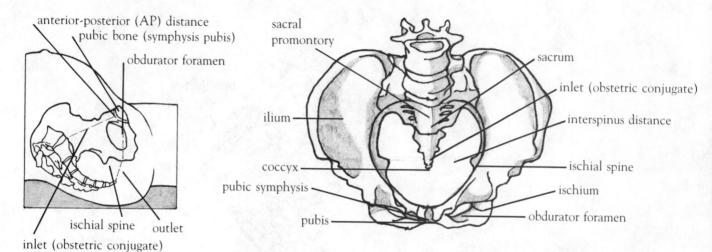

anterior-posterior (AP) distance
pubic bone (symphysis pubis)
obdurator foramen
ischial spine
outlet
inlet (obstetric conjugate)

sacral promontory
ilium
coccyx
pubic symphysis
pubis
sacrum
inlet (obstetric conjugate)
interspinus distance
ischial spine
ischium
obdurator foramen

The pelvis is a hard basket with a hole in the bottom; it is made up of several bones that support the upper body and the organs of the abdomen. During a vaginal delivery the baby passes through the pelvis, fitting between the pubic bone and the sacrum first, then squeezing even more tightly between the spines on either side of the pelvis.

Both the pelvis itself and the hole in the center come in a variety of shapes. Most women have a combination of several of the pure pelvic types shown here.

the bony tunnel or canal the baby must pass through during birth. The distance between the hipbones' *ischial spines* in the middle of the pelvis is called the *inter-spinous diameter*. The ischial spines are bumps that protrude into the birth canal on either side. On the average, both the A-P distance of the inlet and the inter-spinous diameter of the mid-pelvis are greater than 10 centimeters. The distance across the bottom of the pelvic basket is called the *outlet*. It is the final part of the tunnel that the baby must negotiate, and curves around from the bottom of the sacrum to the bottom of the hipbones (*ischial tuberosities*), to the bottom of the pubic bone. The outlet averages more than 8 centimeters. The measure of the mid-pelvis is the most important predictor of whether the pelvis is large enough for a vaginal delivery. The inlet is the second most important measure, and the outlet is the least. The vast majority of women have a pelvis that is adequate for an average-size baby to pass through.

Women's pelves have a variety of shapes, but four "pure" categories are used to describe the shape of the inlet opening. These shapes also give the doctor or midwife a clinical suggestion of whether the mother can deliver vaginally. (1) *Gynecoid*, which is round, is the most common shape and applies to almost half of all women. This shape is the most favorable in terms of a vaginal delivery. (2) *Anthropoid*, which is an oval that is widest from front to back, is the second most common shape. It applies to half of nonwhite women and a quarter of white women. (3) *Android* is heart-shaped. It applies to a third of all white women and a sixth of all nonwhite women. (4)

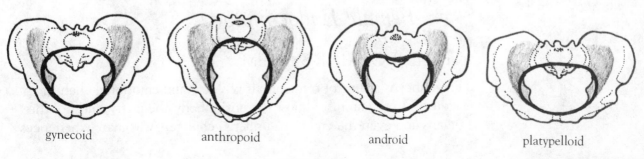

gynecoid   anthropoid   android   platypelloid

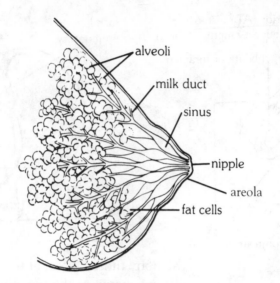

The breast is a specialized organ with thousands of tiny milk glands, which enable a woman to produce milk after the birth of a baby.

Platypelloid, which is the rarest, is an oval that is widest from side to side. It applies to less than 3 percent of all women. In many cases women's pelves reflect a mixture of pure types. The shape of the pelvis, in conjunction with the position the baby is in as it passes through the birth canal, helps determine the particular sensations a woman feels during labor and delivery.

THE BREAST

The female breast is a highly specialized kind of *exocrine gland.* This type of gland, which includes the sweat glands and the digestive glands, makes a substance that is channeled into ducts, accumulated in central storage areas, and released in batches. The breast consists of fifteen to twenty-five branching segments called *lobes.* Between the lobes are fat, connective tissue, lymph vessels, and nerves. Within each lobe are a number of tiny *alveoli,* which are the structures that actually produce the milk. They empty into a common duct. Together the alveoli and the duct are called a *lobule.* Each lobule looks like a tiny branch of cauliflower. Ducts from several lobules join into larger and larger ducts leading toward the nipple. Just behind the nipple are widened areas of the ducts called *lactiferous sinuses.* It is here that milk is temporarily stored. Past the sinuses the ducts narrow again and group together, ending in the nipple.

Female Endocrinology

THE ENDOCRINE SYSTEM

Pregnancy is a time of tremendous physical and emotional change. In addition to the uterus, almost the entire body chemistry, most of the organs and even the emotions undergo change. A woman experiences

How hormones affect body feelings during pregnancy

HORMONE	CHANGES IN BODY	FEELINGS
Estrogen: produced by placenta	Uterus enlarges	Abdomen feels bigger
	Breasts enlarge	Breasts feel tender
	Genitals enlarge	Increased sexual sensitivity
	Decreased stomach acid	Digestive upsets
	Increased production of skin pigment	Darkened genitals and nipples
Progesterone: produced by ovary and placenta	Increase in fatty deposits	Weight gain
	Reduced digestive tract movements in stomach	Heartburn
	Respiratory center more sensitive	Feeling of breathlessness
	Relaxation of smooth muscle tone	Constipation, urinary problems, leg swelling
Human chorionic gonadotropin: produced by placenta	Body temperature is raised .5°C	Increased perspiration and feelings of warmth

these changes as physical sensations, mood alterations, and differences in body habits. Many of the changes are orchestrated and effected by the endocrine glands, which secrete small amounts of chemicals called *hormones* directly into the bloodstream. During pregnancy hormonal fluctuations bring about much greater upheavals than a woman experiences at any other time in her life, including puberty and menopause.

The major control center for the endocrine system is the *hypothalamus*, a structure that is not an endocrine gland but part of the nervous system. The hypothalamus is located near the base of the brain, in the area that controls all the automatic functions such as breathing, heartbeat, and body temperature. It is genetically programed to regulate such long-range processes as puberty, the monthly menstrual cycles, and menopause, as well as pregnancy. These body cycles have evolved over millions of years and show common characteristics that are unique to the human species. Although the hypothal-

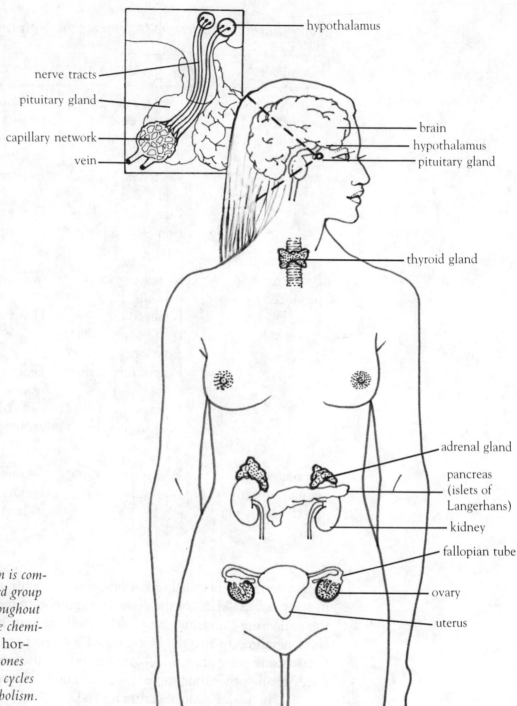

hypothalamus

nerve tracts

pituitary gland

capillary network

vein

brain

hypothalamus

pituitary gland

thyroid gland

adrenal gland

pancreas
(islets of
Langerhans)

kidney

fallopian tube

ovary

uterus

The endocrine system is composed of a complicated group of organs located throughout the body that produce chemical messengers called hormones. These hormones regulate reproductive cycles as well as body metabolism.

amus basically mediates bodily functions that are not under a person's conscious control, it is affected by a person's higher brain centers, conscious thoughts, perceptions, and experiences in the outer world. The hypothalamus sends special chemicals to the *pituitary gland,* the so-called master gland, which controls the rest of the endocrine system. The pituitary is conveniently located directly below the hypothalamus and is connected to it by a stalk.

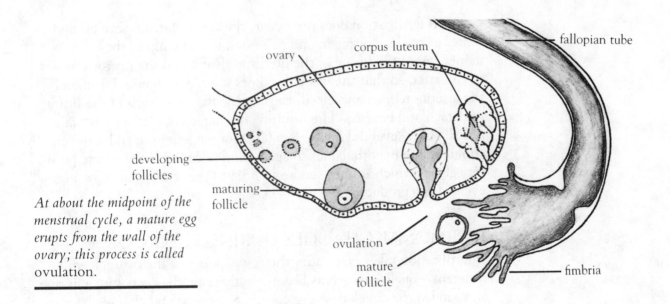

ovary

developing
follicles

maturing
follicle

corpus luteum

fallopian tube

ovulation

mature
follicle

fimbria

*At about the midpoint of the
menstrual cycle, a mature egg
erupts from the wall of the
ovary; this process is called*
ovulation.

THE MENSTRUAL CYCLE

Among the many substances that the hypothalamus gives off that control pituitary output are *releasing* and *inhibiting* hormones that control a woman's ovulatory cycle. At the beginning of the menstrual cycle a releasing hormone from the hypothalamus causes the pituitary to send out *follicle stimulating hormone (FSH)*. FSH causes an immature egg to ripen in the ovary over a period of about fourteen days. As the egg increases in size, the surrounding cells develop into a temporary structure that immediately begins to produce the female hormone *estrogen*. While the egg is ripening, the estrogen causes a number of related changes: the uterine lining thickens, cervical mucus increases and becomes more receptive to sperm, the vaginal lining thickens, and the fallopian tubes contract more actively. All these changes tend to promote fertilization.

Shortly before the midpoint of the ovulatory cycle the hypothalamus sends out a releasing hormone that causes the pituitary gland to secrete a sudden surge of *luteinizing hormone (LH)*. This hormone causes the mature egg to erupt from the wall of the ovary. At this point the temporary structure that had surrounded the developing egg undergoes further growth and transformation, becoming the *corpus luteum*. This altered structure continues to produce estrogen and also begins to produce another hormone, *progesterone*. Progesterone stimulates the estrogen-primed lining of the uterus to thicken further, produce more blood vessels, and manufacture a special sugar within the *uterine glands*. Progesterone also slows down contractions in the uterus and the fallopian tubes, causes the cervical mucus to become thin and impenetrable to sperm, and produces a slight elevation in basal body temperature. This sequence of events facilitates intercourse, fertilization, and the implantation of a fertilized egg.

If fertilization does not occur, the corpus luteum shrivels and ceases to produce estrogen and progesterone. The dip in these hormones causes the lining of the uterus to shrink and the nearby arteries to constrict, so that the lining becomes starved for blood. Ultimately the arteries reopen and bleed, causing the top two-thirds of the lining to detach and be shed. The resulting discharge is called a *menstrual period*. After several days the low levels of progesterone and estrogen stimulate the hypothalamus to again send releasing factor to the pituitary gland, which in turn sends out FSH to the ovary, starting a new cycle of egg production.

HORMONAL CHANGES DURING PREGNANCY

If fertilization takes place after the egg pops out of the ovary, a whole different sequence of events begins. In this case the corpus luteum that surrounded the developing egg continues to grow and change, producing steadily increasing amounts of progesterone. These levels of progesterone are thought to maintain pregnancy in its earliest phases. In fact, the name *progesterone* comes from the Latin word meaning "in favor of gestation."

Meanwhile the fertilized egg grows into a ball of cells and travels into the uterus, where it floats freely for a time and then burrows into the lining of the uterus, attaching itself with fingerlike projections, called the *trophoblast*, which eventually will form the placenta (see p. 58). These microscopic projections play a major role in the endocrinology of pregnancy; within days they begin to manufacture hormones themselves. The trophoblast quickly produces enormous amounts of estrogen. In a single day it causes a pregnant woman's body to produce as much estrogen as a nonpregnant woman's ovaries produce in 3 years. During the course of a normal pregnancy, a pregnant woman produces as much estrogen as a nonpregnant woman would in 150 years!

What is truly remarkable is that most of the estrogen is actually produced by the placenta, not by the mother's ovaries. As early as the seventh week of pregnancy, over half the mother's estrogen levels are placental in origin. But the placenta cannot make estrogen from basic chemicals (cholesterol and acetates), as does the corpus luteum in the mother's ovary. For estrogen production to occur, the placenta needs the help of the fetus. Doctors refer to this remarkable relationship as the *fetoplacental unit*. To make estrogen, the placenta converts a male-like hormone that comes from the adrenal glands of the growing baby (as well as from the mother's adrenals). Not surprisingly, the fetal adrenals are comparatively the largest organs in the baby's body during pregnancy; they are as large as an adult's and produce ten times the amount of hormones that an adult's do. After birth the baby's adrenals shrink considerably, their part in maintaining pregnancy having been completed.

The hormones produced by the placenta in conjunction with the fetus profoundly affect the mother's body. Because the fetoplacental unit, rather than the mother, makes so many of the hormones, some doctors question the extent to which the baby controls the environment in which it is growing. This information certainly gives a new perspective on pregnancy. Most people think in terms of the protected setting and sustenance the mother's body provides the growing baby; in other words, they think of the mother's body as being in charge. But it appears more accurate to think in terms of the mother's body responding to chemical messages from the baby and the placenta. Thus right from the beginning we have a new and more profound sense of the baby as an independent being.

Besides initially promoting fertilization, estrogen has multiple effects on the mother's body throughout gestation. During pregnancy estrogen causes growth and change to occur in the uterus, cervix, vagina, and breasts. Estrogen also causes significant changes in the mother's body metabolism—her salt and water balance, insulin secretion, and ability to break down sugars and carbohydrates. These general physiological changes cause many of the alterations in mood and body sensations that are common to expectant mothers. (We will deal with these changes more specifically in the section on physiology.)

In addition to estrogen, the placenta produces several other hormones. In fact, the placenta produces more progesterone than estrogen, taking over this function from the corpus luteum, which produces progesterone in the days immediately after fertilization. The pregnant mother's progesterone levels become ten times as high as they were before conception. These high levels of progesterone keep the uterus from contracting and encourage the growth and mainte-

(text continues on page 40)

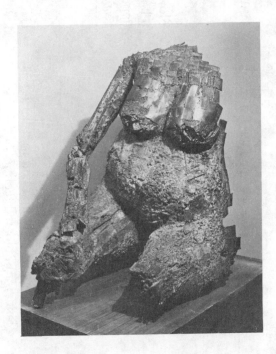

High levels of estrogen and progesterone cause many changes in the pregnant woman's breasts, uterus, and vagina. Torso, Cesar, 1954. Welded iron, 30⅜" x 23⅜" x 27⅛". Collection, The Museum of Modern Art, New York. The Blanchette Rockefeller Fund.

Body feelings during pregnancy

CONDITION	CAUSE	REMEDY
Morning sickness: can occur at any time of day; generally begins between the 2nd and 6th week, and ends by the 14th week.	Unclear. Thought to result from increased HCG hormone. Affected by slowed digestion, emotional lability, and stress.	Frequent, small meals as often as every 2 hours. Eat dry carbohydrates upon awakening and for snacks whenever stomach feels upset. Avoid smelly, spicy, or greasy foods. If severe, doctor may recommend medication, such as Emetrol, rather than Bendectin.
Food cravings for specific foods or unusual combinations of foods.	Unknown.	No treatment necessary unless mother's diet becomes unbalanced or she craves nonfood substances such as clay or starch.
Heartburn: a burning sensation in the esophagus or regurgitating small amounts of acid stomach fluid.	Slowed peristalsis and digestion, and relaxed function of the stomach's upper valve caused by increased progesterone.	Avoid large or fatty meals. Sit erect; don't bend over the stomach. Avoid drinking large quantities of liquids with meals. May be helped by milk or ice cream; if necessary, *low-salt* antacids such as Gelusil or Maalox can be used.
Excess gas, including burping, flatulence, and bloated feeling.	Decreased peristalsis due to increased levels of progesterone.	Avoid gas-producing foods such as cabbage and cauliflower, and avoid large, fatty meals. Chew food thoroughly.
Constipation: infrequent, hard stools.	Slowed peristalsis due to increased progesterone causes more water to be absorbed from the bowel; iron supplements add to the problem.	Increase fluids, fruits (especially prunes), roughage (especially bran). Get regular exercise. Pay attention to bowel signals and try to establish regular bowel habits.
Gingivitis: red, swollen, tender gums which bleed easily. Occasionally little lumps will develop on the gums.	Increased amounts of estrogen stimulate the growth of blood vessels throughout the body.	Maintain good dental hygiene throughout pregnancy, brushing and flossing regularly. The condition normally disappears within several months after delivery.

CONDITION	CAUSE	REMEDY
Hemorrhoids: swollen veins around the anus can cause itching or pain and may protrude after a bowel movement.	Progesterone causes the walls of the veins to relax and expand. As pregnancy progresses, the enlarging uterus presses on the veins, slowing blood flow and causing the veins to expand further. Constipation and squeezing aggravate the problem.	Avoid constipating foods (see above). Soaking in a warm bath relieves discomfort because it increases blood flow, emptying the veins and reducing swelling. Witch hazel or ice packs likewise reduce swelling. Anesthetic ointments also lessen swelling and discomfort. Get moderate exercise. Avoid standing for long periods; rest with hips elevated to increase return blood flow.
Varicose veins: swollen veins in calves, thighs.	Progesterone causes the walls of the veins to relax and expand (as with hemorrhoids). May become worse as pregnancy progresses and the enlarging uterus slows blood flow from the legs. Tends to run in families.	Avoid tight clothing or stockings around the calves. Avoid standing for long periods. Avoid crossing legs at the knee. Rest often with legs elevated. If necessary, wear support hose.
Swollen ankles.	Impaired return of venous blood flow from the legs due to pressure of the enlarging uterus on the veins of the legs.	Avoid tight clothing around the legs. Avoid prolonged standing or sitting. Rest with legs elevated. Rest on either side, not on back, to relieve pressure on the vena cava (see p. 45).
Reddened palms and spider nevi, which are tiny, widened arteries just under the skin.	Increased amounts of estrogen.	Reddened palms normally disappear within a week after birth, while the spiders fade with time, but do not completely disappear.
Oily skin and acne.	Increased amounts of estrogen.	Wash frequently with medicated soaps. Do not use topical or internal vitamin A–related medications (see p. 131). Condition normally disappears after delivery.

(continued)

CONDITION	CAUSE	REMEDY
Faintness or dizziness when standing up or lying down suddenly.	Slowed circulation. Sudden standing causes blood to pool in the legs; lying on the back puts pressure on the vena cava, which slows blood return to the heart.	Avoid sudden position changes and lying flat on back. Get lots of exercise, especially for the legs.
Shortness of breath or difficult breathing.	Increased progesterone speeds breathing to meet the body's increased need for oxygen. As pregnancy progresses, the uterus pushes up the diaphragm, giving a feeling of less room to breathe.	Standing or sitting erect and keeping shoulders back relieves shortness of breath. Raising arms over head lifts the rib cage and gives lungs more space. Avoid hyperventilating by breathing at a normal rate.
Lower back pain.	The enlarging uterus changes a woman's center of gravity and tends to tilt her pelvis forward, straining the muscles of her back. This tilting tends to increase as pregnancy progresses.	Maintain good posture with pelvis tilted back (see p. 104). Do regular abdominal exercises to strengthen muscles that support the uterus. Avoid back strain from excessive bending, lifting, and walking. Always squat rather than bend to lift. Wear low-heeled shoes. Sleep on a hard mattress. If necessary, wear a maternity girdle.
Breast tenderness.	Increased blood vessel and glandular development due to hormonal changes. May be particularly noticeable in early pregnancy.	Warm showers and a well-fitting maternity bra lessen tenderness.
Upper backache.	Most common in first trimester, when breasts increase rapidly in size, putting increased strain on the muscles of the upper back.	A well-fitting maternity bra relieves strain.
Round ligament pain: pain along a diagonal line from the top of the uterus down to either side of the pubic bone.	Stretching and pressure from enlarging uterus on these ligaments.	Support uterus with pillows when lying down; roll out of bed, and push to a sitting position or out of a chair to lessen strain. Warm baths or a heating pad may help, as may a maternity girdle.

CONDITION	CAUSE	REMEDY
Leg cramps.	Increased pressure from the uterus on the nerves and veins going to the legs can cause muscle spasms.	Pull up toes with hands or push heel down on floor or bedboard. Regular exercise and leg elevation help prevent the problem.
Tingling and numbness in the fingertips.	Drooping shoulders and thrusting head forward put pressure on the nerves under the arms.	Good posture with spine and head erect will help alleviate the problem, as will a maternity bra and occasional bed rest.
Urinary frequency and occasional leakage.	Increased pressure from the uterus on the bladder during first trimester; baby drops and presses on the bladder after lightening in late pregnancy.	Before bed or travel, decrease liquids to lessen frequency. Do Kegel exercises to strengthen urinary sphincter and prevent leakage (see p. 102).
Excessive thick vaginal secretions.	Produced by cervix in response to high levels of estrogen. The acidity of the secretion protects the baby against infection.	Follow normal cleanliness routines. Wear absorbent underpants and change frequently. Call doctor if secretion changes color or causes burning or itching. Do not douche unless practitioner advises.
Insomnia.	Initially due to urinary frequency and various discomforts. During the last weeks, anticipation, anxiety, fetal movements, and muscle cramps may interrupt normal sleep.	A firm bed with many pillows arranged to provide support for crucial areas will help to achieve a comfortable position. Warm milk, a warm bath, or relaxation exercises before bed may help to induce sleep. Regular exercise during the day also seems to help.
Fatigue.	Of unknown origin in early pregnancy. May be hormonal; possibly due to disruption of normal sleep cycles due to urinary frequency at night. Fatigue in late pregnancy may be due to insomnia and cumbersome size.	Rest is the only treatment. Early fatigue generally goes away by second trimester. Decrease liquids at night if frequency is a problem. Avoid insomnia-inducing circumstances if possible. Paradoxically, limited amounts of exercise during the day may help.

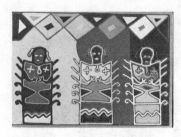

When women first become pregnant, they often do not realize the extent to which their body will undergo change. The Mothers of the Gods, *Huichol Indian, Mexico. The Fine Arts Museums of San Francisco. Gift of Mr. Peter F. Young.*

nance of blood vessels and glands in the uterine lining. In this way progesterone helps to maintain pregnancy and nourish the growing baby.

The placenta is also responsible for making *human chorionic gonadotropin (HCG)* and *placental lactogen (HPL)*. Chorionic gonadotropin initially keeps the corpus luteum from shrinking back in the weeks right after conception. It is one of the first hormones to be made in pregnancy; production begins as soon as the fertilized egg differentiates into diverse kinds of cells. HCG is the chemical that is measured in over-the-counter early pregnancy tests, and it is thought to keep the mother's body from rejecting the embryo as foreign tissue (see pp. 48–49); later in pregnancy it causes boy babies' testes to produce the male hormone *testosterone*. Placental lactogen, the other hormone produced by the placenta, alters the mother's metabolism to make sugars and proteins more available to the growing fetus. It is believed to be the main hormone involved in the baby's growth. Placental lactogen also stimulates the *alveoli* in the mother's breasts to develop and prepare for lactation. It is truly remarkable that the embryo can produce substances related to such varied and time-dependent activities.

Changes in Maternal Anatomy and Physiology During Pregnancy

Before becoming pregnant the first time, few women realize the tremendous extent to which their bodies will undergo change as a result of the experience. The changes fall into two categories: those a woman readily feels and notices, and those that are less readily discerned but can nonetheless be measured scientifically. During pregnancy every organ system in the mother's body is affected. Generally organs increase in activity, but some actually decrease.

CHANGES IN THE REPRODUCTIVE ORGANS

The earliest and most obvious changes brought about by pregnancy occur in the mother's reproductive system. Blood vessels in the uterus and vagina increase in size and length continuously throughout the nine-month period. At the same time veins in the pelvic area enlarge so they can act as a reservoir, thereby keeping the blood flow to the embryo at a constant rate. This blood vessel growth is accompanied by an obvious increase in the size of the uterus. By delivery the uterus has grown to between 500 and 1000 times its nonpregnant size. Before conception the volume of the uterus is about 10 milliliters (roughly 2½ teaspoons); by term the volume ranges from 5 to 10 liters (roughly 1 to 2 gallons). In length, the uterus grows from 6.5 to 32 centimeters

(2½ to 12½ inches). The uterus does not merely stretch; actual growth of muscle fibers is responsible for most of the increase in size. Fibers become 7 to 10 times as long and 2 to 7 times as wide. The muscle cells grow in response to the increased levels of estrogen circulating in the mother's body. As the fibers grow, a network of elastic collagen fibers develops between them, adding considerable strength to the uterine wall.

During the first few months the uterus changes from a small, hard, pear-shape organ to a soft, spherical sac through which the baby can easily be felt. By the end of the third month the uterus begins to expand out of the pelvic cavity, touching the abdominal wall first and later pushing the intestines up and to each side. The uterus continues to grow until by the ninth month it almost touches the mother's liver, just under her bottom right rib. Most mothers readily verify this piece of anatomical information when the baby moves and kicks in late pregnancy. Eventually the diaphragm, which separates the chest from

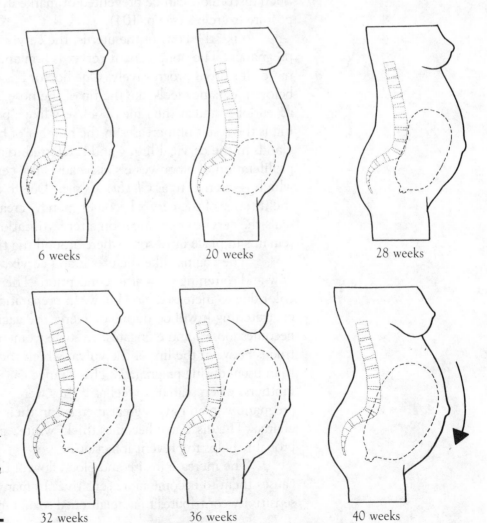

6 weeks   20 weeks   28 weeks

During pregnancy the uterus grows from 500 to 1000 times its nonpregnant size. Changes in the weight and size of the uterus cause corresponding alterations in the mother's posture, resulting in an exaggerated curve in her lower spine.

32 weeks   36 weeks   40 weeks

the abdominal cavity, is pushed up about 4 centimeters by the enlarging uterus. This change actually causes minor alterations in the position of the heart and lungs (see p. 45).

As it expands above the bony pelvic basket, the top of the uterus is no longer supported by the tough pelvic ligaments. Rather, it becomes freely movable, supported by the backbone when a woman is lying down and by the abdominal wall when she is standing. The increase in the size and weight of the uterus causes noticeable changes to take place in the mother's posture. To counterbalance the weight of the uterus leaning on the abdominal wall, the pregnant woman tends to tilt backward which results in an exaggerated curve in her lower spine. She may also tend to tilt her head forward and slump her shoulders slightly. This curvature of the lower spine, coupled with the natural loosening of the pelvic joints, contributes to increased strain on the muscles and ligaments of the lower back and legs, resulting in the common backache and muscle aches that many women experience in the last trimester. Occasionally changes in the mother's head and shoulder positions may even cause numbness and aching in her arms. Such discomfort can be prevented or markedly alleviated by doing posture exercises (see p. 104).

Like the body of the uterus, the cervix shows changes early in pregnancy. The nonpregnant cervix is firm and muscular. During pregnancy it softens progressively. One doctor has observed that the cervix before pregnancy feels like the tip of the nose, at mid-pregnancy like an earlobe, and at the time of delivery like a person's lips. This softening is the result of increases in the number of blood vessels and mucous glands in the cervical lining and is referred to as *Goodell's sign*. The proliferation of blood vessels also causes the cervix to become bluish, which is referred to as *Chadwick's sign*. Due to the increase in glands, the interior of the cervix becomes spongy, creating a *mucous plug* that seals the cervical opening soon after fertilization takes place. This plug remains in place until somewhere around the time labor begins.

The vagina, like the uterus and cervix, shows increased blood flow and softening soon after conception. The vagina takes on a violet color due to increased blood flow. In preparation for the huge amount of stretching it will do during delivery, the vaginal wall thickens, becomes looser, and elongates. In some women the vagina almost protrudes between the lips of the vulva, which themselves may be larger than usual during pregnancy. This change causes some expectant mothers, when seated, to feel as if they were sitting on something. All pregnant women have a great increase in their normal vaginal discharge. The discharge becomes thick, white, and also acidic, which probably helps to prevent infection.

The increase in size and blood flow of the reproductive organs causes them to become more sensitive. In many women this increased sensitivity contributes to a heightened sexual interest and arousal, particularly in the second trimester (see p. 110). In women as in men, sexual excitement depends upon erectile tissues swelling with blood. In a pregnant woman the erectile tissues are continuously in a somewhat swollen state. This condition not only tends to make a woman more easily aroused, it tends to increase the likelihood of her ability to have multiple orgasms. In the last trimester the uterus may even spasm during and after intercourse.

During pregnancy a woman's breasts undergo remarkable changes. Within several weeks after conception—about the time of the first missed menstrual period—many women become aware of tingling, fullness, heaviness, or even soreness in their breasts. These sensations are due to breast engorgement caused by the growth of ducts and milk glands or *alveoli*. High levels of estrogen and progesterone are responsible for these changes, just as they are for the changes in the uterus. Breast tenderness may occur off and on throughout pregnancy, particularly during sexual arousal, when increased blood flow adds to the engorgement of the already swollen tissues.

By the second month of pregnancy the breasts begin to increase noticeably in size and become somewhat lumpy as the alveoli increase. As pregnancy progresses, small veins and stretch marks called *striae* become visible in the skin over the breasts. The *areola*, the pigmented area around the nipples, become wider and darker. Color change tends to be greatest among dark-skinned women. Tiny oil-producing glands in the areola become more prominent and raised. And the nipples themselves become larger, darker, and more erectile. Many women find that individual milk ducts in their nipples become more readily distinguishable. By the end of the tenth week some women begin to notice a discharge from their nipples, particularly if they are squeezed or sucked on. This fluid, called *colostrum*, becomes thicker, creamier, and yellower as pregnancy goes on. It is the same high-protein, high-fat liquid that is produced for about a week after birth, until the mature milk comes in.

CHANGES IN OTHER ORGAN SYSTEMS

A number of skin changes are common during pregnancy. We have already mentioned the appearance of stretch marks or striae on the breasts. Such marks also occur on the abdomen, and even thighs, of over half of all pregnant women. They are caused by a breakdown of the elastic tissue in the lower layers of skin. Generally the striae are slightly sunken and redder or purpler than the surrounding skin. After pregnancy the marks don't disappear completely, but lose their color and become less noticeable as the body returns to its prepregnant size.

Throughout pregnancy hormonal changes lead to greater pigmentation of the skin and sensitivity to sunlight. From the end of the second month until term, there are higher levels of a melanocyte-stimulating hormone (*melanocytes* are cells in the lower layers of skin that produce the pigment that determines skin color). Progesterone and estrogen also stimulate the pigment-producing cells. The most common areas where darkened patches occur are the face and neck, the nipples, and the midline of the abdomen, particularly below the navel. Darkening on the face, neck, and abdomen tends to disappear after pregnancy; darkening of the nipples does not.

During pregnancy two-thirds of Caucasian and Asian women and 10 percent of black women develop tiny red raised dots on their skin that are surrounded by spidery red lines. These marks are made up of small blood vessels and are appropriately called *vascular spiders.* The most common locations for vascular spiders are the face, chest, and arms. They are caused by high levels of estrogen and generally disappear after pregnancy, when estrogen levels drop.

Many of the most interesting changes of pregnancy take place inside the body and are neither seen nor felt by the expectant mother. Nevertheless, they have profound implications for the growth of the baby. During pregnancy the volume of the mother's blood increases remarkably. The volume grows slightly in the first trimester, greatly in the second trimester, and somewhat less in the last trimester. By term the woman's body will have an average of one and one-half times as much blood, ranging up to twice as much. The nonpregnant woman has about $3\frac{1}{2}$ quarts of blood; the pregnant woman at term has about $5\frac{1}{2}$ quarts, not including the baby's blood, which is totally separate. This additional quantity is necessary to fill the blood reservoir of the greatly enlarged uterus and to protect the baby against normal drops in maternal blood pressure, as well as to prepare the mother's body for the normal loss of blood experienced during the birth process.

Of the extra blood volume, almost half a quart is pure red blood cells, which represents a third more than the mother normally has. This increase in addition to the blood produced by the fetus, means that the mother needs to enlarge her iron stores greatly in order to keep her red blood cell count normal toward the end of pregnancy. Without supplementary iron the expectant mother will only make about half as many red blood cells as she would with extra iron. The pregnant woman also makes added amounts of several blood clotting factors in response to elevated levels of estrogen.

With such a significant rise in blood volume, the mother's heart needs to work harder than normal, and it does. During pregnancy a woman's resting heart rate (pulse) rises 10 to 15 beats per minute, from about 80 beats to 90 or 95 beats per minute. In addition to the heart beating more quickly, the amount the heart pumps out with each beat increases. As a result of both these factors, the total output of the mother's heart increases by about one-third. Even under the best training conditions no athlete could expect such a dramatic gain in six to nine months.

Surprisingly, a healthy woman's blood pressure shows only slight differences during pregnancy. However, the large size and weight of the uterus have significant effects on the mother's cardiac output and on blood return from the veins in her legs. When a pregnant woman lies flat on her back, the uterus presses on the *vena cava*, which is the largest vein leading to the heart, thereby slowing the return of blood and reducing the amount the heart can pump with each beat. Such pressure on the vena cava also raises the pressure in the veins of the legs and contributes to the varicose veins and swelling of the legs or *edema* that some women develop during pregnancy. By lying on her side, a woman relieves pressure on the vena cava and the veins of her legs. This simple action may raise the output of her heart by 22 percent or more.

Paralleling the changes in the cardiovascular system are important changes in the respiratory system. We mentioned earlier that the expanding uterus pushes up the diaphragm, the large muscle under the lungs that separates the abdomen from the chest cavity. The elevated diaphragm in turn reduces the space for the lungs, but this loss is compensated for by the expansion of the rib cage. As pregnancy progresses, the mother's ribs actually flare up and out as the angle between her ribs and her backbone widens.

During pregnancy a woman's lungs become more efficient, bringing in extra air and oxygenating additional blood to keep up with the greater volume passing through her heart. Amazingly, this increased efficiency is accomplished without any increase in the size of her lungs or in the number of times she inhales per minute. Each breath simply takes in more air. In fact, during the latter part of pregnancy, each time the mother inhales and exhales, she moves 39 percent more air. Any serious athlete would love to equal such a feat. The increased movement of air makes it possible for the additional red blood cells to carry that much more oxygen to the body.

As a result of all these changes, many women become more aware of their breathing during pregnancy. Some women report that it feels more difficult to breathe. Actually it is no more difficult; they are simply breathing more deeply and moving more air, which requires extra effort. This deeper breathing is automatically regulated by increased levels of progesterone affecting the respiratory center in the mother's brain. By week 24 of gestation, the pressure of the expanding uterus causes a woman to begin to breathe high in her chest rather than from her abdomen. The change often makes women slightly uncomfortable, but it can be helped by abdominal breathing exercises (see p. 103).

Some of the most noticeable changes that take place during pregnancy relate to the digestive tract. As we said earlier, the expanding uterus gradually pushes the intestines and even the stomach up and to the side. The shift in the stomach's position changes the angle at

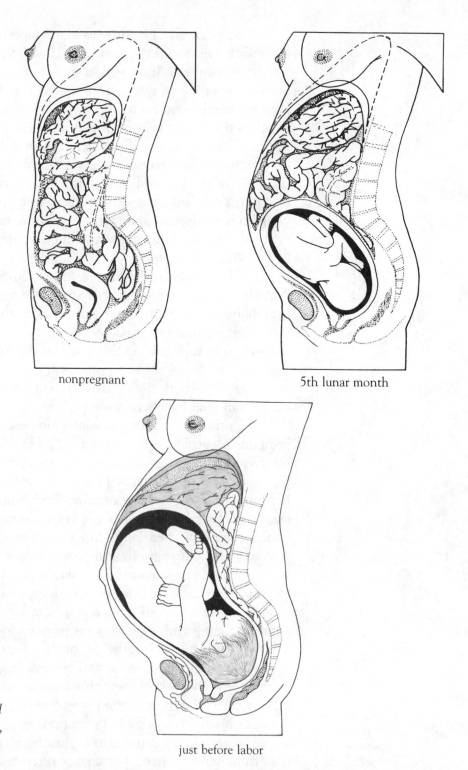

nonpregnant

5th lunar month

just before labor

The expanding uterus and growing baby gradually but significantly shift the mother's intestines, stomach, and diaphragm up or to the side, affecting both her digestion and breathing.

which the esophagus enters the stomach, causing the valve at the top of the stomach to work less efficiently than usual. This change is partly responsible for the common condition called *heartburn,* in which the stomach contents come up into the esophagus. In addition, the high levels of progesterone produced by the fetoplacental unit decrease the muscle tone and motion of smooth muscle throughout the woman's body.

Lowered muscle tone and displacement of the digestive organs contribute to heartburn, indigestion, and constipation, which are among the most common complaints of pregnancy. Since all the muscles and valves in the digestive tract are smooth muscle, the *transit time*, the time it takes food to move through the stomach and intestine, is greatly increased. Because food moves more slowly through the lower intestine, more water is absorbed from the stool, and the stool tends to become harder. The morning sickness that is sometimes experienced in early pregnancy probably has a more complicated cause. It is thought to be due to a combination of longer transit time, poor valve action, anxiety, and a physiological response to human chorionic gonadotropin (see p. 40), the hormone that maintains the mother's estrogen levels in very early pregnancy.

Bleeding gums are another digestive system alteration that is brought about by hormonal changes. Many pregnant women notice that their gums become puffy and red and bleed excessively when brushed. This is nothing to worry about; it is a result of the general blood vessel stimulation caused by higher levels of estrogen. The old myths about losing teeth or getting new cavities with each pregnancy are not true. The growing baby does not rob the mother's teeth of calcium, and puffy gums are just a temporary condition.

Among the most significant changes in pregnancy are those that occur in metabolic processes. At no other time in a woman's life do such tremendous changes take place in her ability to break down food, make energy, and maintain cells. In general, all metabolic processes speed up in response to the increasing needs of the growing baby and the enlarging uterus. During pregnancy women normally store more water than usual—up to 7 quarts in the last month. This water is retained throughout the body, but is especially taken up by the fetus, the placenta, the amniotic fluid, and the mother's increased blood volume, as well as by her enlarged uterus, breasts, and legs.

A pregnant woman also stores much more protein than she does in the nonpregnant state. The mother herself adds about four pounds of protein to her body, and the baby about a pound and a half. These gains require a significant and constant increase in protein intake throughout pregnancy. Fat metabolism is altered during pregnancy as well. Around the second trimester an excess of fat is stored by the mother's body; toward the end of pregnancy this excess is drawn on by the baby.

The mother's carbohydrate needs rise tremendously during pregnancy. Basically the body metabolizes carbohydrates into a simple sugar called glucose, which is used to make energy. The growing baby may use enough glucose to drop the mother's blood sugar levels slightly below normal. At the same time the mother's body makes more *insu-*

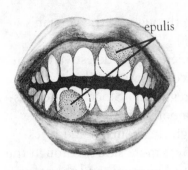

epulis

High levels of estrogen during pregnancy cause the mother's gums to become puffy, bleed easily, and occasionally develop swellings called epulis.

lin, the hormone that is necessary for cells to break down glucose. For reasons that doctors do not understand, this insulin does not work as effectively as usual. The complicated alterations in sugar metabolism that occur during pregnancy occasionally bring on a temporary diabetes that disappears when pregnancy ends.

One of the changes that mothers are most aware of is the significant weight gain brought about by pregnancy. Although there is great variation among healthy women, the average pregnant woman gains about 25 pounds: roughly 3 to 4 pounds in the first trimester, another 12 to 14 pounds in the second trimester, and 8 to 10 more in the third trimester. Of this increase, about 11½ pounds is accounted for by the baby, the placenta, and the amniotic fluid. Thus more than half of the 25 pounds is weight gained by the mother. This additional weight is distributed as follows: 2½ pounds in the uterus, 3 pounds in the breasts, 4 pounds in extra protein stores, 3½ pounds in extra blood, and 4½ pounds in excess fluid.

Not surprisingly, the mother's urinary system undergoes important changes during gestation. First, the system has to process the wastes of both mother and baby. As a result, the amount of material the mother's kidneys filter goes up by as much as 50 percent. Under this tremendous load the kidneys may begin to work less effectively, spilling amino acids (proteinuria), vitamins, and sugar. While this might be a problem in a nonpregnant woman, it is generally not a problem during pregnancy because the kidneys are filtering such large amounts of blood.

Like the digestive tract, the urinary tract is made of smooth muscle, which, as we have said, loses tone during pregnancy due to the high levels of progesterone. As a result, urine tends to move more slowly into and out of the bladder, slightly increasing the chances of urinary infection. Also, the expanding uterus puts pressure on the bladder, decreasing the amount of urine it can hold and causing the expectant mother to have greater frequency of urination. Many women particularly notice this increased frequency at night because it causes them to waken.

Finally, some fascinating changes take place in the pregnant woman's immunological system. Since the fetus is genetically different from the mother, its presence is somewhat like that of a transplanted organ. Normally a person's body will reject a transplant, making antibodies to attack it. Rh incompatibility is an example of the mother's body producing antibodies against the cells of a baby who has a different blood type from her own (see p. 40).

Why the mother's body usually doesn't reject the fetus is still unknown, but several factors seem to play a part. First, the placenta is fairly effective in keeping the baby's cells from entering the mother's bloodstream. Second, doctors have found in animal studies that high levels of progesterone slow down antibody production and delay rejection of skin grafts. Finally, the baby is thought to produce special surface repellent molecules that cross the placenta and coat the mother's *lymphocytes*, the white blood cells that normally produce antibodies, thereby preventing them from attacking the baby's cells.

All of the changes that take place in the expectant mother's anatomy and physiology show how well-prepared her body is to conceive and nurture a baby over a nine-month period. These dramatic transformations result in a wide variety of new sensations. When a woman understands the cause of these sensations, she doesn't worry about them, she develops even greater trust in her body, and she can work more effectively to prevent or alleviate the inevitable minor discomforts that pregnancy brings.

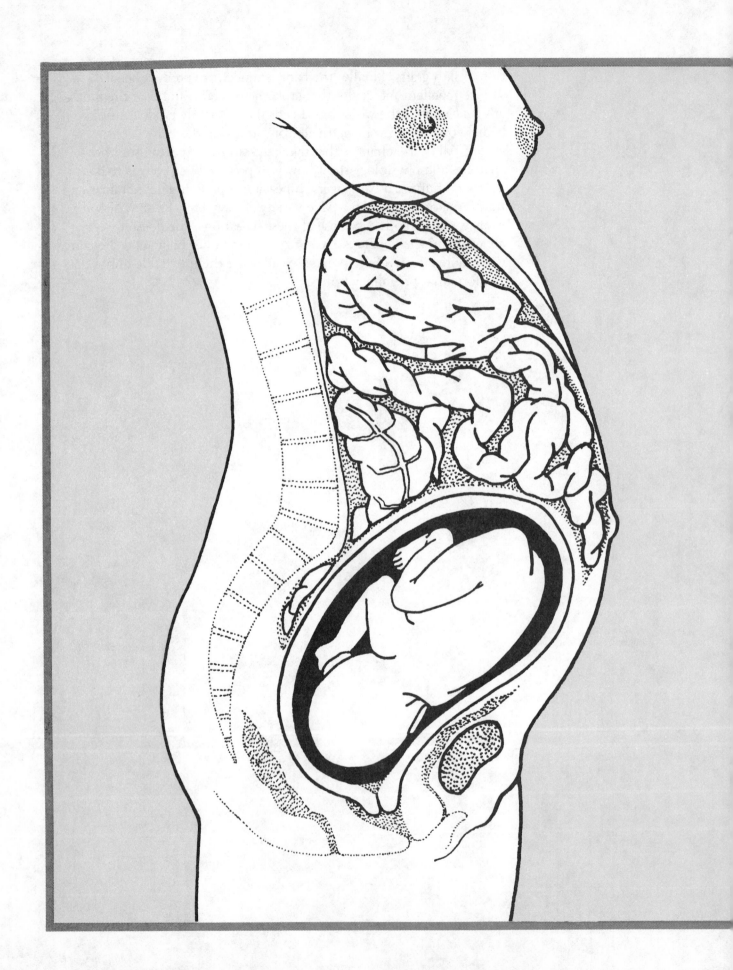

Development of the Baby

Visualizing Development

Once pregnancy is confirmed, parents become extremely curious about what is going on inside the uterus. Unfortunately, such information has traditionally been hard to come by. Much of people's information about pregnancy and prenatal development comes from relatives and friends and tends to be very sketchy. This information may have been augmented over the years by health classes and biology or embryology courses that deal with fetal development in greater detail. But generally the health classes people have taken were at a junior high level and the biology courses dealt with chicks and amphibians. Women who are pregnant often discuss their physical experiences and sensations, but for the most part the baby's development is not visible and not accessible through firsthand experience. Up to now what's been widely available has been unique and arresting photographs of the developing fetus, such as those of Lennart Nielsen. Really specific information has only been available in medical texts that are often impenetrably dense and sometimes alarming.

Just as infants pass through a series of landmarks from birth to age one, so the developing baby in utero passes through an even more complex and miraculous set of landmarks from conception to birth.

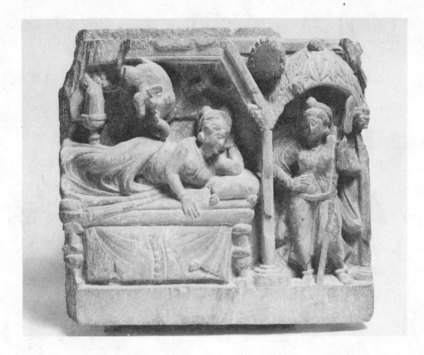

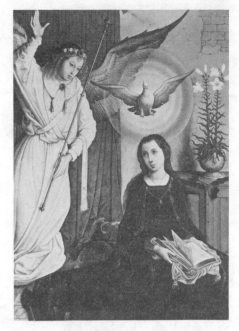

We believe that the more parents understand about the baby's development in the uterus, the more they become involved in their parenting role even before birth. Being able to visualize what's happening gives parents a here-and-now grounding in what initially may seem a rather abstract experience. A vivid mental picture of the events unfolding within the uterus enables expectant parents to feel a special connection to the baby. And it helps to motivate them to act in ways that will ensure that their baby's growth and development is positive right from conception.

Actually a woman does not usually know that she is pregnant until a great deal of development has already occurred. A few women immediately notice subtle changes in their body or have a truly psychic sense that conception has taken place, but most don't suspect they are pregnant until they miss a menstrual period. By that time the baby is already three weeks old and beginning to develop its nervous system. But we will begin at the beginning.

Production of the Egg and Sperm

Human development begins at the moment of fertilization, when the father's sperm makes contact with an egg (or eggs) from the mother. Biologists refer to this way of initiating new life as *sexual reproduction.* It differs fundamentally from *asexual reproduction,* which, in the absence of mutation, produces offspring that are exact copies of the parent organism. Sexual reproduction creates infinite variety by shuffling the genetic material of the mother and father.

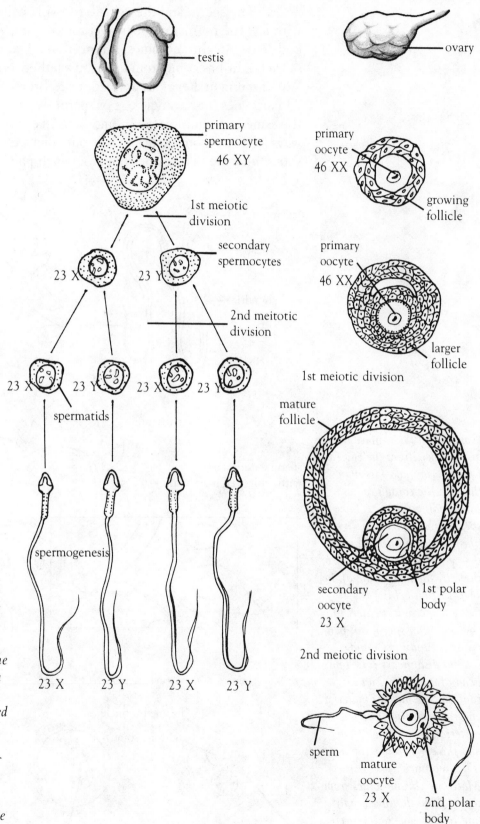

testis

primary
spermocyte
46 XY

1st meiotic
division

secondary
spermocytes

23 X   23 Y

2nd meitotic
division

23 X   23 Y   23 X   23 Y

spermatids

spermogenesis

23 X   23 Y   23 X   23 Y

ovary

primary
oocyte
46 XX

growing
follicle

primary
oocyte
46 XX

larger
follicle

1st meiotic division

mature
follicle

secondary   1st polar
oocyte   body
23 X

2nd meiotic division

sperm

mature
oocyte
23 X

2nd polar
body

*In the formation of both egg
and sperm, two special cell
divisions take place that
leave these cells with half the
number of chromosomes of a
normal human cell. In the
male four sperm are produced
from each original cell. In
the female only one egg is
ultimately produced; half of
each division turns into a
polar body. This process
gives all the cytoplasm to the
one egg that is produced.*

The sperm and the egg are the only cells in the human body with *half* the normal number of chromosomes. All other cells in the body have 46 chromosomes, arranged in 23 complementary pairs. One of each pair has come from a person's father, one from the mother. When sperm and eggs are formed, one chromosome from each of the 23 pairs goes into a single egg or sperm. No egg or sperm gets exactly the same combination of chromosomes, because there are so many ways for the chromosomes to sort out. Picture 23 different pairs of shoes: imagine taking one shoe from each pair, randomly choosing

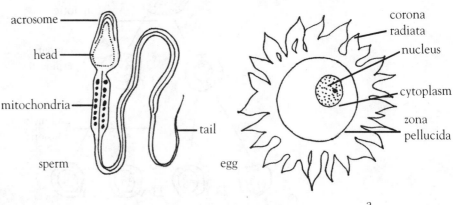

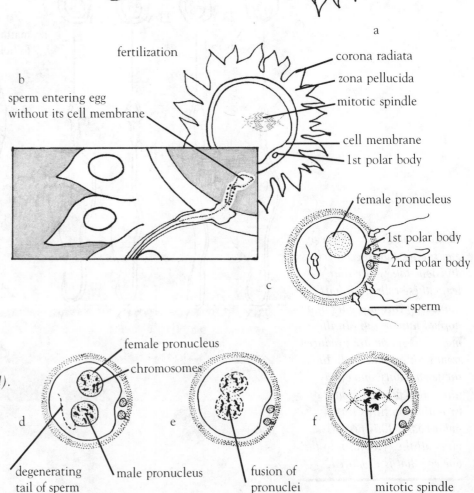

Conception takes place when a sperm fertilizes the egg (a). One sperm makes its way through the corona radiata surrounding the egg. The sperm then pierces the plasma membrane and enters the cytoplasm in the center of the cell; the membrane of the sperm is left behind (b). Once a sperm has entered the egg, no other sperm can penetrate it, and the corona radiata disappears (c). The head of the sperm, which contains the nuclear material, enlarges greatly. The nuclear material of both the sperm and the egg become apparent (d). The two nuclei fuse (e). Matching chromosomes from the egg and the sperm pair and line up for the first cell division (f).

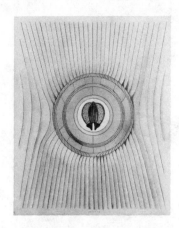

Only one sperm in a million reaches the egg. The Blind Swimmer, *Max Ernst, 1934. Oil on canvas, 36⅜" x 29". Collection, The Museum of Modern Art, New York. Gift of Mrs. Pierre Matisse and the Helena Rubinstein Fund.*

either a right or a left. Repeating this a number of times in a row, you'd never get the same combination of shoes. In essence, this is the way in which the chromosomes are allotted to individual sperm and egg cells.

At birth a woman actually has the cells that are precursors of all the eggs she will ever produce. At 50 days a female embryo has 600,000 of these primitive *germ cells,* or potential eggs. At the peak, during a female embryo's fifth month in the uterus, it has 7 million germ cells. No more are formed, and the number drops continually after this. By puberty a girl only has 30,000 remaining germ cells. Of these only 400 will actually mature in the years between puberty and menopause.

Shortly before a girl is born, her potential eggs start to divide in a special way. Up to this point the germ cells have contained 46 chromosomes, but now they start to divide into cells that will have only 23 chromosomes. Amazingly, this special cell division, called a *reduction division,* stops at an early stage. Surrounding cells produce a substance called *oocyte maturation inhibitor* that keeps the cell division frozen until a girl reaches puberty. Once puberty begins, this special cell division is resumed: one germ cell completes the division into an egg with half the usual number of chromosomes about 38 to 48 hours before ovulation. This process continues on a monthly basis until a woman reaches menopause.

During ovulation the newly divided cell starts to divide a second time. But only if it is fertilized does it complete this second division. Although it is smaller than a dot and has only half the usual number of chromosomes, the mature egg is a giant among cells: it is almost 100,000 times heavier than a sperm. The egg or *ovum* is surrounded by a layer of cells called the *corona radiata.* Inside the corona radiata is a clear membrane called the *zona pellucida.* Within the egg is the control center or *nucleus,* which contains the egg's 23 chromosomes. The nucleus is surrounded by *yolk,* which supplies the ovum and later the embryo with nutrients for several days if fertilization takes place.

Like the female, the male fetus has germ cells present that will remain dormant until puberty. But *unlike* the female, the male germ cells are not suspended in the middle of a reduction division. In a male the reduction divisions do not start until puberty. More important, the male germ cells begin to multiply at puberty, producing new cells daily. Eventually they produce 4 sperm for every germ cell. On the average, a man produces 300 million sperm cells a day.

Each sperm consists of a head and a tail. The head has a cover called the *acrosome* and contains the nucleus, which has 23 chromosomes. Whereas all eggs contain a female chromosome called the X *chromosome,* sperm may contain either an X or a Y *chromosome.* An X from both mother and father produces a girl; an X from the mother

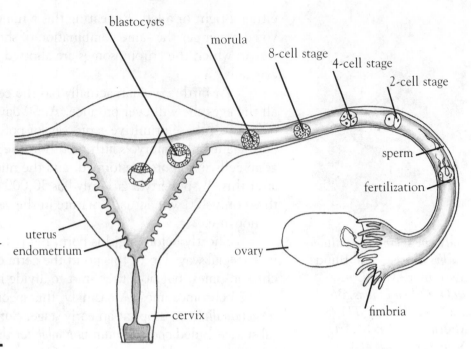

blastocysts

morula

8-cell stage

4-cell stage

2-cell stage

sperm

fertilization

uterus
endometrium

ovary

cervix

fimbria

It takes approximately five days for an egg to erupt from the ovary, pass into the fallopian tube, be fertilized, and then travel on into the uterine cavity. During this time the egg undergoes a number of cell divisions.

and a Y from the father produces a boy. Thus the father's sperm determines the sex of the baby.

Development of the Fetus

CONCEPTION

Around the fourteenth day of a woman's menstrual cycle, a single egg in one ovary undergoes a growth spurt as a result of hormones that are circulating in her bloodstream (see p. 31). The egg swells the side of the ovary and eventually bursts out of it. At this point the egg is briefly free in the abdominal cavity, but then it is swept into the opening of the *fallopian tube* on a wave of abdominal fluid that moves in

The decision to conceive a baby is a momentous choice that opens new areas in a couple's relationship. Two Dreaming The Same Dream, *Constantino Nivola, 1962. Collection of Whitney Museum of American Art, New York. Gift of the Howard and Jean Lipman Foundation.*

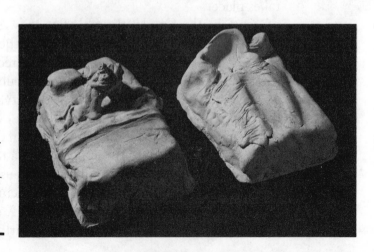

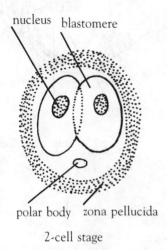

nucleus blastomere

polar body zona pellucida

2-cell stage

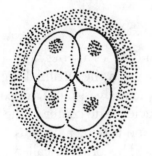

4-cell stage

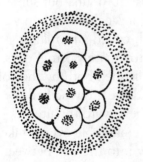

8-cell stage

After fertilization the egg doubles its cell number with each division, passing through a 2-, 4-, and 8-cell stage.

response to the beating of the *fimbriae,* the fingerlike projections at the end of the tube. Once it is in the mouth of the tube, the egg is slowly moved along by muscular contractions of the fallopian tube and by the beating of microscopic projections called *cilia,* which line the tube.

For fertilization to be accomplished, the sperm must begin their journey to meet the egg at about the same time as ovulation occurs. When a man and a woman have intercourse, the man's ejaculation propels the sperm to the back of the woman's vagina, near where the cervix enters the uterus. The average ejaculation consists of 3½ milliliters of *semen,* which contains about 350 million sperm. Although the egg is less than twelve inches from the cervix, and the sperm can cover the distance in as little as five minutes, very few will complete the journey. Several factors work against the sperm: distance, the curves and crannies of the fallopian tube, the presence of an egg in only one of the tubes, and the fact that the fallopian cilia beat in the opposite direction to propel the egg toward the uterus. The result is that only 300 to 500 of the original millions of sperm actually reach the egg—that is, one sperm in a million.

A few factors aid the sperm's journey. Sperm have a powerful energy packet in their tails and are strong swimmers. Around the time of ovulation the vaginal mucus becomes alkaline like the sperm, and the cervical mucus thins, making entrance to the uterus easier. Both the mechanism of a woman's orgasm and chemicals in the semen cause rhythmic contractions in the uterus and fallopian tube, which also help to propel the sperm toward the egg.

Generally conception takes place high up in the middle of the fallopian tube, in the area called the *ampulla.* The first sperm to reach the egg passes through its outer layers, the corona radiata and the zona pellucida. As soon as the first sperm has penetrated the inner membrane, a remarkable series of reactions takes place. Enzymes in the egg radically alter the inner membrane, making it impenetrable to any other sperm. Meanwhile, the successful sperm fuses its membrane with the membrane of the egg that surrounds the yolk and nucleus. Next, the head and tail of the sperm slip out of their covering and move into the center of the egg. Then the sperm's tail dissolves and its nucleus enlarges greatly. The male and female nuclei move toward each other, their membranes dissolve, and their chromosomes intermingle. The fertilized egg now has 46 chromosomes—23 from the father and 23 from the mother—in a combination that has never occurred before. The number of chromosomes necessary for a human baby to develop has been reestablished. This miraculous process of halving the chromosomes in the egg and the sperm and recombining them in the fertilized egg enables the human species to maintain the same chromosome number from generation to generation, but allows for great diversity. The whole process, from the sperm reaching the egg to the chromosomes intermingling, takes about 24 hours and is called *fertilization.*

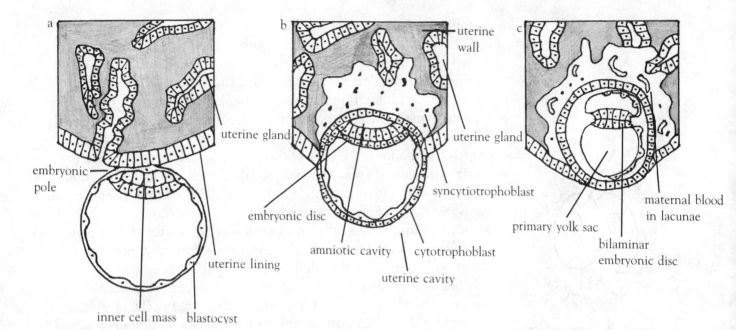

embryonic pole

uterine gland

uterine lining

inner cell mass · blastocyst

uterine wall

embryonic disc

amniotic cavity

uterine cavity

syncytiotrophoblast

cytotrophoblast

uterine gland

primary yolk sac

maternal blood in lacunae

bilaminar embryonic disc

By the time the fertilized egg is ready to implant in the uterine wall, it has formed a hollow ball with a thickening of cells on one side. The thickened side makes contact with the wall of the uterus (a) and develops fingerlike projections that grow into the rich lining of the uterus (b). Eventually the entire growing egg or embryo becomes embedded in the wall of the uterus (c).

THE FIRST TWO WEEKS (0–2 WEEKS)

Over the next several days the fertilized egg undergoes a series of equally extraordinary changes. The chromosomes in the fertilized egg match up by complementary pairs, duplicate themselves, pull to opposite sides of the cell, and form two separate nuclei. The center of the cell then pinches in, dividing the cell in half and leaving a nucleus with 46 chromosomes in each of the new cells. This process, called *cleavage*, occurs again and again, each time doubling the number of cells and also reducing the size of the cells until they are as big as a normal body cell. The first division takes almost 30 hours, but subsequent ones happen faster and faster, producing a 2-cell ball, then a 4-cell ball, and so on until a 12- or 16-cell ball, called a *morula*, is formed. All these changes take place over approximately 3 to 4 days. During this time the dividing ball has been nourished both by the yolk and by fluid secreted by the fallopian tube. And the growing ball of cells has traveled slowly down the fallopian tube toward the uterus.

As the morula enters the uterus, more remarkable events take place. First, fluid from the uterus begins to flow into the ball between the cells, eventually forming a hollow ball with a mass of cells at one end, which is called the *blastocyst*. The cells making up the wall of this ball are referred to as the *trophoblast*, from the Greek word for nutrition. These cells will later give rise to both the membranes that surround the baby and the placenta that nourishes the baby. The group of cells adhering to one side of the wall will develop into the baby itself.

As the blastocyst grows, the zona pellucida, the membrane that had surrounded the egg originally, breaks up and disappears. The zona

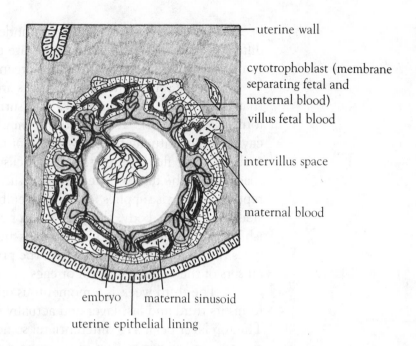

uterine wall

cytotrophoblast (membrane separating fetal and maternal blood)

villus fetal blood

intervillus space

maternal blood

embryo

maternal sinusoid

uterine epithelial lining

After the embryo becomes embedded in the wall of the uterus, fingerlike projections continue to grow out into the uterine lining. They are separated from the mother's blood vessels by a thin membrane. These projections form a rudimentary placenta through which the embryo takes in nutrients and sends out waste products.

pellucida had kept the cells together as a ball and prevented the morula from adhering to the wall of the fallopian tube. With the zona pellucida gone, the sticky outer cells now attach themselves to the wall of the uterus. During days 5 and 6, the outer layer of cells, the trophoblast, develops fingerlike projections that rapidly grow into the rich lining of the uterus, eventually embedding the blastocyst in the wall. As the trophoblast grows into the uterine wall, spaces called *lacunae* form between the projections. These spaces gradually fill with a mixture of maternal blood and secretions from the uterine glands. This fluid mixture will nourish the developing embryo for another week, until the placenta becomes functional.

Blood vessels in the uterine wall, both arteries and veins, now link with the lacunae, and the lacunae themselves become interconnected, assuming a spongelike appearance. Soon the mother's blood starts to flow through these microscopic tunnels, bringing the developing embryo oxygen and food. These nutrients cross the membrane that separates the lacunae from the trophoblast and the embryo. Waste products and carbon dioxide from the embryo cross the membrane in the other direction and are carried away by the mother's bloodstream. Thus although the placenta is not yet fully formed, the embryo is already being nurtured by a primitive system of circulation, which, like the placenta, does not bring the embryo into direct contact with the mother's blood.

THE EMBRYO (2–8 WEEKS)

During the second week the embryo takes advantage of this nutrient supply system and grows very rapidly. The inner cell mass attached to the wall of the blastocyst starts to differentiate, forming two layers and flattening into a *disc.* Up to this point the cells in the embryo have been alike; now, for reasons still not understood, they begin to take on different characteristics that will prepare them for the specialized functions they will perform as the major organ systems develop.

At the same time great changes are taking place in the tissues that will become the membranes that surround the baby. A new space forms above the disc; it is called the *amniotic cavity*. The lining of the cavity will eventually become the *bag of waters* that surrounds the baby with amniotic fluid, protecting it and cushioning it from shock. The space below the disc is called the *yolk sac*. Whereas the yolk sac in reptiles and birds supplies food for an embryo that has to develop outside the mother's body, the yolk sac in humans does not help to nourish the developing embryo. In humans and other primates the yolk sac gives rise to the digestive tract and the primitive germ cells, the precursors of the embryo's sperm or eggs.

The third week is a momentous one for the embryo: the disc forms its third and last layer and actually starts to form the first organs. The top layer begins to differentiate: some of the cells in this layer separate and slowly pile up in the center of the disc, forming a thickening called the *primitive streak*, which is a forerunner of the spinal cord and nervous system. The primitive streak makes apparent an axis by which head and tail and right and left can be identified.

A groove forms in the primitive streak, creating a migratory channel through which cells from the top layer move down and establish a new middle layer between the two older layers. The modified upper layer is called the *ectoderm*; the new middle layer is called the *mesoderm*; and the bottom layer is called the *endoderm*. From these three layers will arise all the cells and organs in the developing embryo. In time, cells from the ectoderm will give rise to the skin, hair, nails, and all the parts of the nervous system. Cells from the mesoderm will give rise to the muscles, bones, blood cells, heart, lungs, and the reproductive and excretory organs. Cells from the endoderm will give rise to the glands and the linings of the lungs and digestive tract.

At about day 16, cells from the mesoderm, the middle layer, begin actively to migrate and differentiate, forming a loosely woven supporting tissue that will act as a scaffold for the developing organs. One group of these cells migrates toward the head end of the embryo, folds in on itself, and forms the *notochord*, which gives rise to the *vertebrae*, the bones of the spine. Cells in the notochord release a chemical that causes great change in the top layer: cells in the ectoderm increase rapidly and form a thickened area called the *neural plate*. This plate soon folds in on itself, giving rise to the spinal cord, the ganglia, and, later, the brain.

The cardiovascular system starts to develop at the same time that the nervous system is unfolding. Another group of cells in the middle layer form clumps called *blood islands*, which develop hollow spaces in the middle. The embryo's first blood cells are produced within these spaces. Eventually the blood islands join together to make blood vessels. Larger clumps form big channels called *heart tubes*, which fuse and give rise to the *primitive heart*. By day 21 all these tubes have become interconnected and have formed a working cardiovascular system within the embryo. Circulation of blood starts by the third week, making this the first organ system to become functional.

While blood vessels were developing in the embryo, others were developing in the trophoblast, the forerunner of the placenta. These blood vessels join with those in the embryo through a tiny stalk. It is this stalk that will develop into the *umbilical cord*, which connects the growing baby with the placenta. At this stage the baby's blood flows from the embryo, through the stalk, and into the primitive placenta, where it flows side by side with the mother's blood, separated by only a thin membrane. This early establishment of a circulatory system is critical to the embryo's survival. The embryo's millions of cells could not continue to grow and develop with only diffusion of nutrients and oxygen from the wall of the uterus.

At about day 20 the mesoderm, the middle layer, begins dividing into matched segments on either side of the spinal column. These blocks of tissue are called *somites*; they will give rise to the bones and muscles of the head and trunk. The somites form slowly in a head-to-tail order. From about day 20 to day 30, 38 pairs of somites will form.

By the end of the third week the embryo is about 2 millimeters long (about ⅛ inch) and has a long, flat, figure-eight shape. It has a working heart and is rapidly developing nervous, skeletal, and digestive systems. The embryo is now totally embedded in the wall of the uterus, suspended by a thin stalk and connected to a large sphere, which is the yolk sac. The embryo lies in a tiny open space, secure and protected like a seed in a pod, surrounded by a network of its own and its mother's blood vessels. At about this stage of development the mother misses her first menstrual period and realizes she may be pregnant. Most parents feel a tremendous sense of excitement when a test or the mother's feelings indicate that she has conceived. Although no visible difference is apparent, both mother and father feel the import of what is to come.

Corresponding to the parents' first awareness of the growing baby is a stage of incredible change and development in the embryo. In the single month between the fourth and the eighth weeks, the baby goes from a primitive shape to one that is becoming recognizably human. It is this period that scientists refer to as the *embryonic stage*. During this time all major internal and external organs and structures will begin their development. So much is elaborated in the embryonic period that scientists literally talk about changes and developments on a day-to-day basis. Starting at about day 22 two arches appear at the head that will become the upper and lower jaws. At about day 24 the

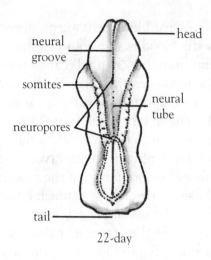

neural groove

head

somites

neural tube

neuropores

tail

22-day

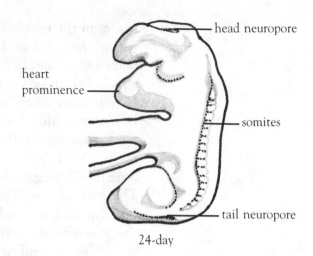

head neuropore

heart prominence

somites

tail neuropore

24-day

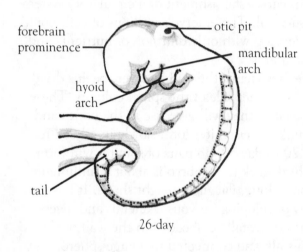

forebrain prominence

otic pit

mandibular arch

hyoid arch

tail

26-day

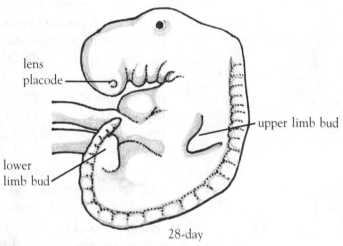

lens placode

upper limb bud

lower limb bud

28-day

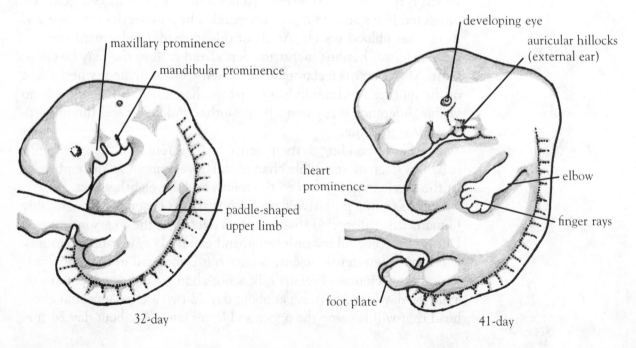

maxillary prominence

mandibular prominence

paddle-shaped upper limb

32-day

developing eye

auricular hillocks (external ear)

heart prominence

elbow

finger rays

foot plate

41-day

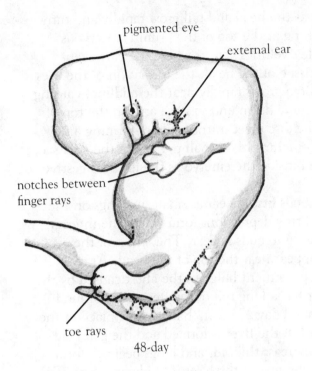

pigmented eye

external ear

notches between
finger rays

toe rays

48-day

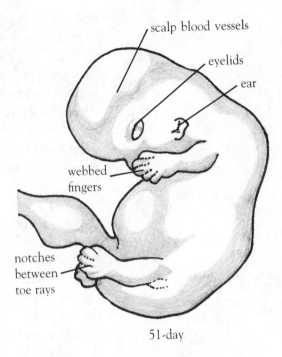

scalp blood vessels

eyelids

ear

webbed
fingers

notches
between
toe rays

51-day

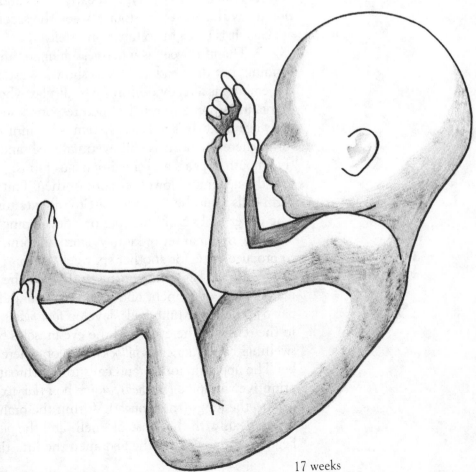

*The growing embryo follows
a carefully timed sequence of
developments. By the time
the baby is 10 weeks old, all
the basic organ system have
been laid out.*

17 weeks

embryo takes on a C shape as the head and tail grow rapidly and turn in on themselves. The opening at the top of the primitive nervous system now closes, and little swellings appear where the ears eventually will be. Within the tissue of the head, the formation of the eyes begins. Meanwhile the embryo grows rapidly near the midline, causing the sides of the flat disc to curve down and squeeze around the top of the yolk sac. The sides of the disc meet in the middle, forming a new cylindrical body shape and pinching off a small portion of the yolk sac, which becomes incorporated inside the embryo as the future digestive tract.

Around day 26 arm buds first appear as small swellings on the upper sides of the body, and tiny depressions form where the internal ears will be. By day 28 lower limb buds appear. The lenses of the eyes form, causing swellings to appear near the top of the head. At this stage the embryo also has a prominent bulge in the chest caused by the relatively large heart, and it has a long tail of somites curled around the lower limb buds. At around day 27 great changes take place in the digestive and excretory systems: the liver is formed and the gall bladder, stomach, intestines, pancreas, thyroid, and lungs begin to form. By early in the fourth week the first of three sets of kidneys forms. This first set is similar to the type in early fishes and never becomes functional. By the end of the fourth week the second set of kidneys appears; it is thought to function briefly.

The fifth week is much less dramatic in terms of new structures forming, but the head and brain show a substantial increase in size and the embryo is already beginning to display whole-body reflex movements in response to touch. Such responses show that even at this early age the baby's nervous system is beginning to function. Nasal pits form where the nostrils will eventually be, and around day 31 a primitive mouth appears and the esophagus forms. The valve that will separate the upper and lower sections of the primitive heart forms, and the germ cells from the yolk sac start to migrate toward the genital area. The upper limbs continue to grow, developing rough *hand plates* by day 33. Now the final set of kidneys starts to form, but they do not begin to produce urine for another six weeks or so.

At the beginning of the sixth week the embryo is about 8 millimeters long, or ⅓ inch, and weighs a thousandth of an ounce. Around day 37, the lower limb buds develop *foot plates.* Pigmentation appears in the retina of the eyes, and the eye muscles begin to form. Tiny swellings called *auricular hillocks* develop where the external ear will be. The upper lip forms, and cells in the throat area give rise to a primitive windpipe (*trachea*), voice box (*larynx*), and tubes that will lead to the lungs (the *bronchi*). Within the brain the *olfactory lobe,* which deals with the sense of smell, and the *pituitary* or master gland begin to form. Within the abdomen the intestines develop, and the primitive germ cells arrive at the genital area. By this time the embryo's muscles are beginning to contract, although the mother is rarely aware of their movement till about sixteen to twenty weeks. At about day 40 the jaws, teeth, and facial muscles start to develop; the diaphragm forms, separating the chest and abdominal cavities; and the heart begins its separation into four chambers. By around day 41 dramatic changes take place in the limbs: first the elbow and wrist curves appear, and then swellings called *finger rays*, which are precursors of the fingers. Several days later similar changes take place in the lower limb buds: knee and ankle indentations appear, followed by *toe rays*.

Until almost the seventh week the baby's sex is not structurally apparent; embryologists refer to this time as the *indifferent period*. The *testes* and the *ovaries* develop from common unspecialized tissue; during this period the tissue can develop into either male or female organs. The male's Y chromosome causes the tissue to develop into testes, whereas the female's two X chromosomes cause the tissue to develop into ovaries. Within several days the cells of the ovaries and testes will be differentiated enough to be microscopically distinguishable. At about day 42 the *nipples* also begin to develop in both sexes.

During week 7 the limbs continue to grow and differentiate: the fingers become distinct and the arms begin to bend at the elbow. Within the primitive connective tissue, cartilage and some bone starts to form. Cartilage is a fast-growing, very flexible tissue that makes a scaffold for bones. Bone is a much slower-growing, denser material that very gradually begins to replace cartilage in those areas where bones will develop. This process continues long past birth, ending between the ages of sixteen and twenty, when a person stops growing.

At about day 44 eyelids begin to take shape and nerve cells form in the *retina* of the eyes. Within the ear the *semicircular canals* that control balance start to develop. Other signs point to the fact that the nervous system is maturing and the baby is becoming more responsive to the environment around it. When the baby's head or upper body is touched, newly developed reflexes specifically cause the baby to turn away. And the earliest measurable brain waves appear about this time. Around day 46 the tip of the nose and the *nasal openings* form, and by day 48 the tongue begins to form.

At the beginning of the eighth week, changes start to take place in the *external genitalia*: the *female clitoris* appears at day 50, and by the end of the week the *scrotum* begins to swell in the male. By day 52 further changes take place in the head as the *external ears, taste buds,* and *palate* form. By the end of this week the embryo has grown to 1¼ inches long from head to buttocks and weighs 1 gram. As the embryonic period ends, all the baby's organ systems are roughly formed; the tail has disappeared as the lower limbs have grown, and the baby is now recognizably human.

THE FETUS (WEEK 9–DELIVERY)

Week 9 begins the *fetal period,* which continues until the baby's birth. Doctors commonly refer to the growing baby as a *fetus* from conception on, but embryologists refer to the baby as an *embryo* until all its systems are formed at the end of the second month. For parents trying to visualize their baby's development, as well as for embryologists, the ninth week marks a true turning point. Until then cells in the baby's body are migrating and undergoing radical transformations, creating new organs and systems almost daily. After the beginning of the ninth week only the reproductive systems will undergo new formation, and this will largely take place during this week. Throughout the rest of the gestational period the baby's organs will simply undergo fine differentiation and growth.

During week 9 the fetus experiences a great spurt in growth, almost doubling its length and more than doubling its weight. Up to this point the baby's head has been as large as the rest of its body; now the body begins to catch up, and the baby begins to attain proportions more like those of a newborn. The baby's bones and muscles are growing rapidly, particularly in the area of the torso. Because of this growth, coupled with changes in proportions, the baby's head no longer is bent tightly against its chest but begins to assume a more upright posture. As the body lengthens, the abdomen becomes less prominent, although the intestines still remain outside the body in the umbilical cord, where they began their development as a pinched-off part of the yolk sac.

All parts of the skin system become more refined during week 9. *Fingernails, toenails,* and *hair follicles* appear; they are all specialized parts of the top layer of skin, the *epidermis.* The skin itself thickens and becomes less transparent. A number of changes also take place around the face. The eyes develop an *iris,* the pigmented area that controls the amount of light admitted to the eye, and the eyelids meet and fuse, remaining closed for the next several months. Meanwhile baby teeth begin to form under the gumline, with the outer *enamel* and the inner *dentine* being laid down.

During week 9 the penis becomes distinguishable, however the female's external genitalia do not become well defined for another month. Like the ovaries and testes, the external genitalia in both sexes develop from the same primitive tissue: the *genital tubercle* becomes the *penis* in the male, the *clitoris* in the female. Swellings on either side of the tubercle become the *scrotum* in the male, the *labia* in the female.

However, some of the internal reproductive organs develop from different sources in the male and the female. The female develops the *fallopian tubes* from remnants of the first set of kidneys, whereas the male develops the *sperm ducts* from remnants of the second set.

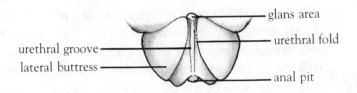

glans area

urethral groove

lateral buttress

urethral fold

anal pit

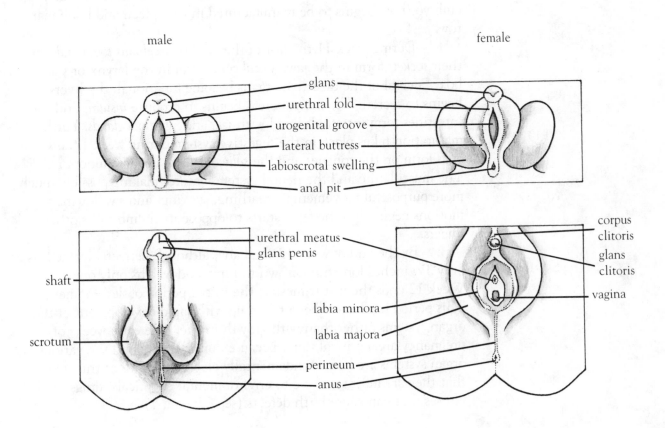

male

female

glans

urethral fold

urogenital groove

lateral buttress

labioscrotal swelling

anal pit

shaft

scrotum

urethral meatus

glans penis

labia minora

labia majora

perineum

anus

corpus clitoris

glans clitoris

vagina

Remarkably, much of the male and female genitalia develop from common tissue. The baby's sex does not become structurally apparent until about week 7; thus the early weeks are referred to as the indifferent *period.*

The male ducts, as well as the penis, actually form in response to chemicals made by the testes. The vagina develops from primitive tissue that gives rise to the bladder and urethra in both sexes. All these sexual developments continue over several weeks until the external genitalia achieve a mature fetal form.

By 10 weeks connections between muscles and nerves in the peripheral nervous system are mature enough to transmit messages to and from the brain. The skin over most of the body is now responsive; that is, touching it will cause the fetus to move. The brain itself has approximately the same overall structure as it will have at birth, although an enormous amount of refinement will take place in succeeding weeks and months. Already the fetus shows certain specific reflexes: it opens its mouth when its face is touched and bends its fingers when its arms are touched.

A number of developments take place in the digestive system during week 10. The hard, bony part of the *palate* forms and the *thyroid, pancreas,* and *gall bladder* complete their formation. The *intestines* now move fully into the abdomen from the umbilical cord, and muscles in the walls of the digestive tract become functional. Fetal blood, which originally was formed in blood islands surrounding the early embryo, now begins to be manufactured in the spleen and bone marrow.

During week 11 the last of the twenty *deciduous tooth buds* and their *sockets* form in the jaw. *Vocal cords* form in the larynx or voice box. Several of the digestive organs become functional: the liver begins to secrete *bile,* the pancreas begins to produce *insulin,* and the intestines form into folds lined with *villi* and *intestinal glands.* Further maturation takes place in the digestive system during week 12: *taste buds* form on the tongue, and the *salivary glands* become functional. The musculature and the neural system mature, making possible much more purposeful movements: breathing, sucking, and swallowing motions begin, and the fetus starts to oppose its thumb to its other fingers.

By the end of week 12 the baby, although perfectly formed, is only 3½ inches long from crown to rump and weighs only one ounce. Week 12 ends the first trimester, the initial period of development. This period has largely been taken up with rapid development of the organ systems rather than with growth in size. The early weeks of pregnancy are a critical time, because during this period the various organ systems are being fundamentally elaborated. It is at this stage that they are most sensitive to environmental chemicals, drugs, and viruses that can cause birth defects (see Chapter 7).

Lunar Month 4* (13–16 Weeks)

The second trimester begins with a month of the most rapid growth that the baby experiences in the uterus. Developmental changes slow to such an extent that they are now spoken of in terms of months rather than weeks or days, as was true in the first trimester. Most of the growth in the fourth month takes place in the body and limbs, not in the head, so that the baby begins to assume proportions more and more like those of a newborn. Whereas at two months the head was as big as the rest of the body, by the end of month four the head accounts for only a third of the baby's total length.

The baby's head position continues to become more upright as its neck and back muscles develop and more and more of its skeleton turns from cartilage to bone. Pads develop on the fingertips and toes,

* A *lunar* month is commonly considered to be 4 weeks or 28 days, as opposed to a calendar month which varies. A true moon cycle is actually 29½ days.

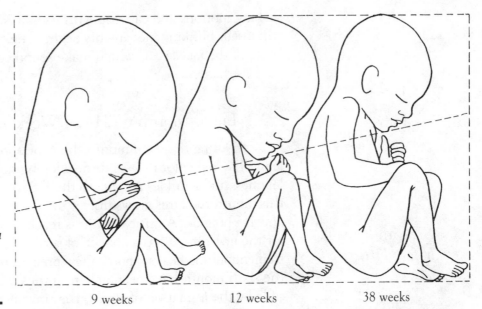

9 weeks   12 weeks   38 weeks

As the baby grows, its proportions as well as its size change radically. Whereas the head is as tall as the rest of the body at 8 weeks, it is a third the size of the body at 12 weeks and a quarter the size at birth.

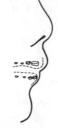

5 months in utero

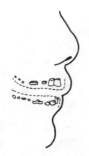

birth

By the fifth month many of the baby's deciduous teeth are well formed under the gums.

giving the baby its own unique fingerprints and footprints. In the female primitive egg cells form in the ovaries in great numbers from the germ cells that have migrated from the yolk sac. And the female reproductive system finishes forming.

During the fourth month the baby's movements become more pronounced and the mother becomes aware of them for the first time (see p. 246). A *fetal water cycle* evolves as the baby begins to swallow and excrete the amniotic fluid. Meanwhile the mother's body absorbs amniotic fluid and produces new fluid at a constant rate. By week 16 *meconium*, the early fecal matter, is beginning to collect in the baby's intestinal tract.

Lunar Month 5 (17–20 Weeks)

During the fifth month the baby begins to appear so well developed that one would think it could survive outside the uterus. Yet it still would not live apart from its mother; several things make survival impossible. First and most important, the baby's lungs are not yet sufficiently developed. Also the digestive system is not fully mature, and the baby cannot maintain its temperature due to lack of specialized fatty tissue that produces heat. This tissue, called *brown fat*, forms in the neck, chest, and crotch area during the fifth month.

Oil glands in the baby's skin begin to secrete the *vernix caseosa*, a fatty substance that mixes with dead skin cells to form a cheesy coating that protects the baby's skin from its prolonged exposure to the amniotic fluid. At about this point the baby develops eyebrows, hair on its head, and *lanugo*, fine hair that covers the whole body. The lanugo may help in temperature regulation and/or may provide an anchor for the vernix caseosa.

By the end of this month the baby becomes capable of its first sucking motions and can grip with its hands. Although the eyelids are still fused, blinking movements begin. The bones of the ear, including those of the *middle ear*, which make sound conduction possible, now ossify or harden.

Lunar Month 6 (21–24 Weeks)

During the sixth month the baby appears red, wrinkled, and lean. The red color reflects its developing skin capillary system; the leanness and wrinkles are due to the lack of body fat under the skin. In this month the fetus grows from 8 inches and ½ pound to 12 inches and 1½ pounds. A critical point is reached in the baby's development: for the first time it has a chance of surviving outside the uterus. Given tremendous medical support, a few premature babies born at the end of the sixth month have been able to survive. Largely, this is made possible by the formation of *alveoli,* the tiny air sacs in the lungs.

By week 24 the lungs have developed both alveoli and surrounding blood vessels that will enable the baby to exchange oxygen and carbon dioxide after it is born. The alveoli begin to manufacture a substance called *surfactant,* which prevents their walls from sticking together. More and more surfactant is produced during the third trimester as well, especially in the two weeks before birth. The number of alveoli continues to increase after birth until about the age of eight years. This is an excellent example of the fact that all development does not end with birth. Rather, birth is an important milestone in the long and gradual process of maturation that is completed when puberty ends and growth ceases.

By the sixth month the nostrils, which, like the eyelids, have been fused, reopen and the baby begins to make muscular breathing movements. The baby's brain wave patterns are now similar to those that would be seen in a full-term newborn. These waves are believed to originate in the more highly evolved part of the brain, the *cortex.* They reflect beginning activity in the baby's hearing and visual systems.

Lunar Month 7 (25–28 Weeks)

The seventh month begins the last trimester. With each day the baby's chances of surviving outside the uterus increase. At about week 26 the baby's eyelids unfuse and reopen. The eyes are completely formed now and perceive light. In addition, the baby can actually hear, smell, and taste, and it has been responsive to touch for some time. The baby shows increased muscle tone, and its sucking and swallowing skills develop further, helping to prepare it for life outside the uterus.

Subcutaneous fat, called *white fat,* forms and fills out the wrin-

Size of the baby before birth

4 weeks:
  ⅕ inch long

8 weeks:
  1 inch long

12 weeks:
  3 inches long,
  ¾ ounce

16 weeks:
  3½ inches long

20 weeks:
  10 inches long,
  8–9 ounces

24 weeks:
  14 inches long,
  2 pounds 8
  ounces

28 weeks:
  16 inches long,
  4–5 pounds

32 weeks:
  18 inches long,
  5–5½ pounds

9th month:
  20 inches long,
  6–9 pounds

Stimulating the baby before birth

By 28 weeks of development, all of the senses of the unborn baby are functional.

MOTHER'S ACTIVITY	EFFECT ON THE BABY
Movements, including dancing, yoga, walking, swimming, and resting Sex, massage Sunbathing, showering	Stimulation of touch perception and balance
Speech and singing, especially the mother's Music and gentle repetitive or rhythmic sounds	Stimulation of hearing
Exposing the mother's belly to direct light, especially the sun	Stimulation of visual perception
Conscious relaxation, meditation, and deep-breathing exercises Interesting and stimulating experiences for the mother, especially ones that have a short period of excitement, followed by a release of tension and by rest. Balance and harmony in the mother's daily life	Stimulation of the baby's whole body

kles in the baby's skin. Red blood cell production shifts entirely to the bone marrow. The fine hair that once covered the whole body now becomes limited to the back and shoulders. In male babies the testes descend from the abdomen down into the *scrotal sac*.

During the seventh month tremendous changes take place in the nervous system. A fatty sheath called *myelin* is laid down around the nerve fibers. This sheath makes the transmission of nerve impulses faster and easier. Although the sheathing process begins now, it is another of the physiological maturational processes that is not complete until long after birth.

During this month the brain grows greatly in size, surface area, and number of cells, causing it to fold in on itself and produce the wrinkles and indentations that are characteristic of the human brain. Neurological functions now localize to specific areas of the brain. The number of nervous circuits grows enormously, making possible increasingly refined movements and more sophisticated learning.

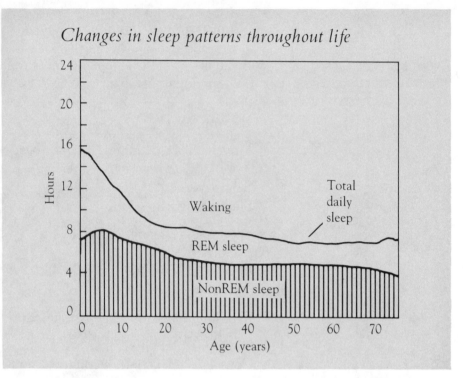

Changes in sleep patterns throughout life

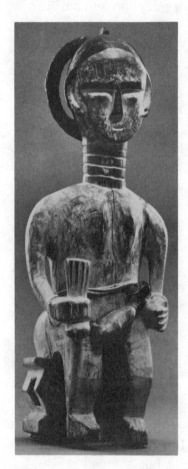

Primitive myths, even more than our scientific theories and observations, sometimes capture the interconnection between mother and developing baby. Mother and Child, Ghana, 19th–20th century. The Metropolitan Museum of Art. The Michael C. Rockefeller Memorial Collection, the Diana Woolman Memorial Collection, 1973.

At this stage the baby's brain is just as advanced as a newborn's. Studies show that the baby actually exhibits all the types of brain waves that adults exhibit, although not in the same sequence or for the same length of time. These waves, which include *rapid eye movement (REM) sleep, deep sleep,* and *alpha (wakeful relaxation),* are associated with definite awake or alert periods and periods of sleeping. Mothers are aware of these periods as times when the baby is active and moving or being still.

Western brain researchers believe that this is the beginning of true consciousness. Premature babies born at this point have the ability to see, hear, remember, and learn. It is interesting to note that people who have reputedly been hypnotized to recall events before their birth can remember back to about the sixth or seventh month. Based on this evidence, some psychiatrists speculate that the *ego,* the "I" of the personality, is already beginning formation.

Lunar Month 8 (29–32 Weeks)

During the eighth month the baby's growth in weight and length slows. New fat makes the baby appear more filled out. Approximately 8 percent of the baby's weight is white fat, especially on the arms and legs. At about week 30 the baby's pupillary light reflex appears as the iris becomes capable of closing down in response to light.

Lunar Months 9 and 10 (33–40 Weeks)

The last weeks of gestation are referred to as the *finishing period*. Growth slows even more, but the baby continues to gain in white fat. During the immediate weeks before birth the baby gains about 14 grams a day in white fat, which generally means the baby has a plump look at term. By the middle of the last month the average baby weighs about 6 to 8 pounds and is 14 to 15 inches long from crown to rump.

The skin of Caucasian and Oriental babies has become white or bluish pink. The fingernails and toenails have grown to the ends of the digits, and most of the lanugo has disappeared. Generally only the back remains covered with the waxy vernix caseosa. Due to stimulation of hormones in the placenta that prepare the mother's breasts for nursing, the breasts swell in both boy and girl babies. The baby also receives antibodies from the mother that assist its immature immune system. These antibodies protect against bacteria and viruses such as German measles, influenza, mumps, whooping cough, and strep.

Despite all that scientists have learned about perinatal development, much of what happens to the baby in the uterus remains a mystery. But Western science is coming to realize and appreciate how alive and aware the developing infant is, and how greatly the mother and her environment affect the baby before birth. Researchers describe fetal development as they have been able to measure it, and that description of necessity only partially conveys the miraculous nature of what takes place. It tends to stress observation of an external phenomenon, rather than participation in an interconnected experience between mother and baby. Primitive peoples have sometimes captured the spirit of the phenomenon more successfully in their legends and stories.

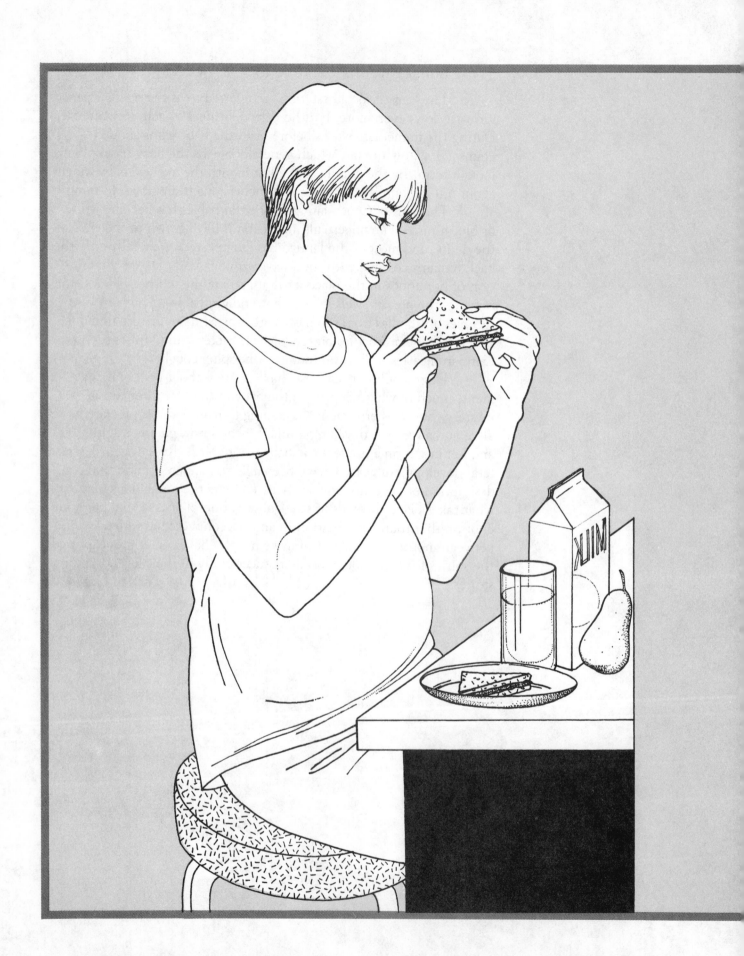

Nutrition During Pregnancy

Dietary Guidelines

Throughout history different cultures have had special guidelines for what a pregnant mother should or should not eat. People have always had the belief that the mother's diet had an effect on the developing baby, either in terms of esthetics or health. Often dietary prescriptions were tied to spiritual taboos, such as a Philippine tribe's belief that eating green mangoes can cause a miscarriage. While such taboos are not substantiated, they are farsighted in holding that food, like other environmental factors, has important effects on the developing baby. The fact that primitive dietary restrictions and advice were integrated with behavioral and spiritual advice indicates that many primitive cultures had an intuitive concept of the multiple factors that affect both the development of the baby and complications of pregnancy. It is only in the last fifty years that Western medicine has come to recognize the impact of both nutrition and other environmental factors on the baby.

Generally, the dietary suggestions of primitive peoples are quite specific. For example, certain Philippino tribes believe that eating twin bananas can cause twins, that eating squid or eggplant can cause

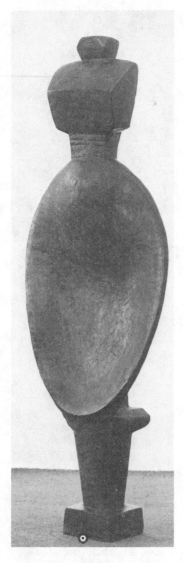

All cultures have placed importance on the pregnant woman's diet, believing it had significant effects on her pregnancy. Spoon Woman, Alberto Giacometti, 1926. Solomon R. Guggenheim Museum, New York.

the baby to be born with dark skin, and that eating slippery foods like eel can cause the uterus to drop after birth. Although many such dietary dictums seem purely superstitious, some of them overlap with the advice of modern nutritionists, if for different reasons. For example, the Philippinos believe that eating salted fish will cause the baby to have less amniotic fluid and that eating sugar will make the baby too big. For many years Western obstetricians advised pregnant women to restrict their salt intake, believing that salt caused them to retain more water and contributed to toxemia. Although this restriction has been tempered, obstetricians continue to advise pregnant women to eat sugar in moderation because it causes weight gain without any nutritional benefit for the baby or the mother.

Since the eighteenth century the major dietary thrust of Western obstetrics has been to restrict the mother's food intake in order to keep her from gaining too much weight during her pregnancy. At that time in Europe diseases of malnutrition, particularly rickets, caused many women to develop a narrow, misshapen pelvis during childhood. Such a pelvis made it dangerous or impossible to deliver normal-size babies. In order to save the lives of these babies and mothers, physicians encouraged *all* mothers to limit the amount of weight they gained. Thus in 1888 the German obstetrician Ludwig Prochownick wrote, "Semi-starvation of the mother is really a blessing in disguise because curtailment of food would produce a small light-weight baby easier to deliver."[1] He proposed a pregnancy diet that was severely limited in calories, carbohydrates, protein, and salt.

Sue Rodwell Williams, a well-known nutritionist, has commented about the policy of limited weight gain, "Incredible as it now seems in retrospect, in the light of advanced knowledge and research, despite any scientific evidence to support such ideas, this general view became implanted in obstetrical textbooks and practice, and passed from one generation of physicians to the next."[2] Even as late as the latter part of the 1960s, limiting weight gain was advocated by obstetricians in most university centers and is still promoted by some doctors who were not recently trained.

Low-Birth-Weight Babies

As far back as the 1940s, studies began to show that limiting the pregnant mother's weight gain negatively affected the growing baby. Not only was the baby likely to weigh less, it would probably be in poorer condition at birth. Such babies are referred to as *low-birth-weight babies, growth-retarded babies,* or *intrauterine growth retarded (IUGR) babies.* In addition to babies who are premature this group includes full-term babies who have low birth weights for their gestational age. Currently babies who weigh under 6 pounds 10 ounces

(2999 grams) are considered to be low-birth-weight babies from the standpoint of malnutrition. This group has three times the infant mortality rate of babies weighing over that amount.

The distinction between prematurity and low birth weight is important because until these studies came out, it had been assumed that all low-birth-weight babies were premature and that a baby's size was simply a matter of how long it had been developing in the uterus. This view was based on the belief that the growing baby, like a parasite, would get whatever it needed from the mother's body in order for it to grow. For example, it was thought that the baby would draw calcium from the mother's teeth if she didn't eat enough dairy products.

The so-called parasite theory has been proved wrong in several important ways. A group of studies done by Burke at Harvard in the 1940s showed that mothers who had nutritious diets tended to give birth to heavy babies (8 lbs. 8 oz. on the average) that were judged to be in excellent condition. Those women who had poor diets tended to give birth to lightweight babies in poor condition. Prematurity and

For several hundred years obstetricians advocated a policy of limited weight gain, but it has been found that women who gain very little weight are more likely to have low-birth-weight babies. Still Life, *Henri Fantin-Latour, 1866. National Gallery of Art, Washington, D.C. Chester Dale Collection, 1962.*

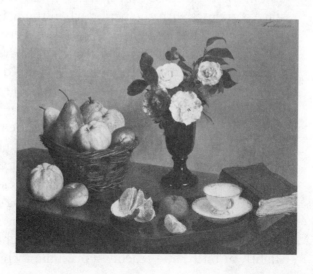

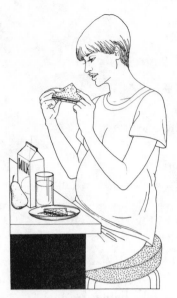

Doctors no longer recommend that women limit their weight gain during pregnancy.

even infant death were definitely shown to be associated with poorly nourished mothers.

A second group of studies showed the parasite theory to be false in another way. These studies dealt with pregnant women in Holland and Leningrad who were malnourished because of food shortages during World War II. It was found that babies who were born during the period of famine were not only much lighter on the average, they had twice the fetal mortality rate. These findings, though tragic, were important because they also showed that the effects of malnutrition on the baby varied with the stage of pregnancy during which the mother was deprived of good nutrition. Poor nutrition in the *first trimester* correlated with higher incidences of congenital malformations and stillbirths, whereas poor nutrition in the *second half* of pregnancy correlated with higher incidences of low-birth-weight babies.

Going a step further, more recent studies have been designed to study the effects of supplementing the diet of one group of mothers while leaving unchanged the poor diets of a control group of mothers. Not only did these studies support the earlier conclusions, they showed that food supplements and dietary advice tended to reverse the ill effects of poor nutrition and result in lower incidences of serious newborn problems. These studies reveal a direct correlation between the amount of calories the mother consumed and the birth weight of the baby.

Nutrition and Fetal Growth

The parasite theory was further discredited by Winick, whose animal studies showed that fetal development takes place in three basic stages. In the first stage the cells in the baby's body and the placenta increase in *number*; in the second stage they increase in both *number and size*; and in the third stage they increase in *size* only. In humans the first stage correlates with the period when the major features and organ systems are being formed. This period covers roughly the first trimester, although it varies with different organ systems. The first stage of development is crucial, because if the fetus does not attain enough cells in a given system or systems at this point, the effects are irreversible.

The second stage correlates with the period when the basic systems are already laid down but are being elaborated upon and are growing in size. This period covers much of the rest of pregnancy and for many organs extends through the first year or two of life. The third stage, in which the system is simply growing in size of cells and external size, occurs mostly after birth in humans. For example, the number of cells in the brain keeps increasing throughout pregnancy, slows slightly at birth, and reaches a maximum when a baby is 18 months old. Growth in brain cell size starts at about 7 months in utero and continues until about 3 years of age. If the baby stops getting sufficient nourishment during the third stage, when the cells are simply increasing in size, the particular organ systems affected will be perfectly formed but will be smaller than average. It is interesting to note that studies have shown that small cell size appears to be reversible with later feeding. Thus the type, severity, and reversibility of damage caused by poor nutrition depend upon the stage at which it occurs.

Based on animal studies, intrauterine growth retardation has been separated into two broad categories. The animal babies in one category are small but normally proportioned. These babies have an irreversible 15 to 20 percent fewer cells in the brain, liver, and other organs. This reduction in cells is caused by a lack of calories and protein *throughout* pregnancy. In the other category the babies have a normal size head and body, but they have very little muscle or fat on their frame. This is caused by malnutrition during the final weeks of gestation or by problems with the placenta, which supplies the baby with nutrients.

The most significant and upsetting finding in the research just

Factors that can compromise a mother's nutrition

- Poverty: high stress and lack of nutritious foods
- Living alone: lack of balanced meals
- Working: increased stress, neglect of nutrition, fatigue
- Frequent eating out: high-calorie, high-fat, low-protein, low-nutrition foods
- Vegetarian diets: low protein and vitamin B_{12} content unless carefully planned
- Frequent weight reduction or "crash" dieting: low protein, and blood becomes acid, which is dangerous to the baby
- Heavy exercise combined with restrictive diets: less protein for the baby
- Previous pregnancy within a year: lowered stores of iron and other nutrients in mother's body
- Severe morning sickness: loss of nutrients or reduced intake of adequate foods
- Smoking: reduces baby's ability to make use of nutrients
- Alcohol use: inadequate nutrition for the mother and decreased ability of baby to use nutrients
- Very low or high prepregnancy weight: poor dietary habits
- Very low weight gain during pregnancy: inadequate intake of protein and calories for baby's growth
- Severe emotional stress on mother: poor utilization of nutrients

discussed is the reduction in cells, particularly brain cells, that results from long-term malnutrition throughout pregnancy. Should serious malnourishment of an animal continue after birth, studies have shown that the deprived offspring can have up to 60 percent fewer brain cells than well-nourished babies. Animal studies have also shown that the offspring of nutritionally deprived babies are hampered after birth by lowered ability to absorb both protein and carbohydrates through their intestinal wall. As a result, light-birth-weight animal babies have a harder time gaining weight in a normal way, further retarding their growth in cell size and number.

Although brain cell counts have not been done on human children, cell-number studies have been made on human placentas. Among animals the weight and number of cells in the placenta is proportional to the weight and number of cells in other organs, including the brain. Thus it is considered very significant that among babies who are light for their gestational age at birth, the placentas are 15 to 20 percent smaller than normal in weight and cell number.

A balanced maternal diet that is rich in proteins and carbohydrates has been shown to be necessary for the organs of the developing baby to attain normal size and cell number.

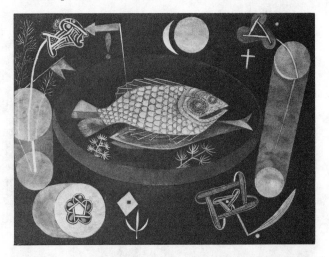

Around the Fish, *Paul Klee, 1926. Oil on canvas, 18⅜″ x 25⅛″. Collection, The Museum of Modern Art, New York. Abby Aldrich Rockefeller Fund.*

The Breakfast Room, *Pierre Bonnard, 1931. Oil on canvas, 62⅞″ x 44⅞″. Collection, The Museum of Modern Art, New York.*

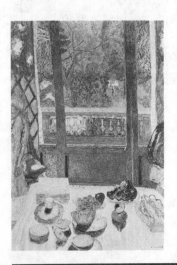

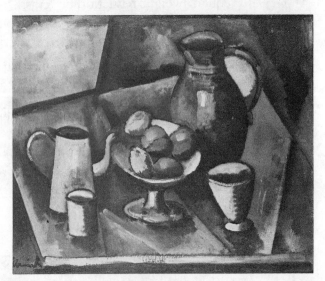

Still Life With Lemons, *Maurice de Vlaminck, 1913. National Gallery of Art, Washington, D.C. Chester Dale Collection.*

Studies have shown that women who eat poorly during pregnancy tend to have placentas that are smaller and lighter by 15 percent.

When a pregnant animal does not eat enough protein or calories, there are not enough amino acid building blocks to make either DNA, the material in cells that transmits genetic information, or the enzymes that are necessary to direct digestion and growth, and there is not enough energy or nutrients to make the existing cells grow. Thus cell functions break down, and normal growth cannot occur. Not surprisingly, such deprivation is most damaging when the cells are undergoing rapid growth and division.

During the first trimester of pregnancy very radical changes are taking place in the fetus, but it doesn't require very much energy or nutrition because it is so small. Nevertheless, serious malnutrition during this stage can cause malformations or spontaneous abortions. During the second and third trimesters the growing baby has much greater requirements for both nutrients and energy. These requirements peak in the last trimester, when the baby's cells are increasing rapidly in both number and size. The baby's needs are so great that they can only be met by a maternal diet that has high levels of all the basic nutrients.

Not only do cell number and growth appear to be directly affected by the quality of nutrition, but intelligence seems to be affected in a similar manner in animals and humans. Analysis of a group of seven-year-olds who had been balanced for maternal age, number of siblings, and social class shows disturbing trends for low-birth-weight babies. Neurological impairment, lower IQ, and mental retardation had a higher than average incidence among the low-birth-weight group. Similarly, poor reading ability and poor visual-motor performance were more frequent among these children. The only variables other than low birth weight that relate as strongly to neurological performance are maternal smoking (see p. 122) and toxemia during pregnancy (see p. 265).

Another nutritional factor that has been shown to affect babies' intelligence is the way mothers metabolize the food they eat. As we've discussed earlier, pregnant women have different metabolic patterns than nonpregnant women (see p. 47). In particular, they process sugar differently. When a pregnant woman does not eat for a period of time, her body begins to break down stored fat for energy more quickly than normal. As a result, pregnant women are more susceptible to producing high blood levels of acetone, a metabolic by-product that is ultimately spilled in the urine. Acetone is toxic to the nervous system of the developing baby; studies have shown that women who had a history of spilling acetone tended to have children of significantly lower IQs than did mothers without such a history. Spilling of acetone can arise within six hours of not eating. Thus it's very important that pregnant women not skip meals.

The Present Focus of Nutrition for Expectant Mothers

All these studies on nutrition and birth weight have been of great concern to researchers in preventive medicine and to the Department of Health, Education and Welfare. At present in the United States an astonishing 80,000 to 120,000 babies are born each year with a birth weight under 5½ pounds as a result of poor maternal nutrition. The incidence is no lower today than it was in the 1920s. The United States ranks thirteenth in the world in infant mortality and has twice as many low-birth-weight babies per capita as does Sweden, which ranks lowest in number of infant deaths. Concern over these statistics has led the U.S. Public Health Service to make nutritional counseling its number-one priority in its efforts to improve the health of newborns.

It is encouraging to note that studies have shown that nutritional supplements and education can have a significant impact upon the nutritional status of expectant mothers and the condition of their babies at birth. A striking study in Guatemala has shown that when disadvantaged high-risk mothers were given nutritional supplements

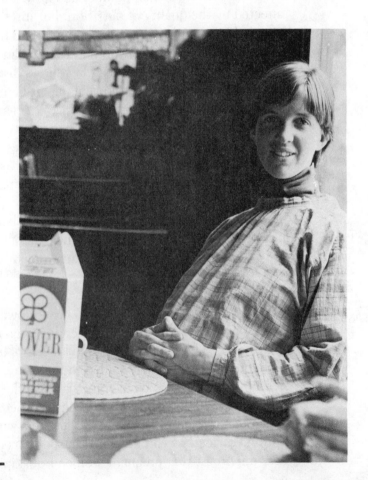

Each pregnant woman has her own food habits and is therefore unique from a nutritional point of view. Photo by Michael Samuels.

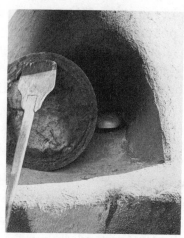

Nutritional supplements have been shown to increase the birth weights of babies born to disadvantaged mothers. Pueblo Indian Bread Oven. *Photo by Michael Samuels.*

and counseling, those who incorporated the help showed a consistent increase in the birth weight of their babies. For every 10,000 calories ingested by the mother, the birth weight of the baby increased by 50 grams. Mothers who ate high amounts of the supplement had half the number of low-birth-weight babies. Interestingly enough, it did not seem to matter whether the mother was given supplemental protein or calories. Apparently there was sufficient protein in their normal diet, but without supplementation of some sort, the protein was not available for cell growth and was used for energy production. Thus either additional calories or additional protein could supply the energy that was needed.

A food-supplement study done in Canada showed that supplementation and counseling could work just as well among high-risk poor mothers in an affluent nation. Giving mothers milk, eggs, and oranges, as well as intensive nutritional education, resulted in babies with birth weights and infant mortality figures that were dramatically improved.

NUTRITIONAL ASSESSMENT FOR PREGNANT WOMEN

Each pregnant mother is unique from a nutritional point of view. Each one enters pregnancy with particular dietary habits, body build, and metabolic patterns. Based on these differences and on recent research, nutritionists are now giving very specific advice to expectant mothers.

The first step in any nutritional program for pregnancy is to figure out a woman's status. This process is called *nutritional assessment.* It is typically divided into a history and a physical exam. The point of the assessment is not only to individualize a woman's dietary guidelines but to identify those women whose babies may be at nutritional risk. Such mothers can benefit most from dietary advice.

Life situation appears to be one of the most important factors in a woman's nutritional status. Women who are poor are least likely to get an adequate diet. The average middle-class educated woman who eats a balanced diet is unlikely to be at risk, but even she may be, depending upon her dietary habits. In any case, expectant mothers can optimize their baby's development if they follow the guidelines for an enriched diet.

Other factors that affect a mother's diet, though not necessarily in a negative way, are whether the mother lives alone, whether she works, whether she eats out frequently, whether she adheres to any weight reduction diets, whether she follows any specialized food regimens such as vegetarianism, and whether she exercises regularly. Women who live alone or who work and eat on the run may find that their diet is not well balanced, either because they skip meals or don't take time to select foods that supply a variety of nutrients. Women who are vegetarians, especially those who do not eat eggs or milk products, may find that they need to pay special attention to getting enough complete protein.

If a woman has a long history of dieting for weight loss, she may find it emotionally difficult to accept the weight gain that is now considered adequate in pregnancy. Likewise, if a woman is very slender and very conscious of her weight, she may feel ambivalent about gaining weight. Women who exercise in a serious, disciplined way may also have difficulty with the idea of weight gain.

Past reproductive history is another factor that affects a woman's nutritional status. If a mother has been pregnant or has nursed a baby within the previous year, her nutritional stores, particularly iron, are more likely to be low. If a woman has previously had a low-birth-weight baby, she is automatically considered to be at nutritional risk.

Besides life-style and diet, other factors in the present pregnancy can also put a mother at nutritional risk. Both regular smoking and alcohol consumption (see pp. 122–27) are associated with light-weight babies and definitely put a mother at greater nutritional risk. Smoking affects a mother's utilization of calories, while alcohol is likely to substitute for more nutritious liquids like milk. Severe or continued morning sickness can undermine a woman's best nutritional efforts, as can life stress (see Chapter 8). Finally, ambivalent attitudes toward the baby can lower a mother's motivation to maintain a high-level diet. Even women who are happy to be pregnant may feel unhappy or resentful at changes that pregnancy brings, such as altered shape, or changes pregnancy necessitates, such as giving up cigarettes or alcohol. Such ambivalent feelings can affect a woman's eating habits without her being aware of it.

During the first prenatal exam the doctor or midwife will be checking the mother's initial pregnant weight. Although this check is thought to be merely routine by many women, it is actually very important from a nutritional point of view. A number of studies have shown that women who are either underweight or quite overweight at the start of pregnancy are at increased risk of having a low-birth-weight baby. Women who are 5 percent or more underweight not only have increased incidences of low-birth-weight babies, they also tend to have more complications during pregnancy. The more underweight a woman is, the greater the risk.

The highest number of low-birth-weight babies are born to mothers who not only are underweight before the pregnancy but who also gain very little during pregnancy. The increasing number of middle-class well-educated mothers who strenuously exercise and tend to be underweight can fall into this category if they do not modify their life-style for pregnancy. Women who are substantially overweight often tend to diet or eat lightly during pregnancy in an attempt to

Desirable weights for nonpregnant women (pounds)*

HEIGHT BAREFOOT	SMALL FRAME	MEDIUM FRAME	LARGE FRAME
4'10"	92–98	96–107	104–119
5'	96–104	98–110	106–122
5'1"	99–107	100–113	109–125
5'2"	102–110	107–119	115–131
5'3"	105–113	110–122	118–134
5'4"	108–116	113–126	121–138
5'5"	111–119	116–130	125–142
5'6"	114–123	120–135	129–146
5'7"	118–127	124–139	133–150
5'8"	122–131	128–143	137–154
5'9"	126–135	132–147	141–158
5'10"	130–140	136–151	145–163
5'11"	134–144	140–155	149–168

* With indoor clothing

keep from gaining weight that they will only have to lose after the baby is born. Overweight mothers who eat a restricted diet are at risk of having light-birth-weight babies if their diet is low in protein or carbohydrates.

Both underweight and overweight mothers can be reassured that the body has natural homeostatic mechanisms that tend to return a mother to her previous weight within a matter of months after the baby is born. In addition to changing her fat metabolism after birth, the mother loses a great deal of weight with the delivery (see p. 406) and with nursing.

How to calculate frame size

HEIGHT BAREFOOT	WRIST SIZE (IN INCHES)		
	SMALL FRAME	MEDIUM FRAME	LARGE FRAME
Up to 5'3"	5.5	5.5–5.75	+ 5.75
5'3"–5'4"	6	6–6.25	+ 6.25
5'4" and up	6.25	6.25–6.5	+ 6.5

How to calculate calorie and protein requirements

DESIR-ABLE WEIGHT	LOW ACTIVITY		MODERATE ACTIVITY		HIGH ACTIVITY	
	CALO-RIES	PROTEIN	CALO-RIES	PROTEIN	CALO-RIES	PROTEIN
80	1600	40	1900	40	2400	40
85	1650	43	1950	43	2450	43
90	1700	45	2000	45	2500	45
95	1750	48	2050	48	2550	48
100	1800	50	2100	50	2600	50
110	1950	53	2250	53	2750	53
115	2025	54	2325	54	2825	54
120	2100	55	2400	55	2900	55
125	2150	57	2450	57	2950	57
130	2200	58	2500	58	3000	58
135	2250	59	2550	59	3050	59
140	2300	60	2600	60	3100	60
145	2350	63	2650	63	3150	63
150	2400	65	2700	65	3500	65
155	2450	68	2750	68	3250	68

Nutritional Advice for Pregnant Women

At present the most highly recommended and popular dietary guideline for pregnant women is the Montreal Diet Dispensary Method, designed by Mrs. Agnes Higgins. The program was used in the study cited earlier concerning the effect of supplementary foods on the birth weight of babies in Canada; it determines an expectant mother's protein and calorie needs by taking into consideration her *present weight*, her *ideal weight*, and her *typical activity level*.

The mother's initial intake levels are considered to be adequate for the first 20 weeks of pregnancy, unless she is underweight or undernourished. If a woman is undernourished, she will be told by a nutritionist what she needs to eat to achieve ideal levels. For example, if a

A typical food record for a diet history

FOODS YOU EAT				
Meal or snack	Time	Place	Food eaten	Food amount

medium-framed woman is 5 feet 5 inches tall, weighs an ideal 125 pounds, and is moderately active, her ideal prepregnant levels would be 2450 calories and 57 grams of protein a day. If her diet assessment showed that she averaged only 2000 calories and 30 grams of protein, she would be advised to add an additional 450 calories and 27 grams of protein a day. If the woman was underweight by more than 5 percent (in this case, 6¾ pounds), she would be advised to eat an additional 20 grams of protein and 500 calories a day. The object would be to have her make up the number of pounds she was underweight by gaining about one extra pound a week until she was no longer underweight.

Finally, if a mother is under any kind of nutritional stress, she is advised to add an extra 200 calories and 20 grams of protein per stress per day, with a maximum of 400 calories and 40 grams extra a day. The Montreal method defines nutritional stress as (1) frequent vomiting, (2) another pregnancy less than a year earlier, (3) a poor obstetrical history of any kind, (4) failure to gain 10 pounds by 20 weeks, or (5) any kind of serious emotional upset in a woman's life.

At 20 weeks of gestation the Montreal method advises a mother to add 25 grams of protein and 500 calories a day to her diet for the duration of pregnancy. These increases are dictated by the needs of the now rapidly growing baby.

As complicated as the calculations may be, and as confusing as the dictums sound, the diet can be implemented in a simple way. Rather than radically altering her normal diet, a mother is advised to make as few food changes as possible. Instead she is advised to add certain foods to ensure that she achieves the calorie and protein intake that she needs. Milk alone can virtually make up the additional requirements. Peanut butter, cheese, bread, and eggs are also high in protein and calories. For example, if a mother simply added to her daily diet a quart of whole milk, a glass of orange juice, and one egg, she would be getting an additional 700 calories and 40 grams of protein. This would be enough to meet the additional needs of pregnancy

A pregnant woman needs to supplement her diet in order to assure that she gets enough protein and calories to nourish the baby properly. In a real sense, she is eating for two. Photos by Michael Samuels.

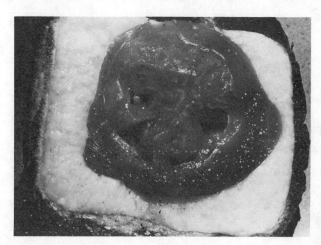

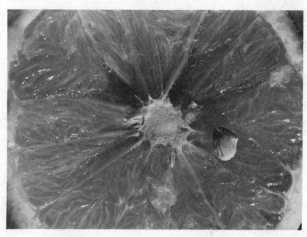

Increased nutritional demands of pregnancy

NUTRIENT	PREPREGNANT NEED	PREGNANT NEED	HOW THE NUTRIENT IS USED	FOODS SUPPLYING THE NUTRIENT	RECOMMENDED DAILY AMOUNTS*
Protein	46 g	75–100 g	Rapid growth of baby, amniotic fluid, placenta, uterus, breasts, and blood volume	Dairy products: Milk, Cheese, Eggs, Yogurt	1 qt 2 oz or ½ cup 2 ½ cup
			Storage reserves for labor, delivery, and lactation	Meat, fish, and fowl	2 servings (6–8 oz)
				Grains, legumes, nuts, bread, cereal, dried beans, rice, pasta	1–2 servings by choice
Calories	2100	2400	Increased metabolism and energy needs Conserve protein	All foods, particularly carbohydrates and fats	Supplied by the recommended amounts of all the foods
MINERALS					
Calcium	800 mg	1200 mg	Formation of baby's bones and teeth, and increased maternal needs	Milk, cheese, grains, eggs yolks Leafy vegetables	As above 1 serving
Phosphorus	800 mg	1200 mg	Formation of baby's bones and teeth, and increased maternal needs	Milk, cheese, lean meats	As above

Increased nutritional demands of pregnancy

Iron	18 mg	18 mg, plus 30–60 mg supplement	Increased maternal blood volume, and fetal liver storage	Liver or organ meats	1–2 servings per week
				Other meats, eggs, grains, leafy vegetables, nuts, dried fruits	As above
Iodine	100 micrograms	125 micrograms	Increased maternal metabolism and production of thyroid hormone	Iodized salt	Daily in cooking
				Seafood	1–2 servings per week
Magnesium	300 mg	450 mg	Enzymes in energy production and muscle action	Nuts, soybeans, cocoa, seafood, dried peas and beans	Occasional servings

VITAMINS

A	4000 IUs	5000 IUs	Cell, tooth, and bone growth of the baby	Butter, cream, fortified margarine	2 tbs
				Leafy vegetables, liver, egg yolk	As above
D	0	400 IUs	Absorption of calcium and phosphorus for teeth and bones	Fortified milk, fortified margarine	As above
E	12 IUs	15 IUs	Growth and maintenance of red blood cells	Vegetable oils, leafy vegetables, cereals, meat, eggs, milk	Supplied by recommended amounts above

(continued)

Increased nutritional demands of pregnancy

NUTRIENT	PREPREGNANT NEED	PREGNANT NEED	HOW THE NUTRIENT IS USED	FOODS SUPPLYING THE NUTRIENT	RECOMMENDED DAILY AMOUNTS*
C	45 mg	60 mg	Growth, formation of connective tissue and blood vessels, aide in iron absorption	Citrus fruits, strawberries, melons, papayas	1–2 servings
				Broccoli, green peppers, tomatoes, chili peppers, potatoes	Occasional servings
Folic acid	400 micrograms	800 micrograms, plus 200–400 supplement	Increased maternal metabolism	Liver, green vegetables, lentils, nuts	1 serving
			Prevention of a rare form of anemia		
			Formation of red blood cells and cell nuclei		
B complex	Different for each B vitamin	Slightly higher	Increased energy metabolism	Meat, beans, milk, cheese	As above

* The recommended daily amounts or their equivalents, *taken together*, supply the average needs of a pregnant woman.

after 20 weeks and to compensate for poor nutrition, low weight, or one stress factor. Some doctors feel that 2-percent-fat milk is preferable to whole milk if a mother is gaining weight adequately.

Mrs. Higgins has reinstated the old idea that a pregnant woman has to eat for two, stating that it is as important to feed the baby during pregnancy as it is after birth. She cautions that just as a mother wouldn't skip a baby's feeding after it's born, she shouldn't skip a "feeding" while she's pregnant. Thinking of it in these terms may help a woman who doesn't particularly like milk or who's feeling a little put out with all the changes she's having to deal with. Mrs. Higgins even suggests that mothers who have trouble remembering to drink their milk mark a quart container with a large *B* for baby to remind them. Paying careful attention to her nutrition is one of the most important things a mother can do to take active responsibility for the baby while she is pregnant. It is an essential form of prenatal parenting.

Another valuable approach to nutrition during pregnancy comes out of the work of nutritionist Dr. Sue Williams. She groups foods into three basic categories. The first group, *protein-rich foods*, includes milk, eggs, meat, grains, nuts, and beans. The second group, *mineral-rich foods*, includes milk, grains, green leafy vegetables, and seafood. The third group is the *vitamin-rich foods*, including margarine, liver, vegetables, and fruits. Williams recommends getting a certain daily amount of nutrients from each group, which basically means one quart of milk, two eggs, two portions of meat or mixed-grain substitutes, four or five slices of whole-grain bread, one or two servings of green vegetables, two tablespoons of butter, and one or two servings of fruit (preferably citrus) per day. Williams also advises one yellow or orange vegetable and liver or seafood several times a week, as well as iodized table salt to taste.

The Williams diet corresponds closely with the work of obstetrician Dr. Tom Brewer, who specializes in nutrition and has written the influential *What Every Pregnant Woman Should Know: The Truth About Diets and Drugs in Pregnancy*. Both Williams and Brewer emphasize that women do not need to change their basic cultural food habits; rather, they should simply make substitutions within the food groups they normally eat, because the fewer changes, the more likely they are to adhere to them. For example, it's perfectly reasonable to substitute rice and beans for meat, pasta for bread, or bamboo shoots for green vegetables within their guidelines. Williams gives extensive lists of substitutions for various ethnic and racial groups such as Mexican, Chinese, Philippino, and black, in her *Handbook of Maternal and Infant Nutrition*.

In addition to these general dietary recommendations, most nutritionists agree that women should receive supplemental iron (30 to 60 mg.) every day during the second and third trimesters, in order to

Guide for pregnant women who are vegetarians

Eat a wide variety of foods to meet increased protein, vitamin, and mineral needs.

Combine grains, legumes, nuts, and seeds to obtain whole protein.

Use iodized salt or supplement iodine.

If no milk is used, supplement calcium and vitamins B_{12} and D.

make enough red blood cells for both themselves and the baby. Often the reason mothers need supplemental iron is that their stores have been reduced by previous pregnancies and/or nursing. Iron is the one nutritional substance that the baby will receive at the expense of the mother. Vitamin C (250 milligrams) is usually given at the same time to enhance the absorption of the iron. It is also recommended that most women get extra folic acid (200 to 400 micrograms per day), simply because this is the vitamin pregnant women are most commonly deficient in. The need for these supplemental vitamins is not universally agreed upon by all nutritional researchers but most would recommend them.

Based on recent research, the old concepts of limiting weight gain and restricting salt intake (to prevent toxemia, see p. 265) have been totally discarded. Williams goes so far as to say that under no condition should a pregnant woman's food intake be limited. When weight gain is not restricted, the average gain during pregnancy is 25 to 30 pounds. Perhaps a more useful index is the *rate of gain*. The average woman gains 2 to 4 pounds during the first three months, 5 to 7 pounds in the fourth month, and thereafter roughly a pound a week for the remainder of her pregnancy. Williams considers a weight gain of less than 9 pounds in the first 20 weeks to be considered a nutritional alert signal.

The current concept of nutrition for pregnancy is based on the idea of supplying the developing baby with the building blocks neces-

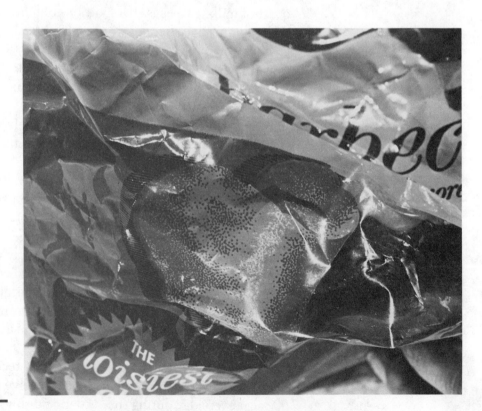

Junk food and fast foods are often very high in calories and low in nutrition. Junk Food, *photo by Michael Samuels.*

How weight gain is distributed in pregnancy

	WEIGHT (AVERAGES)
The baby	7.5 pounds
The placenta	1.0
The amniotic fluid	2.0
Increase in uterus's weight	2.5
Increase in breasts' weight	3.0
Increase in mother's blood	4.0
Increase in mother's fat stores needed for energy	4.0–8.0
Total	**24–28 pounds**

sary for optimum growth. Protein-rich foods are needed because they supply the amino acids from which cells are made. Protein is the only supplier of nitrogen, and during pregnancy both the baby and placenta require large quantities of nitrogen (60 grams and 17 grams, respectively). The increase in the mother's breasts requires another 17 grams of nitrogen, the uterus, 40 grams, and increased blood volume and storage reserves, 350 grams.

Obviously this enormous amount of cell building requires energy—at least 15 percent more energy than normal—and this energy is supplied by calories. The cumulative extra energy output necessitated by pregnancy has been estimated at 80,000 calories. Only vitamin- and mineral-rich foods supply the raw materials, such as calcium, that are needed for cell growth and for the regulatory enzymes, like vitamin D, which help to regulate the use of calcium.

Today there is a new understanding of the importance of good maternal nutrition for the growth and well-being of the developing baby. Each expectant mother should evaluate her diet in terms of its strengths and weaknesses. Initially the mother simply needs to maintain an adequate balanced diet, but during the second and third trimesters she needs to supplement her diet with additional carbohydrates and protein to meet the requirements of her growing baby. Often examining her diet during pregnancy will result in altered nutritional habits that will lead to lifelong improvements in the mother's health and well-being.

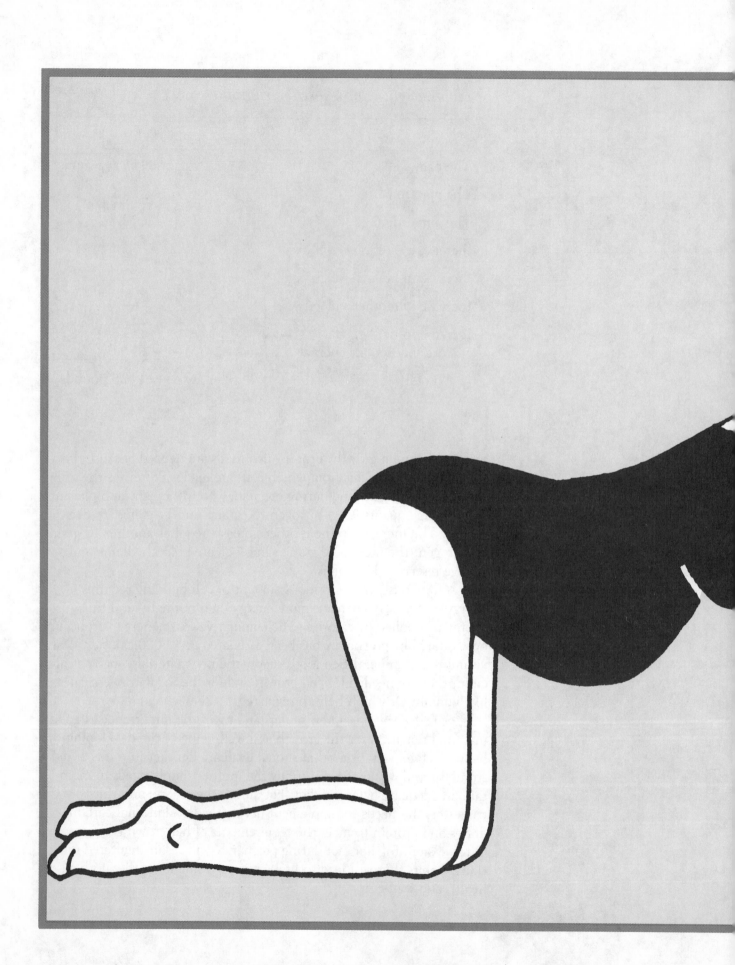

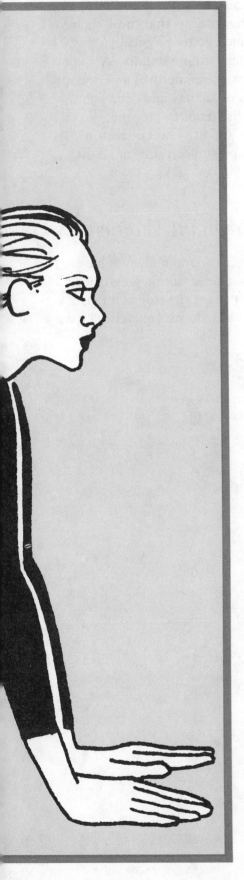

Exercise and Sex During Pregnancy

The General Value of Exercise

In the last ten to fifteen years people have become increasingly aware of the value of regular exercise for adults as well as for children and teenagers. Twenty years ago the vast majority of men and women stopped exercising when they stopped going to school. All too often they associated exercise with mandatory school requirements, not with physical or mental well-being. Recently there has been a great change in many adults' exercise habits and consciousness. Currently it is estimated that 72 percent of adults engage in regular exercise, and of these, 10 percent exercise for over an hour a day.

Doctors, too, have come to see the importance of regular exercise. Over the last decade or so many broad-based studies have shown that people who exercise regularly have a lower risk of coronary-artery disease. Poffenbarger, a respected exercise researcher at Stanford, found that Harvard graduates who did some form of weekly exercise had a 64 percent lower chance of heart attack and a lower incidence of hypertension than did graduates who got no exercise. A dramatic study in Sweden showed that heart attacks were much more likely to be associated with people in poor physical shape who had lower work capacities, higher breathing rates, and lower ability of the heart to rise to meet exercise needs.

Although lowering the risk of heart disease is the reason most adults take up regular exercise, there are other reasons that cause them to continue it. Most people find they feel much better physically. Equally as important, they find they feel much better mentally. A number of studies have shown that regular exercise improves a person's outlook and actually helps relieve symptoms of anxiety and depression. Finally, by toning the muscles, regular exercise tends to prevent weight gain and keeps a person looking trim and fit. This last reason may involve an element of vanity, but it's a great motivator for adults of all ages.

Effects of Exercise on Pregnant Women

In recent years childbirth educators, obstetricians, and midwives have begun to feel strongly that exercise should not cease during pregnancy, only to be resumed briefly after birth in order to get the stomach muscles back in shape. In fact, pregnancy isn't a time to stop exercising;

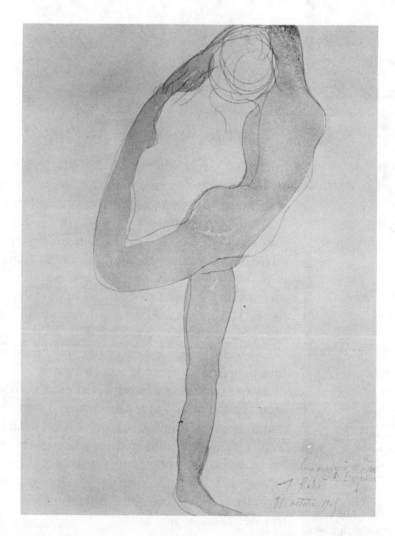

Exercise is just as important during pregnancy as before. Dancing Figure, *Auguste Rodin. National Gallery of Art, Washington, D.C. Gift of Mrs. John W. Simpson.*

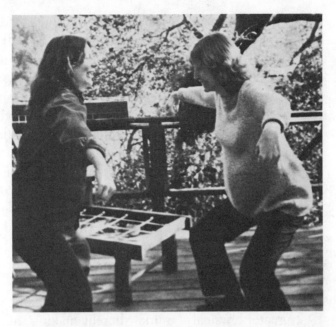

Exercise during pregnancy helps a woman bond with her body and get in shape for labor and delivery. Photo by Ken Levin.

it's an ideal time for women who don't exercise regularly to start.

Exercise during pregnancy has specific advantages in addition to long-range health. With exercise the expectant mother immediately has more energy and feels better. Low energy and lethargy are very common complaints during pregnancy, along with a number of other symptoms, such as backache, leg cramps, breathlessness, heartburn, and constipation. Exercise and regular movement prevent or help alle-

How prenatal exercise affects the pregnant woman and her baby

SHORT TERM:

- Increases mother's energy
- Relieves backache characteristic of pregnancy
- Relieves leg cramps
- Relieves breathlessness
- Stimulates the baby
- Conditions the mother for the physical exertion of labor

LONG TERM:

- Prevents dropped uterus
- Maintains tone of vagina
- Prevents urinary incontinence
- Prevents lower back pain after pregnancy
- Maintains abdominal muscle tone
- Helps mother stay fit

viate all these problems, which has the added effect of making the expectant mother feel better mentally as well as physically.

Prenatal exercise has important medium- as well as short-range effects. According to Elizabeth Noble, a physiotherapist who specializes in exercise for pregnant women, expectant mothers who exercise regularly develop more awareness of their bodies, greater firsthand knowledge of physiological changes their bodies are undergoing, and, ultimately, increased confidence in the physiological functioning of their bodies. Noble suggests that these learnings help a woman create a "bond with her body" that allows her to "trust her uterus and 'let go' during labor."[1] Much like the pioneering English obstetrician Grantley Dick-Read, Noble believes that labor and delivery are involuntary processes and that a profound, basic trust in her body and an acceptance of natural events is more important for a mother than any "contrived" techniques of natural childbirth.

Regular exercise also helps expectant mothers to develop greater physical stamina, thereby making them better able to meet the intense energy demands of labor and delivery, especially if they have a long or difficult birth. Noble observes that "most couples who experience natural childbirth report that a lack of energy is a more common difficulty during labor than unbearable pain."[2]

Several studies have been done on the relationship between exercise and length of labor. Earlier studies had shown a shorter labor in women athletes and a shorter second or third stage of labor for mothers who were fit (see p. 284), but more recent studies have not shown any particular link between exercise and length of labor or the condition of the newborn. However, it should be pointed out that the latter studies were all small. No matter what the length of labor, many doctors and midwives feel that fit mothers are better able to handle labor.

Exercise physiology provides an explanation for why fit women are better able to deal with labor without becoming unduly exhausted. *Aerobic exercise*, that is, exercise that requires increased, sustained oxygen consumption, results in a number of long-term physiological changes that allow the body to process more oxygen than normal. First, the heart becomes stronger, enabling each beat to pump more blood. This allows the heart to deliver more oxygen with less beats, no matter how strenuously the body is working. The more oxygen the heart can deliver with each beat, the less quickly the waste products of fatigue build up in the muscle cells of the body. Thus women who are in good aerobic shape can do a given amount of work with much less increase in heart rate and less muscle fatigue than can women who are not in good shape.

Aside from general long-term effects, specific exercises can benefit the pregnant woman in special ways over a number of years. Pregnancy and childbirth place extra stress on the muscles of the

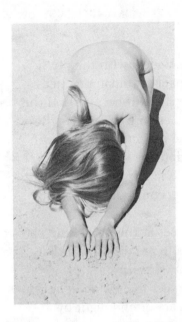

Every woman needs to pick the time, place, and form of exercise that suits her best. Sun Greeting, *photo by Michael Samuels.*

abdomen and the pelvic floor (see p. 27). If these muscles are not strengthened during and after pregnancy, future problems can develop. Many older women think that certain bladder and back symptoms are simply the outcome of having children, but in fact they can often be prevented or cured with proper exercise.

Effects of Exercise on the Unborn Baby

One of the newest and most interesting concepts concerning maternal exercise is how it affects the baby. When an expectant mother exercises, her baby's heart rate, like her own, goes up slightly. The baby's normal heart range is 120 to 160 beats per minute. With maternal exercise the baby's mean resting rate goes from 144 to 148. Researchers speculate that this gentle increase may simply be the result of arousing the baby to an alert state in the uterus (see p. 72). However, the baby's heart rate does not go up as much in response to exertion if a pregnant woman is very fit. This may be because a mother who is in good condition is able to maintain a higher level of oxygen in her blood. Such a response might be important if a baby were under stress during labor or delivery.

Maternal exercise definitely excites the baby physically, causing it to move. Such movement stimulates the baby's developing muscles and nerves and its sense of touch. Studies of chick embryos have shown that fetal movement is necessary in order to evoke proper growth. It's a gratifying and not altogether farfetched idea to think that a pregnant woman's exercise helps to stimulate her baby to grow.

When people exercise they experience a slight increase in blood levels of *epinephrine,* the fight-or-flight hormone that primes the body for strenuous work. This small transient increase, along with a slight increase in natural opiates called *endorphins,* is thought to be the reason people feel better during and after exercise. In a pregnant woman these hormones cross the placenta in small amounts and cause similar physiological responses in the baby.

It is interesting to note that by the seventh month in utero, the baby's developing senses are functional and it can actually hear the increase in maternal heartbeat and breathing that exercise causes. It is also known that the baby can learn in utero. Based on these two pieces of information, one can speculate that the older fetus learns to associate the mother's movements with the alterations in her heart rate and breathing, as well as with changes in epinephrine and endorphin levels. In this way maternal exercise may actually have lifelong conditioning effects on the baby, much as it is thought that the baby's reaction to stress may be conditioned during its time in the uterus (see p. 141). Thus for a number of reasons exercise may be a positive prenatal parenting activity for the expectant mother to engage in.

Exercising for Pregnancy

The following exercises are designed primarily to deal with the physical changes and stresses of pregnancy. The longer a woman practices these exercises, the stronger and more flexible she will become and the more she will build up her aerobic capacity. Therefore the earlier these exercises are begun in pregnancy, the more the expectant mother will benefit from them. In fact, they can even be done by women who are not pregnant but planning to be. It is never too late in pregnancy to begin the exercises, and it's just as important to continue them in the postpartum period as well (see p. 432).

Some mothers diligently do their exercises at the same time every day; others may prefer to fit the exercises in at convenient times. Many mothers find they are most faithful about exercising if they join a pregnancy exercise class, either because they like the sociability of it or because they need the routine. Such classes are often taught by obstetric-gynecologic physical therapists in programs that are run by doctors, hospitals, fitness centers, or exercise groups. Childbirth educators also deal with exercise, but usually not on a continuing basis.

A typical pregnancy exercise class lasts about an hour and a half and includes a warm-up phase, an aerobic workout (optional), a stretching and strengthening period, and a relaxation period. Unlike regular aerobic classes, pregnancy classes have a longer and slower warm-up. The exercises themselves are done more smoothly, and a special effort is made to avoid bouncing, jerking, or straining, which can hurt a woman's back muscles more easily when she is pregnant. Emphasis is put on balance and on toning muscles of the abdomen and pelvic floor. If an aerobic workout is included, it is usually done at a somewhat slower, "conversational" pace. The suggested target pulse rate is 120 beats per minute. The relaxation period at the end is often quite long, since relaxation is an important part of most prepared childbirth methods.

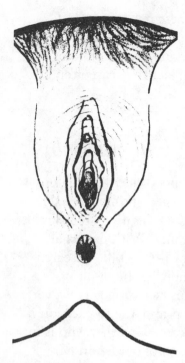

During pregnancy and delivery the muscles of the pelvic floor stretch considerably. Kegel exercises make the mother more comfortable before, during, and after the birth.

Exercise tips for pregnant women

- Start out easily and build up gradually to more strenuous exercises.
- Do each exercise slowly and gently.
- Do not strain at any time.
- Exercise often and make each session short to prevent becoming overtired.
- Stop and rest when feeling breathless, dizzy, or fatigued.
- Avoid breath holding during exercises, because it reduces blood flow to the baby.

When to do pelvic floor exercises (Kegels)

- While working at a counter
- While watching television
- While waiting in line
- While brushing teeth
- In the car at traffic lights

A number of specific exercises are generally included in any pregnancy program. We will describe them briefly, but for those who are interested, the exercises are described at greater length in both the Canadian government's booklet *Fitness and Pregnancy* and in Elizabeth Noble's excellent book, *Essential Exercises for the Childbearing Year.* Exercise therapists divide exercises into several categories, depending on what purpose they serve. The main categories in pregnancy classes are pelvic floor muscles, abdominal muscles, posture, breathing, and aerobics.

EXERCISING THE PELVIC FLOOR

Noble and most other exercise physiologists feel that the pelvic floor is the most important area for pregnant women to work on. As we described in the chapter on anatomy, the pelvic floor consists of the muscles that form a figure eight around the vagina and the anus (see p. 28). These muscles make up the bottom of the pelvic basket and support the bladder, uterus, and intestines. Proper functioning of the urinary and rectal sphincters depends upon these muscles.

The muscles of the pelvic floor are not contracted by normal sports or exercise classes. During pregnancy the weight of the enlarging uterus presses down on the muscles of the pelvic floor, often causing them to sag. This sagging can even reach the point at which the pregnant woman feels as if she's sitting *on* something when she sits down. As Noble remarks, since you can't lighten the baby, you have to strengthen the pelvic floor. Not only does good pelvic floor tone make a mother more comfortable during pregnancy, it increases her bladder control and helps prepare her for a vaginal delivery. Noble points out that a strong pelvic floor is more likely to stretch without tearing during delivery, and it will return to its prepregnant state more quickly following birth.

If a stretched pelvic floor is allowed to continue sagging after delivery, it permits the uterus and bladder to tilt backward and eventually push down on the vagina, particularly when a woman coughs, laughs, jumps, or strains. Too often the results are persistent problems with urinary incontinence, a sagging uterus, and/or a flabby vagina. Any woman who has ever had urine leak during pregnancy or in the weeks following childbirth will have some idea of how uncomfortable a problem incontinence is. A sagging uterus is a more subtle problem, causing vague lower abdominal aches and pains. Finally, a flabby vagina can be the cause of a decrease in sexual satisfaction after childbirth. Vaginal looseness has nothing to do with the way an episiotomy is repaired (see p. 337); the stitches only affect the ring around the opening of the vagina, not the muscle tone or diameter of the vaginal tube itself.

The tissues of the pelvic floor are composed of thin sheets of both *voluntary* and *involuntary* muscle. Unlike large voluntary muscles that are under conscious control, these mixed muscles cannot be contracted for very long, and they tend to fatigue much more quickly. Thus in doing the following exercises, it is important not to try to squeeze too long, too quickly, or too many times in a row. Rather, it is preferable that a woman do the exercises at frequent intervals for 5 seconds at a time, four or five times in a row. Many people in the United States call pelvic floor contractions "Kegels" after the UCLA professor of obstetrics who pioneered their use to prevent the common "female" problems that he found among older women.

There are several ways for a woman to become familiar with the sensation of contracting the muscles of the pelvic floor. For instance, when a woman is having a vaginal exam, she may be asked to squeeze and tighten her vagina around the doctor's or midwife's fingers. A woman can also do this herself, either in the bathtub or in bed. Another way to become aware of the Kegel sensation—and one of the best ways for a woman to judge how strongly she is contracting —is to intentionally stop the flow of urine several times while urinating. Noble cautions against trying this the first thing in the morning when the bladder is very full, or when very tired. She feels that at such times the woman may actually strain the muscles, decreasing rather than increasing muscle tone.

Noble also suggests that a woman practice what she calls sexercises, by contracting the pelvic floor muscles around her partner's penis during intercourse. Some women find they can contract the muscles more effectively immediately after their partner's ejaculation. Most men enjoy the sensation, and they can help the woman by letting her know when she is no longer able to squeeze as tightly. Noble points out that these movements are described in such books as the Indian *Kama Sutra* and *The Arabian Nights* and that among certain cultures the ability to contract the pelvic floor muscles is highly prized.

EXERCISING THE ABDOMINAL MUSCLES

Strong abdominal muscles are important during pregnancy and during the second stage of labor, when a woman is actively pushing the baby out. As we've discussed, the abdominal muscles stretch tremendously

The rectus abdominus, two broad bands of muscles that reach from the rib cage to the pubic bone, often tend to separate during pregnancy. Abdominal exercises help to minimize such separation and prevent backache.

rectus abdominus muscle

separation (diastesis)

during pregnancy to accommodate the growing size of the uterus, especially during the third trimester (see p. 41). If the abdominal muscles are not strong enough to support the baby adequately in the front, there are several results. The mother's center of gravity shifts forward excessively, and her pelvis tends to rock forward. This shift-and-rock sequence puts great strain on the muscles of the back and frequently results in chronic low backaches during pregnancy and even later in life.

Occasionally the topmost abdominal muscles, the *rectus abdominus,* two parallel bands that run from the rib cage to the pubic bone, separate more than usual during pregnancy, especially around the navel. The separation is caused by hormonal softening of the fibrous center between the muscles, as well as by the stretching of pregnancy. If unusual separation, which is referred to as *diastasis recti,* is not prevented or corrected, it will persist through subsequent pregnancies and add to a woman's backache problems.

Immediately after the baby is born, a woman can actually see how much her abdominal muscles have been stretched: her waistline will generally be nonexistent, and her tummy will tend to be flabby and hang down. Exercise, not just weight loss, is the only way a woman can regain a firm, flat stomach.

The basic idea of all abdominal exercises for pregnant women is to strengthen the muscles without putting strain on the back. The simplest exercise is *abdominal breathing and contraction.* Lying on her back, a woman inhales, letting her abdomen expand outward. Then she exhales slowly and forcibly, tightening her abdominal muscles as she does so.

The *pelvic tilt* is the major abdominal exercise. The pelvis is rocked backward, flattening the small of the back against a horizontal or vertical support, and then the muscles of the abdomen and the buttocks are tightened as a woman breathes out. A pregnant woman should do the pelvic tilt in a number of positions: lying on her back or

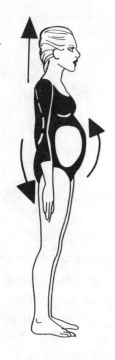

side, sitting in a chair, and kneeling on all fours. To avoid strain, it's very important that the back always be kept flat and the legs slightly bent. In addition to relieving backache, this exercise improves a woman's posture.

Another good abdominal exercise is what Noble calls the *leg slide*. First, a woman lies on her back with her knees pulled up and the small of her back pressed against the floor by tilting her pelvis backward. Then she slowly slides her heels out as far as she can and back. This exercise replaces leg lifts or double leg raising, both of which should not be done during pregnancy because they put too much strain on the back.

The final abdominal exercises are *curl-ups*. Again, the woman begins by lying on her back with her knees pulled up, keeping the small of her back pressed against the floor. Then she slowly and smoothly brings her head as far up toward her chest as possible—about 8 inches. This exercise can also be done with the mother turned on her side. Curl-ups are a substitute for regular *sit-ups*, which are another exercise that tends to put too much strain on the back during pregnancy.

EXERCISING FOR GOOD POSTURE

Posture itself can be a problem during pregnancy because a woman's body, center of gravity, balance, and muscles are changing so quickly and so drastically. Entering pregnancy with bad posture habits tends to make the changes more troublesome. Noble considers pregnancy a time of postural reeducation for all women.

In addition to the abdominal exercises, particularly the pelvic tilt, there are several exercises that Noble recommends for improving posture. Basically, these are *stretching exercises* designed to reduce pressure on the spinal column. In the first exercise the woman lies on her back, flattening her neck and the small of her back against the floor. In this position she points her toes up, stretches her heels out, pushes her knees down, and tightens her abdominal muscles.

Another postural exercise called *bridging* helps to keep the pelvis at a good angle. A woman lies on her back, either with her knees pulled up or with her feet elevated on a stool. By contracting the abdominal muscles and the buttocks simultaneously, she lifts her bottom slightly off the floor, still keeping her back and thighs in a straight line.

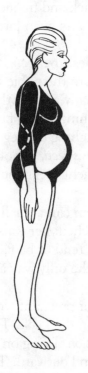

Good posture is very important during pregnancy because it helps to prevent backache and fatigue. Tucking the bottom under and lifting the neck and chin keeps the back in a straight line.

MISCELLANEOUS EXERCISES

There are several exercises that are designed to promote blood flow to the legs and relieve cramps as well as to prevent swelling and varicose veins. In one exercise the toes and foot are alternately bent backward

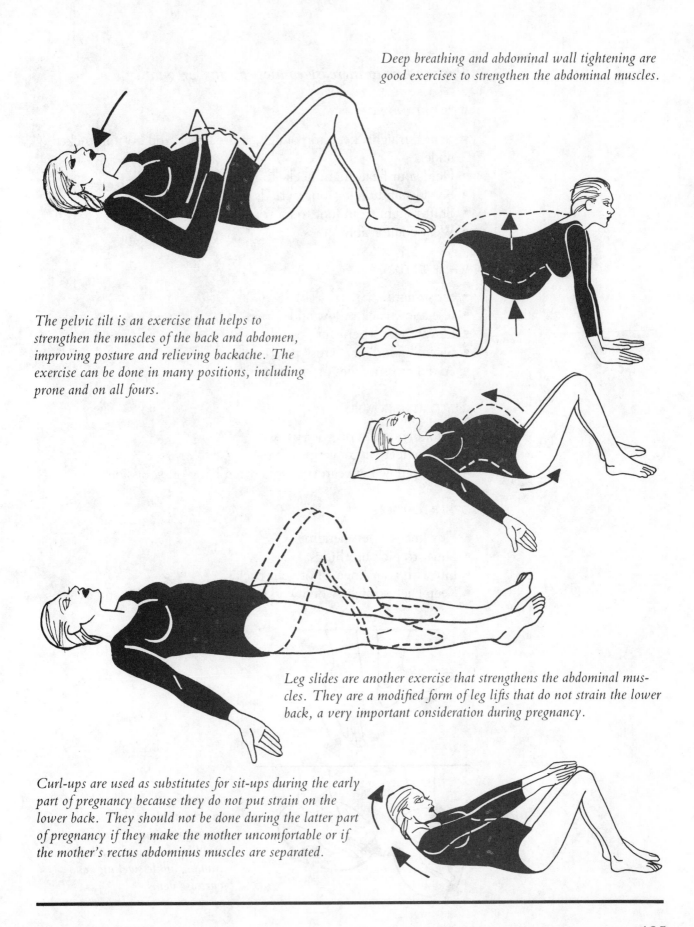

Deep breathing and abdominal wall tightening are good exercises to strengthen the abdominal muscles.

The pelvic tilt is an exercise that helps to strengthen the muscles of the back and abdomen, improving posture and relieving backache. The exercise can be done in many positions, including prone and on all fours.

Leg slides are another exercise that strengthens the abdominal muscles. They are a modified form of leg lifts that do not strain the lower back, a very important consideration during pregnancy.

Curl-ups are used as substitutes for sit-ups during the early part of pregnancy because they do not put strain on the lower back. They should not be done during the latter part of pregnancy if they make the mother uncomfortable or if the mother's rectus abdominus muscles are separated.

Posture tips to increase comfort during pregnancy

WHILE STANDING:

- Stand straight: keep top of pelvis tilted back and bottom tucked under.
- Hold your head high: neck straight, chin up.
- Avoid standing for long periods of time.
- Shift weight from foot to foot.
- Wear comfortable shoes.

WHILE SITTING:

- Sit straight.
- Use a low back pillow and a footrest.
- Elevate feet whenever possible.
- Sit in "tailor" or "lotus" position.
- Avoid crossing feet or knees.

WHILE LYING DOWN:

- Avoid lying flat on your back.
- Elevate feet whenever possible.
- Use a pillow between your legs when lying on your side.

OTHER POSITIONS:

- Flex knees when bending.
- Squat to pick up things.
- Lift with your knees, not your back.
- Keep back straight when working at counters; don't bend over.

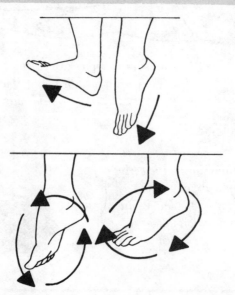

Stretching the feet and bending the ankles aids blood return from the lower legs and helps to minimize leg cramps, ankle swelling, and varicose veins.

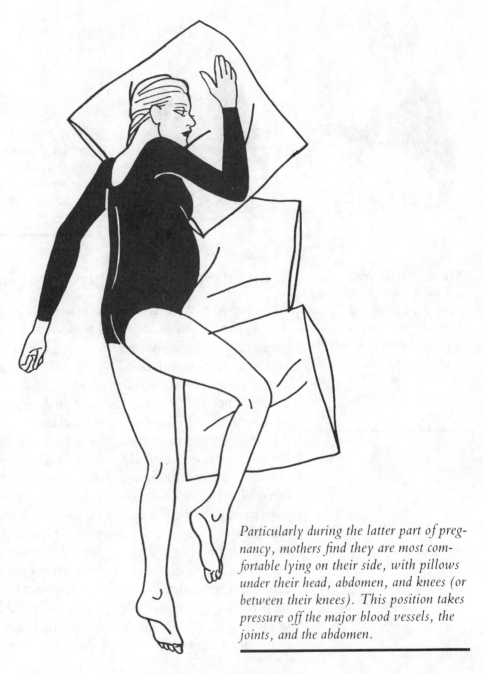

Particularly during the latter part of pregnancy, mothers find they are most comfortable lying on their side, with pillows under their head, abdomen, and knees (or between their knees). This position takes pressure off the major blood vessels, the joints, and the abdomen.

as far as possible, then stretched forward and down to make an arch. Another exercise simply involves rotating the ankles around and around in circles. Finally, Noble suggests a runner's exercise to prevent or alleviate leg cramps. The pregnant woman stands with one foot about two feet in front of the other. In this position she shifts her weight onto her front foot, bending her front leg at the knee. At the same time, she keeps her back leg in a straight position with her heel on the floor. This exercise causes a noticeable stretching in the calves and should be done alternating one foot and the other in the forward position.

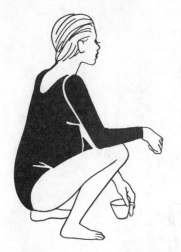 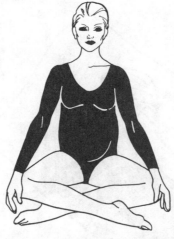

Many pregnant women find it very comfortable to sit in "tailor position," with both knees bent. Exercise physiologists recommend this position because it is good for the lower back and stretches the thigh muscles.

Squatting is the ideal position from which to lift, especially during pregnancy. Squatting minimizes back strain by making the muscles of the legs, not the back, do the work; squatting is also a more stable position than stooping.

AEROBIC FITNESS DURING PREGNANCY

The final part of many exercise classes for pregnant women is aerobics. As we've said earlier, aerobics is sustained exercise that requires greater than normal amounts of oxygen and builds up the heart, lungs, and peripheral circulation. Aerobic exercise includes jogging, bicycling, lap swimming, brisk walking, and cross-country skiing, as well as the skipping, jumping, dancing, and running-in-place combinations that are taught in aerobic exercise classes.

For some years there has been a controversy as to how much aerobic exercise is actually good for pregnant women. In the past obstetricians were concerned that sustained strenuous exercise might cause blood to be shunted away from the uterus to the large muscles, thereby decreasing the baby's supply of oxygen. Recent studies do not support this theory. They show that expectant mothers who did not exercise before pregnancy but who did exercise during pregnancy became significantly *more* fit. One study found that on the average, an exercise regimen increased the oxygen intake of expectant mothers by 18 percent per minute. This gain is comparable to the training results of nonpregnant women. A control group of pregnant women who did not begin an exercise program showed a 4 percent decline in their

Aerobic exercises for pregnancy

- Jogging
- Walking
- Bicycling
- Lap swimming
- Cross-country skiing
- Aerobic dance
- Running in place

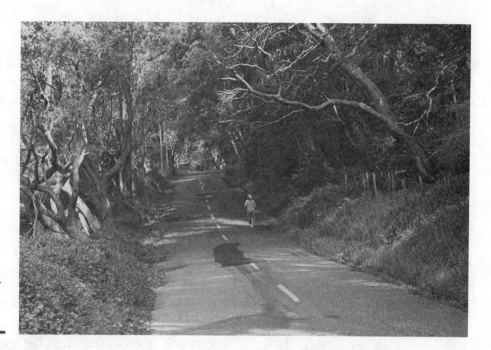

Aerobic exercise increases a pregnant woman's stamina by building up her heart, lungs, and circulation. Running, *photo by Michael Samuels.*

ability to take in oxygen by the middle of the third trimester. Finally, the women in the exercise group showed no ill effects from their exercise. There was no difference in the length of their labor or in the size or condition of their babies.

In spite of the favorable results of studies such as these and the fact that there are a growing number of women who have run marathons while pregnant and shown no detrimental effects, most exercise physiologists still advise women not to overdo aerobic exercise during pregnancy. Generally, they caution mothers to keep their pulse at or below the usual target range for their age and condition. The highly respected Canadian Fitness Program recommends a *maximum pulse rate* of 120 beats per minute, or that a woman still be able to carry on a conversation at maximum exertion. They also suggest that pregnant women keep their head level and hold their tummy with their hands while jogging. This tends to minimize the effects of bouncing on the baby. Many doctors advise women not to *begin* a jogging program during pregnancy, unless they are very careful and build up slowly.

Noble offers no specific restraints except to say that expectant mothers should not continue jogging programs if they experience pelvic pain while walking, since that may signal excessive loosening of ligaments in the central pubic area (see p. 28). Like all exercise physiologists, she recommends that women do warm-up and cool-down stretches before and after aerobic exercise. Noble encourages pregnant women to participate in any kind of aerobic exercise that brings them outdoors into the sunshine and fresh air. She feels that aerobic exercise during pregnancy promotes better overall body function, including greater endurance and circulation, improved balance, and better adaptation to increases in weight.

Sex During Pregnancy

There is an extremely wide range of sexual response among individual pregnant women. Several studies have reported different patterns, but all show great variation in sexual responsiveness at different times during and shortly after pregnancy. Elizabeth Bing, author of *Making Love During Pregnancy*, found the most common pattern was a steady increase in women's interest during the first two trimesters, followed by a decline in interest during the last trimester. Sex researchers Masters and Johnson reported an initial decline in interest during the first trimester, followed by an increase in the second and a decline again in the third. Another study showed a linear decline in interest from the time pregnancy was discovered. One of the largest studies, done by James Mill in 1981, dealt with over ten thousand pregnant women in Israel. His research did not deal with interest as such but with the number of women who actually had intercourse during any given month in pregnancy. His findings tended to agree with Masters and Johnson's, reporting intercourse rates of 90 percent in the first month, 87 percent in the second, 90 percent in the third, 95 percent in the fourth, 95 percent in the fifth, 94 percent in the sixth, 89 percent in the seventh, 66 percent in the eighth, and 36 percent in the ninth. There was general agreement among all the studies that the majority of women experience a decline in sexual desire and activity during the last few months of pregnancy.

There is a wide range of sexual responsiveness among women during pregnancy. It varies with the individual mother, her sense of well-being, and her stage of pregnancy.

Mithuna couple, Indian, 12th century. The Metropolitan Museum of Art. Florence Waterbury Fund, 1970.

Samvara, Tibet, 17th century. Asian Art Museum of San Francisco. The Avery Brundage Collection.

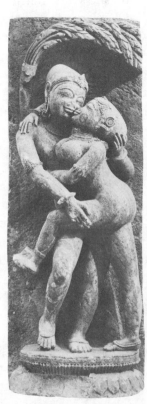

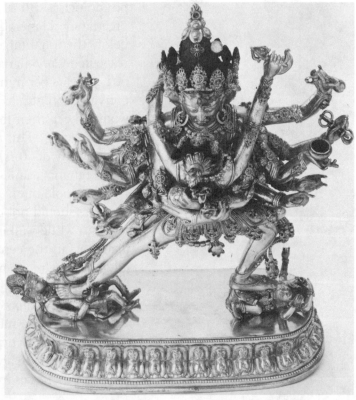

Pregnant women's interest in lovemaking is influenced by a number of factors: their attitudes toward themselves, their attitudes toward sex, physical changes during pregnancy, and their information about sex during pregnancy. For many women there may be a sharp rise in interest when they learn they are pregnant because they are suddenly freed from having to deal with contraception. Women who have been attempting to get pregnant may feel renewed interest because of a profound relief at no longer having to schedule intercourse at the most likely times for conception. On the other hand, women who experience significant nausea or fatigue are likely to be less interested in sex during the first trimester. So are women who have ambivalent feelings about their pregnancy or who are not getting along well with their partners, either because of the pregnancy or for other reasons.

One of the most common reasons for women to become disinterested in sex at any point in pregnancy is fear of causing a miscarriage. This fear is most frequent among women who have a history of miscarriage or who experience spotting. Spotting can be a result of the egg embedding in the uterine wall or of deep-penetration sexual positions that tend to abrade the cervix, which becomes softer and more engorged with pregnancy (see p. 42). Most doctors advise women to refrain from sex during the first trimester if they experience real bleeding and cramps.

The great majority of women will be reassured by their doctor or midwife as to the safety of having intercourse, and will often have an increase in sexual interest. Over all, most women find that if their fears are allayed and they feel well, their interest in sex will be normal or greater during the first trimester. Many pregnant women enjoy deep, positive feelings of sexiness, femininity, and fecundity—a profound sense of marveling at and being proud of their body's ability to create new life.

The positive body feelings that women often experience are augmented by important physical changes that begin to take place in the second trimester. By this stage of pregnancy the entire pelvic area, especially the vagina, experiences significantly increased blood flow in response to the rise in estrogen levels (see p. 35). As nearby veins widen, the lower part of the vagina and the labia minora reach a continuous, slightly swollen state. This area, which is called the *orgasmic platform,* is normally only swollen before orgasm when a woman is sexually excited. During the second trimester the orgasmic platform becomes so engorged that it shifts downward and protrudes. After orgasm the congested veins in the area do not drain as well and the swelling does not subside completely. As a result, during the second trimester most women are in a constant physiological state of semi-arousal. They are therefore more easily brought to full arousal and more likely to have multiple orgasms than at any other time in

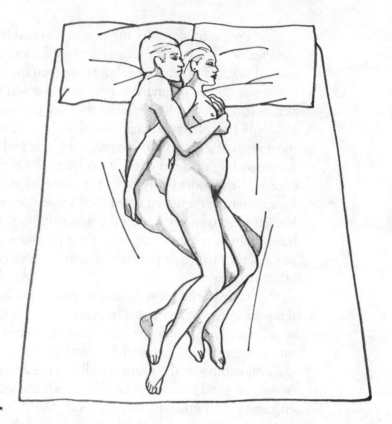

Pregnancy requires couples to make adjustments in their lovemaking. In the latter part of pregnancy many prefer the man to lie behind the woman, because this position does not put pressure on her abdomen.

their entire reproductive cycle. Other physical factors also tend to enhance a woman's sexual pleasure during this period. A woman's breasts, like the orgasmic platform, are vascular tissue and also tend to be engorged and more sensitive.

Additional blood flow to the vagina causes women to have increased vaginal secretion. This added discharge is beneficial in terms of lubrication, but it generally has a much stronger odor, which may be disturbing to a woman's partner during oral sex. Unfortunately, bathing does little to change the quality of the odor. In reference to oral sex, it's important to point out that air should never be blown forcefully into the vagina during pregnancy. Late in pregnancy, when the cervix has begun to open, air bubbles or emboli can enter the mother's bloodstream. For this reason doctors warn against the practice, although they do not consider oral sex itself to be dangerous during pregnancy.

The second trimester for most women is the time they feel the best during pregnancy. Problems of nausea or fatigue are usually resolved, and women have not yet become so big that their size has begun to bother them. Nevertheless, some women cannot release their fears about hurting the baby, or are too engorged to be comfortable during sex. Also, many husbands and wives begin to feel that the baby is almost like a third party watching or joining them in sexual play. While some couples enjoy this and feel it brings them closer to the baby, others are made anxious and uncomfortable by it.

During the third trimester pregnant women begin to experience changes that tend to diminish their interest in sex. Just the size of their abdomen becomes a factor to reckon with, and many women find that sex is no longer comfortable in their usual positions. While some husbands and wives readily adapt to these alterations, others have trouble. Certainly it helps if women are at ease communicating with their partner about sexual matters and if he, in turn, is flexible about making changes in their sexual routines.

At some point in the second or third trimester most women begin to find it uncomfortable to have the man on top because the pressure on their abdomen makes them worry about the baby. Many women find they are more comfortable on top, not only because it takes pressure off their abdomen but also because it allows them to control the angle and depth of their partner's penetration. Having the husband enter from the rear, either with the woman standing or lying on her side, is another alternative that works for some couples. As the woman's size increases and she becomes less adept at moving, she may also prefer a side-by-side position, because it allows her to be more passive and lets her husband be the more active partner.

As their due date approaches, most women find themselves less and less interested in sex, although a few enjoy sex right up until the time of delivery. In part, this decline in interest may be due to a decrease in orgasms. One study has shown that by the ninth month the majority of women had dropped from having orgasms three out of four times to one out of four times, although the orgasmic platform is still swollen. By late in the third trimester some women find themselves too tired to be very interested in sex, and/or increasingly uncomfortable because of their size and shape. Many men find their wives less physically arousing toward the end of pregnancy, and as the

Most obstetricians and midwives feel that intercourse is safe for the mother and baby throughout pregnancy unless there is a specific medical problem.

Couples copulating, Peru, 0–200 A.D. The Metropolitan Museum of Art. Gift of Nathan Cummings, 1965.

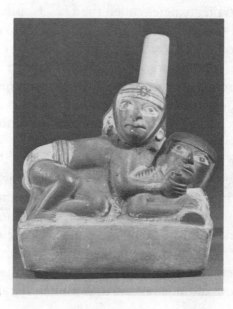
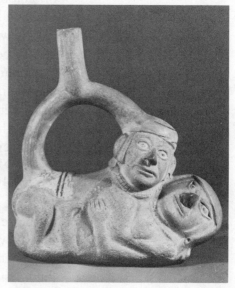

baby begins to move about more, many women and their partners again become concerned that intercourse may hurt the baby.

A decrease in interest and frequency of intercourse and orgasm leads to a natural period of abstinence for most couples as the date of delivery nears. This does not necessarily mean that the couple feels estranged or that sexual tensions mount in an uncomfortable way. Many couples enjoy simply lying together, snuggling, massaging each other, kissing, and walking arm-in-arm. This gives them a lot of touching and skin-to-skin contact, and seems to be pleasurable to both mother and father. Such gestures apparently fulfill each partner's needs for the other's love and support as the culmination of pregnancy looms and they look forward, joyfully and nervously, to birth and the realities of parenting to come.

MEDICAL CONCERNS ABOUT INTERCOURSE

Up until the 1950s pregnancy textbooks and obstetricians warned against intercourse in the last trimester on the basis that it might cause premature deliveries or maternal infections. This restriction was modified or downplayed after a 1953 study failed to demonstrate any connection between premature delivery and recent intercourse. For roughly the next twenty years most doctors viewed intercourse as safe unless a mother had medical complications such as bleeding, abdominal pain, or threatened miscarriage.

Then in 1971 a small study by Goodlin questioned the safety of a pregnant woman experiencing orgasm during the third trimester. It has long been known that orgasm can cause the uterus to contract or spasm. Goodlin's study showed a slight increase in premature delivery among women who had had orgasm after 32 weeks of pregnancy.

In 1979 Dr. Richard Naeye studied the data from a huge report on 26,886 pregnancies called the *U.S. Collaborative Perinatal Project.* He found that infection of the amniotic fluid occurred more often among women who had had intercourse more than once a week in the month before delivery, as opposed to women who abstained from intercourse during the last month. More significant, the mortality rate among infected babies was over four times as high in mothers who'd had intercourse as in those who had not. From this data Naeye concluded that intercourse during pregnancy "may increase the frequency and severity of amniotic fluid infections. . . ."[3]

Naeye noted that the greatest effect was seen among women who had intercourse after week 37. By this time the mucous plug that seals the uterus may be loose or gone, and the cervix has often ripened or shortened considerably (see p. 42). Naeye theorized that seminal fluid may have enzymes that can pass through the mucous plug, and that bacteria attached to the sperm could thus penetrate the amniotic fluid. Naeye did not suggest that women refrain from intercourse unless future clinical trials confirmed his theories. In fact, Naeye was so concerned that abstinence might add to marital discord at this time that he only recommended abstinence for women of "poor reproductive history" or for those who had premature "ripening" of the cervix (see p. 282).

Other studies have not agreed with Naeye's results, and some researchers have called the study's methods into question. Naeye used an unusual technique to determine infection, and he did not balance the 1959 mortality rates with the lower current figures, which some researchers consider crucial. A large-scale study by Mills did not specifically study amniotic fluid, but it did consider intercourse in relation to complications of pregnancy and condition of the baby at birth. Mills's results challenge the view that intercourse in the latter part of pregnancy may be harmful to the baby. He found no greater risk of premature ruptured membranes, low birth weight, or infant mortality before or after delivery.

These two conflicting studies leave obstetricians with questions about what advice to give their patients. In 1979 an editorial in the *New England Journal of Medicine* questioned Naeye's methods and stated that the data does not permit a dogmatic conclusion, but agreed with Naeye's suggestion of "avoidance of intercourse and orgasm in the third trimester in women with a poor reproductive history or in those who, on pelvic examination, have premature ripening of the cervix . . ." The editorial also observes that, fortunately, this is not a problem for most women.

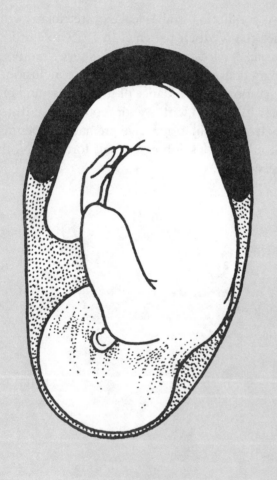

Environmental Agents That Affect the Baby During Pregnancy

The Baby Is Not Isolated

Before the 1940s it was believed that the baby was in a protected state as long as it was in the uterus. This concept of uterine isolation was referred to as the *placental barrier theory.* It held, in effect, that the uterus was a glass bubble that totally separated the baby from the outside world. As a result, birth defects were considered chance occurrences of unknown cause. Typically, people associated birth defects with *events* rather than *agents,* in a manner not unlike primitive peoples' belief that supernatural spirits were the source of such defects.

Today we know that not only nutrients and oxygen but many *environmental agents* cross over the placenta and affect the developing baby to varying degrees. The breakdown of the uterine isolation theory began in the early 1940s, when a pediatrician from Melbourne, Australia, made a connection between babies who were born with heart, eye, and ear defects and mothers who had contracted German measles during a rubella epidemic in their first trimester. The defects caused by German measles are examples of how *infectious agents* can affect an unborn baby.

The second piece of evidence that caused doctors to question the theory of uterine isolation was the results of the atomic bombs dropped on Hiroshima and Nagasaki during World War II. Radiation released by the bombs caused birth defects in babies whose mothers were exposed to the radiation early in their pregnancy. These defects were an example of a *physical agent* affecting the unborn baby.

Finally, during the early 1960s the effects that *chemical agents* could have on the unborn baby became known through the *thalidomide* tragedy. Over a period of several years seven thousand babies were born with limb defects caused when the tranquilizer-sedative was taken by their mothers during the early part of pregnancy. Once thalidomide was identified as the cause of these birth defects, researchers began to study some of the thousands of chemical agents that could affect a baby in the uterus.

The understanding gained from these three tragic events made doctors realize that birth defects actually had causes that were scientifically explainable, and, even more important, that many birth defects could be prevented by avoiding exposure to certain agents. This realization led obstetricians to immunize mothers against rubella when a vaccine became available, to take steps to avoid unnecessary exposure to X-ray radiation, and to attempt to identify and avoid chemical agents that might be dangerous to the baby. Thus the theory of uterine isolation was supplanted by one of *fetal susceptibility*, which dictated avoidance of exposure to any agent that might have negative effects on the unborn baby.

In 1979 the U.S. Surgeon General's Report *Healthy People* identified five major risk factors as causes of infant mortality in this country: smoking, misuse of alcohol, misuse of drugs, occupational hazards, and injuries. Of these, the first four involve agents that cross the placenta by voluntary use. Thus the incidence of infant mortality and illness could be decreased significantly through life-style changes made by pregnant women. The fact that mothers can actually lower the risks to their baby is a positive concept for expectant parents who

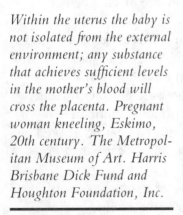

Within the uterus the baby is not isolated from the external environment; any substance that achieves sufficient levels in the mother's blood will cross the placenta. Pregnant woman kneeling, Eskimo, 20th century. The Metropolitan Museum of Art. Harris Brisbane Dick Fund and Houghton Foundation, Inc.

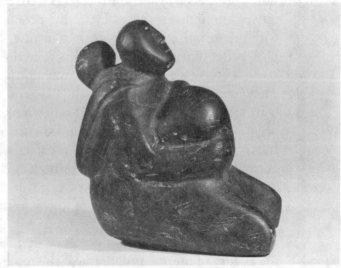

are concerned with their baby's health. It emphasizes the idea of pre-birth parenting. But mothers can only make these changes if they understand how chemicals affect infant development and which chemicals are dangerous.

The basic mechanism by which environmental agents affect uterine development is simple. Substances in the mother's blood are readily transferred from the mother's uterine arteries, across the placental membrane, into the baby's umbilical vein, and then to the baby's entire body. Pharmacologist Charlotte Catz notes that "any substance, if present in sufficient concentration on the maternal side, will eventually reach the fetus," either by simple diffusion or by active transport.[1]

Critical Periods in Development

In terms of the kinds of effects environmental agents have on the baby, there are three basic periods or stages in fetal development. The first period occurs during *fertilization and implantation*, which comprises approximately the first 17 days of pregnancy. *Teratogens*, agents that are associated with birth defects, will usually prevent proper implantation during the first 17 days and will eventually cause the fetus to be spontaneously aborted.

The second stage is the *embryonic period*, which goes from day 18 to day 55 after conception. As we discussed earlier, this is the time of greatest differentiation, when organs are undergoing their most

Critical periods when the baby is most sensitive to chemicals and radiation

ORGAN SYSTEM	HIGHLY SENSITIVE PERIOD (IN WEEKS)	LESS SENSITIVE PERIOD (IN WEEKS)
Central nervous system	3–5.5	5.5–full term
Heart	2.5–6.5	6.5–8
Limbs	3.5–7	7–8
Eyes	3.5–7.5	7.5–full term
Ears	3.5–8.5	8.5–9.5
Teeth	6.5–8	8–full term
Palate	6.5–8.5	8.5–9
Genitalia	6.5–8.5	8.5–full term

rapid and extensive changes. Thus it is also the period when teratogens are most likely to cause severe structural or functional birth defects. Although each organ system is most susceptible during this critical time, they remain susceptible for a varying period thereafter, depending on how long differentiation normally continues. The central nervous system, for example, is susceptible to major defects from week 3 to week 6, but it remains susceptible to minor defects until after the baby is born (see p. 241). The heart, on the other hand, is also most susceptible from week 3 to week 6, but it only remains susceptible to minor defects until week 8, when its basic structure is completed.

The third developmental period is the *fetal stage*, which goes from day 56 of pregnancy to delivery. It is the period of rapid cell growth. Teratogens which affect the baby during this period do not produce major structural defects except in the brain or eyes, which are still undergoing change.

Evaluating the Risks

Teratogens vary greatly in their ability to affect the developing baby. Some are powerful, others are weak. Some teratogens, like thalidomide, affect a high percentage of those babies who are exposed. Thus they are considered *high-risk factors*. But inexplicably, most teratogens affect relatively few babies who are exposed to them. Some chemicals affect so few babies that it has thus far been difficult to prove their effects. These chemicals are considered *low-risk factors*. A number of teratogens act along with other agents; some act independently. Some teratogens may affect a number of organ systems, while other agents may affect only a single system. Conversely, some organ systems are susceptible to many environmental agents, others to only a few. Because of these variables, and because humans are not always affected in the same way as research animals, it is often impossible to predict the outcome of a mother's exposure to a particular chemical or to trace back the cause of a particular birth defect. The problem is made even more complicated by the fact that various defects can be caused by genetic mutation in the sperm or egg before conception ever takes place.

To put all this information in perspective, it's important to look at the statistics on birth defects. Only about 3 to 5 percent of babies born in the United States today have any kind of birth defect. Of these, 60 percent are of unknown origin; approximately 20 percent are caused by diseases such as PKU, which are due to gene mutations; 5 percent are caused by aberrations in chromosomal structure or number, such as Down's syndrome. Only 10 percent of birth defects are due to various teratogens, including environmental agents such as

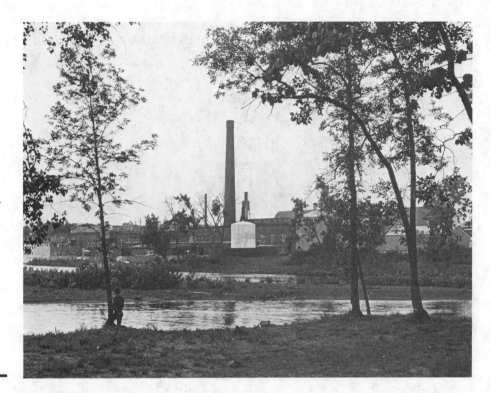

Despite the direct link between chemicals and birth defects, less than five babies in a thousand have problems associated with chemical or drug exposure. Damage tends to be greatest if the baby is affected between day 18 and day 55, when its organ systems are just being differentiated. PCB Plant on the Hudson, *photo by Michael Samuels.*

radiation, infections, and chemicals; and 1 to 3 percent are specifically due to teratogenic drugs taken during pregnancy.

In the last ten to fifteen years researchers have come to realize that there are also a whole group of environmental agents that do not cause major congenital malformations but that result in low-birth-weight babies, developmental delays, diseases such as cancer that do not develop for a long time, and neurological and behavioral problems that can affect bonding and later development. These problems are thought to be caused by chemicals other than known teratogens or by teratogens taken late in pregnancy or in low doses. Such problems pose fundamental questions about when an exposure took place, how often it took place, and in what quantities.

The environmental agents that an expectant mother is exposed to fall into three basic categories: medical agents that are considered necessary for the health of the mother or the baby, agents the mother deliberately chooses as part of her life-style, and agents the mother is unaware of that are in her food, water, and so on. Obviously the easiest ones for the mother to control are the ones she chooses, such as cigarettes, alcohol, caffeine, and over-the-counter drugs. The environmental agents that a mother is unaware or uncertain of are, of course, more difficult to control. The medical drugs that a mother is exposed to depend on the health of the mother-and-baby diad. The necessity of specific drugs and medical procedures must be thoughtfully evaluated with the doctor or nurse-practitioner in terms of their risks versus their benefits.

Generally a woman is pregnant for several weeks before she is

Drugs known to cause or suspected of causing birth defects

DRUG	BIRTH DEFECT
KNOWN:	
Thalidomide	Limb defects
Dilantin	Mental retardation and facial deformities
Coumadin (Warfarin)	Facial and skeletal abnormalities
Tridone	Mental retardation and heart defects
Alcohol	Mental retardation and facial defects
Aminopterin	Mental retardation and facial defects
SUSPECTED:	
Lithium	Heart defects
Streptomycin	Hearing defects
Kanamycin	Hearing defects
Barbiturates	Numerous abnormalities
Propylthiouracil	Mental retardation
Valium	Cleft palate
Brompheniramine	Numerous abnormalities
Tetracycline	Tooth discoloration
Amphetamines	Heart abnormalities
Sulfa drugs	Facial and skeletal abnormalities

certain of it. This means that even the most careful woman, while still unaware that she is pregnant, may be exposed to or choose to use agents that are potentially harmful to the fetus. Fortunately, the fetus is minimally susceptible during the first two weeks, although it becomes increasingly susceptible during the third, fourth, and fifth weeks. Thus any woman who *suspects* she may be pregnant or who misses a period should act as if she is pregnant until proved otherwise. Environmental health researchers go so far as to say that the safest course is to have women of childbearing age avoid all exposure to known hazardous chemicals.

Effects of Smoking During Pregnancy

By smoking, women take a number of chemicals into their bodies. Whereas chemicals in food are absorbed into the bloodstream through the digestive tract, chemicals in smoke are absorbed through the lungs. Just as oxygen crosses the placenta, so do the chemicals in smoke. Studies have clearly demonstrated that smoking reduces blood flow in the placenta during the time the cigarette is being smoked and for up to fifteen minutes thereafter. Researchers theorize that blood vessels in the placenta actually clamp down in response to the chemicals in cigarette smoke. Smoking has other negative effects as well, including association with significant increases in the level of stress hormones in the mother's and baby's bloodstreams.

There are an astounding sixty-eight thousand toxic chemicals in cigarette smoke. Several of these—carbon monoxide, cyanide (hydrocyanic acid), and nicotine—have been studied in detail. Cyanide crosses the placenta and lowers the baby's ability to use vitamin B_{12}, which is vital to the cells' production of fundamental proteins, as well as the formation of red blood cells. Both these factors are important to the growth of the baby. Nicotine, which also crosses the placenta, causes profound physiological changes in both mother and baby, including increase in heart rate, rise in blood pressure, and constriction of blood vessels. The rapid drop in uterine and placental blood flow caused by constriction of blood vessels causes the baby's heart rate to go up in an effort to maintain its oxygen levels.

Smoking mothers have elevated levels of carbon monoxide in their blood, while their unborn babies, for reasons not yet understood, have even higher levels. Studies show that babies of smokers have a carbon monoxide level that leads to about a 20 percent reduction in their blood levels of oxygen. Not only is carbon monoxide transferred directly to the fetus, it is taken up by the hemoglobin in the baby's red blood cells in preference to oxygen. To combat the resulting reduction in oxygen, the baby has to make extra hemoglobin, as if it were living at a very high altitude.

Numerous studies have proved beyond any doubt that smoking during pregnancy is associated with a reduction of 5 to 8 ounces (150–250 grams) in the birth weight of babies. Statistically, the newborn's weight drops sharply with the first few cigarettes smoked by the mother each day. Thus only 10 cigarettes per day result in an average drop in weight of about 7 ounces—almost half a pound. At a pack a day (20 cigarettes), the average drop in weight is almost 9 ounces. Differences

Effects of smoking on the growing fetus

- Increased carbon monoxide levels in baby's blood
- Decreased oxygen levels in baby's blood
- Increased fetal heart rate
- Increased levels of stress hormones in baby's blood
- Decreased blood flow to mother's uterus
- Increased chance of low birth weight
- Increased incidence of serious illness and death
- Increased incidence of spontaneous abortion

in the placenta help to explain how the baby's weight is affected by smoking. Among mothers who smoke, the placentas are lighter and have fewer blood vessels. In this respect they are similar to placentas that function poorly due to structural defects.

Smoking seems to stunt the unborn baby's growth in other ways, too. It is associated with a slower growth rate in the baby's head diameter from about 18 weeks on, and the overall length of smokers' babies is less on the average. Smoking is associated with a definite increase in the rate of spontaneous abortion: smoking up to 10 cigarettes a day increases the chance of such an event by 46 percent above that of nonsmokers. Smoking also increases the risks of premature delivery and perinatal mortality. The perinatal mortality risks increase by 20 percent at less than one pack a day and by 35 percent at over a pack a day.

Finally, smoking has both immediate and long-range effects on the neurological development and intellectual maturation of children whose mothers smoked during pregnancy. One study found that newborns of smokers showed different behavior when evaluated by the Brazelton Neonatal Behavioral Assessment Scale. In particular, these babies were less responsive to sound and less easily consoled by soothing sounds. Later studies showed that at the ages of seven and eleven, children of smoking mothers showed slight but definite lags in growth, and poor scores in reading and math.

All these statistics are so alarming that the *American Journal of Public Health* stated, in a 1983 editorial, that in addition to saying, "Cigarette smoking can be dangerous to your health," cigarette packages should also state, "Cigarette smoking could be harmful to the fetus."[2]

We realize that it is difficult for most smokers to quit. Some fortunate women find that cigarettes become distasteful to them as soon as they become pregnant. For those mothers who aren't so lucky, the relaxation exercises for pregnancy (see p. 159) and a support group such as Smokenders may help them give up smoking. At present most doctors and midwives are doing intensive counseling with their patients because of an unprecedented emphasis on the dangers of smoking in reports in current medical literature. Pregnant women have to deal with a number of life changes, but they have an especially good reason to quit smoking: the health of their babies is at stake. For many women this is a more immediate and compelling reason for stopping than fears of developing cancer, heart disease, or emphysema in later life.

The good news is that studies have shown that quitting has dramatic effects: within forty-eight hours after an expectant mother stops smoking, her blood will carry 8 percent more oxygen to the baby. Some researchers believe this rise is so important that even if mothers cannot give up smoking during pregnancy, they should at least stop around the time of delivery, since oxygen to the baby is normally reduced during contractions. One way to look at all this is that just as a mother would not give a cigarette to a newborn, why would she give it to her unborn baby?

Although maternal smoking has not been found to have specific effects on the baby *after* birth, the nicotine in smoke is known to lower the mother's milk production and interfere with her letdown reflex (see p. 414). And *passive smoking,* the presence of cigarette smoke in the air the newborn breathes, has recently been shown by itself to result in high levels of a nicotine metabolite in the baby's blood.

Effects of Alcohol During Pregnancy

During the 1800s English doctors who observed the babies of jailed alcoholic mothers questioned the effects of large amounts of alcohol on the developing baby. But no significant studies were done and the questions were dropped, not to be revived for over a hundred years. Until the 1970s only a few researchers expressed concern over the idea of a pregnant woman drinking alcohol. Wine and beer were considered by most people to be table beverages of no special import to the expectant mother. More recently it has been found that alcohol crosses the placenta freely and attains blood levels in the baby that are similar to those in the mother.

In 1973 Jones and Smith identified a frightening group of congenital malformations that were the result of heavy maternal alcohol consumption during pregnancy. These malformations included overall growth retardation *before* and *after* birth, mental retardation and developmental delays, and various congenital malformations of the

---

Medical classification of alcohol consumption

Heavy drinker	More than 45 drinks per month, or more than 5 drinks per occasion
Moderate drinker	Between 1 and 45 drinks per month, never more than 5 drinks per occasion
Light or rare drinker	Less than one drink per month

One drink is equal to .5 ounces of alcohol, or:

- One beer
- 4 ounces of wine
- 1.2 ounces of liquor

head, face, skeleton, and heart. Jones and Smith named this set of symptoms the *fetal alcohol syndrome.* In addition to the symptoms cited, these babies are likely to be premature, of low birth weight, hyperirritable, and have neurological defects and poor muscle tone. There is also over thirty times the incidence of *microcephaly,* a condition in which the baby has a small skull and brain, as well as being mentally retarded. The syndrome is also associated with higher infant mortality statistics.

The fetal alcohol syndrome is *dose dependent;* that is, the more alcohol a mother ingests, the more likely her baby is to have the syndrome. Studies show that babies have a 10 percent risk if their mothers drink more than 1 ounce (30 milliliters) a day or five or more drinks at any one time, and a 20 percent risk if the mothers drink more than 2 ounces (60 milliliters) per day.

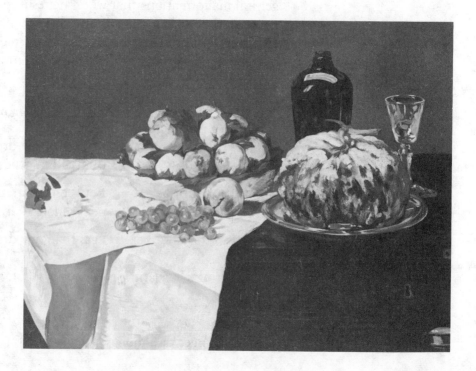

In recent years heavy maternal drinking has been found to be associated with fetal alcohol syndrome, of which mental retardation is the most common symptom. Still Life With Melon and Peaches, Edouard Manet, 1866. National Gallery of Art, Washington, D.C. Gift of Eugene and Agnes Meyer.

While the fetal alcohol syndrome has definitely been associated with women who drink heavily or who drink in binges, especially in the early part of pregnancy, the effects of moderate drinking during pregnancy are not clear. Although studies vary in their definitions, most researchers tend to define moderate drinking as 1 ounce (roughly 2 drinks) a day or 10 drinks a week. Studies of mothers in the moderate drinking category showed that their babies did not have any increase in congenital malformations but weighed an average of 3 ounces less than babies whose mothers didn't drink at all, and might show some of the symptoms of fetal alcohol syndrome, such as tremors or poor neurological response at birth. More subtle behavioral differences have also been found among these babies. Although they appeared otherwise normal, they showed lower arousal and slower learning characteristics on Brazelton's newborn behavior test (see p. 154). To date, studies have not shown any statistical differences between babies whose mothers drank under 1 ounce a day and babies whose mothers did not drink at all. But studies in this area are not yet definitive.

A more recent and disturbing study by Judy Kline shows a direct relationship between drinking and spontaneous abortion. This study is particularly upsetting because it shows that even very low amounts of alcohol ingested in any given month during pregnancy had a low but definite statistical effect. Among 2,800 mothers in New York City, Kline found that the odds of spontaneous abortion went up 3 percent with each additional day that alcohol was consumed, beginning with as little as one drink. The odds of spontaneous abortion for a woman who drinks every day are 2.53 times greater than the odds are for a woman who neither drinks nor smokes. For a woman who drinks and also smokes a pack of cigarettes a day, odds of spontaneous abortion go up to 4.08 times that of a nonsmoking, nondrinking expectant mother.

The present U.S. Public Health Service guidelines recommend that pregnant women drink *no alcohol* during pregnancy. Even light drinking is now believed to be a low-risk factor for the unborn baby.

Effects of Caffeine During Pregnancy

Caffeine is one of the most widely used drugs in the world and is found in over-the-counter prescriptions as well as in so-called foods such as coffee, cocoa, chocolate, and many teas and soft drinks (see chart). Although most people do not think of caffeine as a drug, it is a nervous system *stimulant* that increases heartbeat and metabolic rate. In high doses caffeine causes restlessness, heart palpitations, and irritation of the digestive tract. Caffeine also causes a marked rise in the stress hormone *epinephrine* and essentially puts both mother and baby

Caffeine content of common foods and drugs

FOOD	CAFFEINE IN MILLIGRAMS
Decaffeinated coffee (cup)	2
Instant coffee (cup)	66
Percolated coffee (cup)	110
Tab (can)	44
Dr. Pepper (can)	38
Pepsi-Cola (can)	37
Coca-Cola (can)	34
Mountain Dew (can)	52
Cocoa (cup)	10
One ounce milk chocolate	6
One ounce dark chocolate	20
One tea bag brewed 1 minute	21
One tea bag brewed 5 minutes	40
Iced tea (can)	36
DRUGS	
NoDoz	200
Anacin	64
Excedrin	130
Dristan	32
Sinarest	30
Dexatrim	200

under stress. Elevated levels of epinephrine reduce blood flow to the uterus, thereby lowering the flow of oxygen and nutrients to the baby.

The average person in the United States gets 206 to 210 milligrams of caffeine a day—roughly the equivalent of 1½ cups of coffee. The average pregnant woman gets 144 milligrams. Caffeine not only crosses the placenta, it attains higher levels in the baby's bloodstream than in the mother's. In part this is because the baby's liver is unable to process caffeine as quickly as the mother's, so it tends to remain in the baby's system for a longer time. As it is, caffeine remains in the bloodstream of pregnant women much longer than it does in nonpregnant women.

The first inkling that there might be problems with caffeine came from animal studies that demonstrated that the offspring of animals that had been fed high levels of caffeine showed prematurity, postmaturity, growth retardation, and congenital malformations such as cleft palate. As opposed to gross congenital malformations, low doses of caffeine given to pregnant rats have been shown to cause slower learning ability and lower activity among offspring.

No human malformations have been directly linked to caffeine. However, very high levels of caffeine (approximately 8 or more cups a day) have shown a statistical correlation with fetal death. One study of pregnant mothers who took in more than 600 milligrams of coffee (4 strong cups) a day showed an increase in spontaneous abortions and stillbirths, although other studies have not confirmed these findings. Based on this somewhat confusing information, the Food and Drug Administration has warned mothers to minimize their intake of caffeine during pregnancy. Researchers recommend that expectant mothers have less than 2 cups of coffee or its equivalent per day.

Effects of Life-style Drugs During Pregnancy

Along with the study of various other chemicals that could cause birth defects, researchers have begun to study the ways in which so-called recreational drugs affect the unborn baby. There is a growing concern about the effects such drugs may have on newborn behavior and neurological function, as well as how they affect birth weight and the incidence of congenital malformations.

Marijuana has long been known to have broad effects on the offspring of pregnant animals. Like cigarettes, the chemicals in marijuana cross the placenta and attain significant blood levels in the fetus. Physiologically, the effects of marijuana are somewhat like steroids. Marijuana affects hormonal balance in the fetus as well as in the mother: changes are seen in the mother's ovarian function, uterine contractility, and prolactin secretion during pregnancy.

One study done on home-delivery mothers who smoked marijuana showed a slight increase in labors that didn't progress normally and an increase in the number of babies who had fetal distress as measured by meconium staining (see p. 201). *Meconium* is the name for the normal stool of newborns. Babies who have had a bowel movement while still in the uterus are known to have twice the neonatal mortality risk of babies who are not meconium stained. In a study of hospital births in Los Angeles, the incidence of meconium staining was found to be 57 percent among mothers who smoked marijuana approximately once a week or more, as opposed to 25 percent among nonusers. The same study found that mothers who used marijuana had a higher proportion of labor problems.

A 1983 Israeli study found a higher incidence of low-birthweight and premature babies and a higher number of congenital malformations in babies born to marijuana users. The increase was not great enough to constitute statistical proof, but the researchers felt that until more studies were done, expectant mothers should not smoke marijuana during pregnancy.

Cocaine has been shown to cause spontaneous abortions, low birth weights, and congenital malformations among offspring in animal studies, but its effects on pregnant women and their babies is unknown. For many years it has been known that babies born to *heroin* addicts experience a life-threatening narcotic withdrawal after birth that requires intensive medical treatment. Addicted babies also tend to have low birth weight, premature delivery, and increased fetal distress and perinatal mortality.

Effects of Medical Drugs During Pregnancy

Since the thalidomide tragedy of the 1960s, the effects of prescription drugs on the unborn baby have come under intense scrutiny. At this point literally thousands of drugs and chemicals have been shown by studies to be teratogenic among animal offspring. Ironically, the average pregnant woman takes 3.7 potentially teratogenic prescription drugs during the course of her pregnancy. In Scotland a study found that 97 percent of all expectant mothers had taken some kind of prescribed drug and 65 percent had taken some form of over-the-counter drug.

Although most researchers believe that prescription drugs cause less than 5 percent of all congenital malformations, the figure remains suspect because it is based on crude estimates of the few human teratogens that have been definitely proven. Researchers are worried that medical teratogens may interact with each other and/or with environmental chemicals to produce a higher rate of malformations than is presently suspected. Also, researchers increasingly question whether certain chemicals may be associated with subtle behavioral changes or with long-range changes that do not become evident for many years, such as cancer.

Two kinds of drug studies are routinely undertaken, both of which have yielded relevant information. The first kind deals with a large number of mothers and identifies any drugs they have taken during pregnancy as well as any malformations or changes seen in their newborns. On the whole, these studies have shown that mothers who had taken prescription or nonprescription drugs during pregnancy were more likely to have babies with malformations. One such study done at Yale University in 1981 found that maternal use of one or more prescription drugs was associated with 30 percent more malformations than was the use of no drugs. Of the drugs used, antidepressants, nar-

Drugs taken by the pregnant woman that affect the growing baby

NAME OF SUBSTANCE	EFFECT ON BABY
Heroin	Withdrawal symptoms, depressed breathing
Demerol	Decreased breathing, depression
Morphine	Depressed newborn
Salicylates (aspirin)	Newborn bleeding
Ampicillin	No adverse effects noted
Erythromycin	No adverse effects noted
Flagyl	Not recommended in first trimester
Penicillin	No adverse effects noted
Streptomycin	Deafness
Sulfonamides	Liver problems
Amphetamines	Possible birth defects
Tetracycline	Discoloration of teeth
Thyroid drugs	Possible goiters
Barbiturates	Cross the placenta; baby receives greater concentrations than mother
Thalidomide	Birth defects
Valium	Possible congenital anomalies
Lithium	Alters functions of heart and thyroid; causes congenital anomalies
Methotrexate (for psoriasis)	Birth defects
LSD	Chromosomal damage and possible limb malformations
Alkylating agents	Birth defects
Dilantin	Congenital anomalies
DES (diethylstilbestrol)	Increased incidence of cancer of the vagina
Podophyllin (in laxatives)	Birth defects
Estrogens	Possible masculinization of female babies
Oral contraceptives with progestin and estrogen	Possible congenital anomalies
Vitamin A (very high doses such as in acne medications)	Birth defects
Vitamin C	Minimum daily requirement has no adverse effects reported
Warfarin	Birth defects

cotic-analgesics, and tranquilizers were the most likely to be associated with problems.

The second kind of drug study deals with a sudden increase in a particular defect thought to be connected with known use of a particular drug. It is through this type of study that all the proved human teratogens have been identified, the most graphic example being the

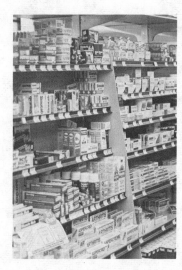

During pregnancy women should not take prescription or over-the-counter drugs without the advice of their practitioner. Photo by Michael Samuels.

thalidomide studies. In that case researchers were able to pinpoint effects to the days the mothers had taken the drug.

As a result of both kinds of studies, medical drugs are now classified into four basic categories (see charts). The first group, *established teratogens*, consists of drugs that are unquestionably known to produce higher incidences of defects and perinatal mortality. The second category, *suspected teratogens*, contains drugs that have apparently caused an increase of defects in a small number of babies, though there may be alternative explanations. The third category, *possibly toxic*, includes drugs on which data is meager and which have only occasionally been implicated in human studies, even though animal studies show a strong association. The fourth and final category, *not toxic under likely conditions of usage*, includes drugs that have been studied extensively and used by pregnant women over many years with no apparent problems.

Since the great majority of drugs fall into the last three categories, it is often unclear exactly what pregnant women should do about taking medical drugs. For this reason most researchers recommend that mothers take *no drugs* during their pregnancy unless it is absolutely necessary. At the same time, mothers can be reassured by the fact that only a small percentage of all birth defects are thought to be caused by medical drugs, and that very few drugs have been identified as being really dangerous. A woman who has to take a drug during pregnancy, particularly if it is from the fourth category or even the third, runs a very low risk of adversely affecting her baby.

Effects of Environmental Chemicals During Pregnancy

In recent years thousands of newly manufactured chemicals have flooded our environment with a host of unknown risk factors for human health. What effect these chemicals may have on developing infants is still largely unknown, but many of them are proved animal teratogens and are known to cross the placenta in humans as well as animals. A significant number of these chemicals, in addition to causing major birth defects, are known to cause growth retardation and neurological changes among offspring of animals who have been exposed to them.

Many of these chemicals are now in our food, our air, and our water. In addition to such accidental exposure, pregnant women may be brought into contact with particular chemicals depending on where they work, what chemicals are used around their home, and what chemicals their husbands are exposed to at work. At present there is a growing sense that pregnant women should not be exposed to any hazardous chemicals, not necessarily because of definitive studies link-

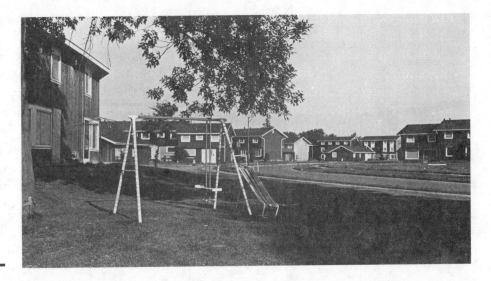

There is a growing concern that pregnant women should not be exposed to hazardous environmental chemicals. Abandoned Housing At Love Canal, *photo by Michael Samuels.*

Chemicals known to affect the reproductive process

Alcohol
Aminopterin
Anesthetic gases
Busulfan
Carbon disulfide
DDT
DES
Diphenylhydantoin
Ethylene dibromide
    (EDB)
Hexachlorobenzene
    (HCB)
Kepone
Lead
Methotrexate
Methyl mercury
Pesticides
PCBs
Tobacco smoke
Vinyl chloride

ing these chemicals to birth defects but based on the realization of how sensitive the fetus is to any toxic chemical.

Concerned women can do much to avoid potentially harmful chemicals. To decrease exposure to chemicals in food, mothers should eat a low-fat diet, wash all fruits and vegetables carefully, and use bottled water if the water supply in their area is known to be high in chemicals. Around the home women should avoid using paints, solvents, oven cleaners, and pesticides. A mother stripping baby furniture in a garage is exposed to thousands of times the chemical levels set by the U.S. Occupational Health and Safety Administration for workplace safety. Women whose gardens are sprayed with pesticides often come into contact with higher levels of these chemicals than do farm workers.

Studies have shown that women whose jobs involve lab work, anesthesia, and soldering have greater numbers of spontaneous abortions and malformations among their pregnancies. If a woman comes into contact with chemicals because of her job, she should think seriously of switching assignments in the early part of pregnancy or stopping work early. For women who are not subject to occupational

Chemicals known to affect function of placenta

CHEMICAL	EFFECT
Carbon monoxide	Lowered oxygen transfer
Lead, cadmium	Suppressed metabolism
Mercury	Delayed cell division
Organachlorine pesticides	Transferred to fetus
Cigarette smoke	Changes enzymes, lowers oxygen

exposure and who avoid the use of chemicals at home, the risks to their babies are very low.

Given the new knowledge of the extent to which the baby in utero is affected by external agents, an expectant mother can do much to protect the health of the developing baby. By not smoking or drinking during pregnancy, and by minimizing drugs and occupational hazards, she can do a great deal to avoid birth defects and prevent a wide range of newborn problems. Just as a woman would not expose her baby to environmental dangers after birth, she can protect the baby while it is in the uterus. Although some life-style changes may be difficult for the expectant mother, they are of extraordinary value to her future health as well as the baby's.

Occupational hazards for women of childbearing age

OCCUPATION	HAZARDOUS SUBSTANCES
Textile and garment workers	Cotton and fiber dusts, noise, formaldehyde, dyes, heat, asbestos, solvents, flame retardants
Health personnel	Anesthetic gases, X-rays, alcohol, noise, laboratory chemicals
Electronic assemblers	Lead, tin, antimony, trichloroethylene, methylene chloride, resins
Hair dressers and cosmetologists	Hair-spray resins, aerosol propellants, solvents, and dyes
Cleaning personnel	Soaps, detergents, heat, enzymes, solvents
Launderers of industrially-contaminated clothing	Various industrial chemicals
Photographic processors	Caustics, bromides, iodides, silver nitrate
Plastic workers	Acrylonitrile, formaldehyde, vinyl chloride
Transportation personnel	Carbon monoxide, polynucleararomatics, lead, vibration, microwaves
Painters	Lead, titanium, toluene

Clerks/clerical workers	Trichloroethylene, carbon tetrachloride, formaldehyde, asbestos, cigarette smoke
Printing personnel	Ink mists, methanol, carbon tetrachloride, lead, noise, solvents, trichloroethylene

NOTE: From Samuels and Bennett, *Well Body, Well Earth*, 1983.

Environmental chemicals and drugs affecting male reproduction

CHEMICAL	EFFECT
Anesthetic gases	Congenital anomalies in offspring
Carbon disulfide	Impotence, loss of sex drive
Chloroprene	Decreased sperm count and motility, increased miscarriages among wives
Cigarette smoke	Abnormally shaped sperm
Dibromochloropropane	Decreased sperm count and infertility
Hydrocarbons	Offspring with higher cancer risk
Kepone	Decreased fertility
Lead	Decreased sperm count and motility, abnormally shaped sperm
Vinyl chloride	Excess fetal loss
Alcohol	Abnormal testes
Anti-amoeba drugs	Decreased motility of sperm, abnormally shaped sperm
Anticonvulsants	Developmental disabilities in offspring
Iodine	Atrophy of testes
Testosterone enanthate	Sterility

NOTE: From Samuels and Bennett, *Well Body, Well Earth*, 1983.

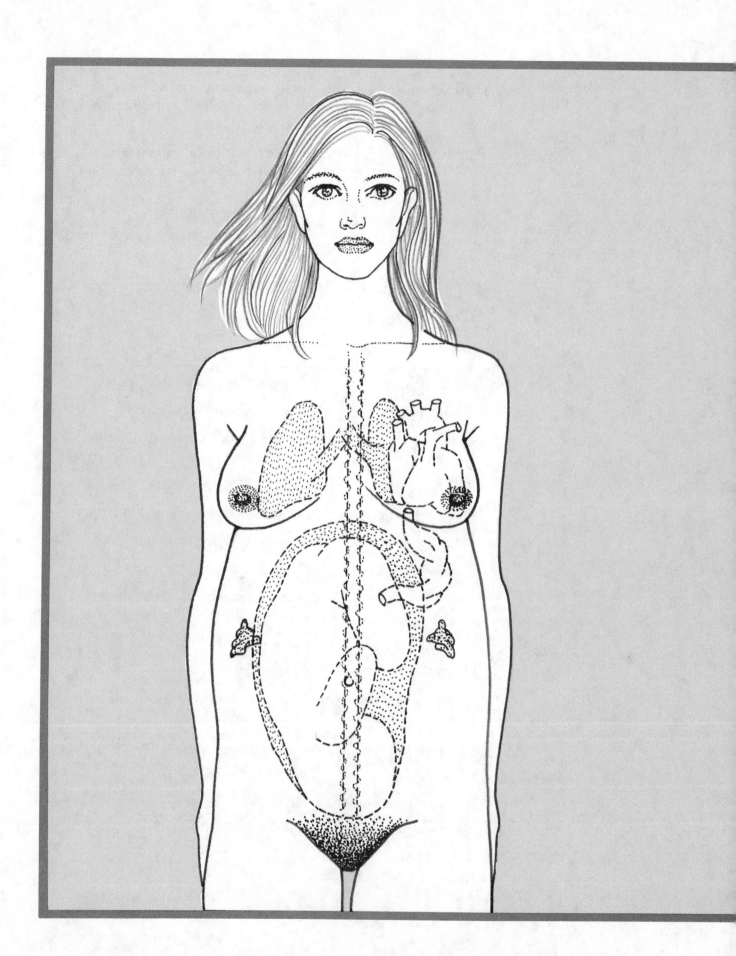

Stress
During Pregnancy

Pregnancy—A Transformative Experience

Pregnancy—especially a first pregnancy—brings profound changes to most women's lives. The majority of expectant mothers sense this intuitively and find that it is corroborated by their physical and emotional feelings. Pregnancy is a momentous, exciting, joyful, and challenging occurrence, perhaps more so now than ever before. Today the average woman is pregnant only twice, not many times as used to be the case, which gives each part of the experience a heightened intensity. This intensity is reinforced by two facts: today many mothers tend to be older when they first become pregnant, and pregnancy is now a more conscious choice because of improvements in contraception instead of an inevitable and unquestioned event that follows marriage. Often pregnancy is a long-considered, long-awaited condition, and when it finally happens, it has greater significance in terms of the psychic energy that has gone into it.

Given the drop in the number of babies per family, the rise in average maternal age, and the likelihood that a woman has been a member of the work force, the expectant mother of today comes to pregnancy with a different background and a different set of expectations than her mother did. First, she has chosen motherhood at a time when many women around her are choosing not to become pregnant or to postpone it. Often, the deliberateness of this choice leads expectant mothers to have high expectations about their performance and to be motivated to learn as much as they can about being pregnant. At the same time, they may have little firsthand experience with pregnant women and newborns. This lack of experience may add to women's feelings of ignorance and insecurity, as well as to their romantic visions of the perfect pregnancy. And a mother's sense of uncertainty may be increased by the prevalent—though poorly supported—notion that mothers over age thirty or thirty-five are likely to have a more difficult or complicated pregnancy (see p. 250).

Not only physically but in every respect, pregnancy becomes a transformative experience, changing the mother and causing her to look differently at her daily life and the roles she plays. Although most pregnant women go about their usual routines, they always have in mind the overwhelming realization that they are pregnant and that that fact makes everything different.

Stress and the Autonomic Nervous System

Tribal cultures have always held that the pregnant woman must be surrounded by a calm atmosphere, based on their profound belief that fear and emotional upsets affect the baby's growth and delivery. Ironically, Western medicine is just coming to recognize stress as an important factor in maternal-infant health. Studies have shown that women who experienced a number of different medical problems during pregnancy and labor had much higher anxiety levels throughout their pregnancy. These studies have also shown that support, attitude, emotional state, and life events that require great adaptation have significant effects on the expectant mother and her baby.

Stress is defined as any situation or event that causes a person to become upset, consciously or unconsciously. Response to stress is a normal human reaction that has an important survival value in evolutionary terms, because it primes people for action when necessary. The initial use of the term *stress* came from Hans Selye's studies on the physiology of the *fight-or-flight reaction* in the 1950s. When people (or animals) encounter a situation they perceive as dangerous, a series of predictable changes occurs in their body. Anxious thoughts excite nerve cells in the brain, which in turn send impulses out through a special part of the nervous system called the *autonomic nervous system*. Autonomic nerves go to virtually every part of the body—the digestive system, the heart and blood vessels, the uterus, and, most important, to the adrenal glands (see pp. 31–32 and 276).

The autonomic nervous system has two parts: the part called the *sympathetic* is stimulated during stress, or fight and flight; the part called the *parasympathetic* is stimulated during relaxed, calm periods. All of us have experienced sympathetic arousal, both acute and chronic. A sudden fight-or-flight sensation is triggered when we feel we're about to fall off a ladder or get into a car accident. Such rapid sympathetic arousal enables people to mobilize themselves physically and mentally in a situation that requires quick action. Throwing a spear at a lion during a hunt or running from a charging elephant are archetypal images of fight or flight. Modern life has replaced lions and elephants with job and family crises. Often such problems produce gnawing worries and "dis-ease" that are the symptoms of chronic sympathetic arousal. Long-standing sympathetic arousal not only keeps the body constantly at the ready, it causes physiological changes that can lead to illness. Parasympathetic arousal, on the other hand, results from quiet, pleasurable activities like lying in the sun or listening to soft music. It leads to warm, tranquil, relaxed feelings that cause physiological changes that promote health and prevent illness.

The arousal of either part of the autonomic nervous system affects the body's adrenal glands, which in turn produce hormones that sustain the response. During fight or flight the core of the adrenals produces *adrenaline (epinephrine)*, which keeps a person galvanized for action. During relaxation the outer portion of the adrenals produces *steroids*, which aid in keeping the body balanced in a healthy, smoothly functioning state.

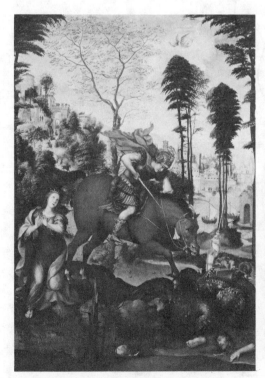

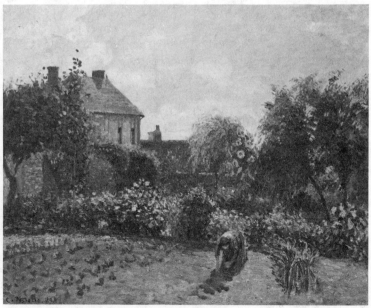

Stress and Disease

Over the last thirty years doctors have learned a great deal about how stress wears the body down and helps cause illness. In terms of infectious diseases and heart disease, the way in which stress promotes illness is well understood. When people perceive themselves as under stress, their sympathetic nerves cause their heart rate and blood pressure to rise, which eventually leads to tears and abrasions in their artery walls. Fatty acids released by the liver become lodged in the tears. Eventually arteries can become blocked if the stress is frequent or long-lasting, causing heart attacks and strokes. Several factors, including smoking, lack of exercise, high-cholesterol diet, and inherited inability to handle cholesterol, add to these effects.

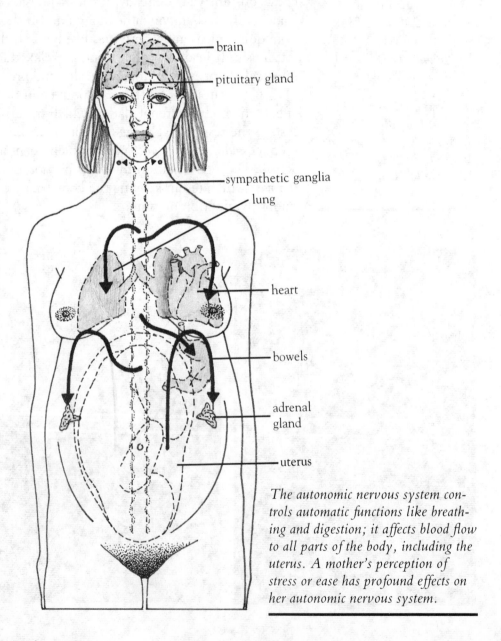

brain
pituitary gland
sympathetic ganglia
lung
heart
bowels
adrenal gland
uterus

The autonomic nervous system controls automatic functions like breathing and digestion; it affects blood flow to all parts of the body, including the uterus. A mother's perception of stress or ease has profound effects on her autonomic nervous system.

Stress also plays a critical role in infectious disease. In addition to a particular germ, infectious illness depends on the *susceptibility* of the person's own body (the *host*). Stress hormones lower the white blood cells' ability to recognize germs and produce antibodies against them. Thus stress, as well as diet, exercise, and genetics, determines how well a person's immune system will function in fighting a particular infection.

Stress and the Baby

Although doctors have been studying the role of stress in heart disease and infection since the 1940s, it is only recently that researchers have begun to demonstrate the many ways in which stress affects the pregnant mother and the developing baby. To grasp this association it is necessary to understand the connection between the autonomic nervous system and the reproductive organs. Like the heart and the digestive system, the uterus and ovaries are richly innervated by the autonomic nervous system and receive blood levels of adrenal hormones.

In response to sympathetic arousal, the reproductive organs tend to receive less blood and to slow their muscular contractions. These reactions are part of bioprograms that have evolved over millions of years to divert great amounts of blood to those organs that are directly involved in the fight-or-flight reaction: the brain, the heart, and the voluntary muscles in the arms, legs, and trunk.

When a pregnant woman feels stress, the blood vessels of the uterus itself constrict, causing blood flow to the uterus to drop even more. Animal studies have shown that anxiety in a mother can cause blood flow to the uterus to drop by 60 percent or more. Another animal study has shown that maternal anxiety causes the baby's heartbeat to drop radically, also resulting in lower oxygenation of the baby's blood. Normally the baby has ample resources to handle a drop in

---

How stress affects the pregnant woman and her baby

- Blood flow to arms and legs increases.
- Blood flow to uterus decreases.
- Blood vessels of uterus contract.
- Blood flow to baby decreases.
- Baby receives less oxygen and nutrients.
- Stress hormones produced by mother are transmitted to baby through placenta.
- Baby's heartbeat increases.

blood flow, but lower oxygenation and lower nutrients over a *long* period can negatively affect the baby's ability to grow.

The fetus not only depends on blood flow for food, oxygen, and removal of waste products, it is constantly affected by the rise and fall of hormones in the mother's blood. Epinephrine, the stress hormone, crosses the placenta in the same manner as food or oxygen. This means that whenever the mother is under stress, the baby is directly under stress as well. High levels of stress hormones affect the developing baby in many ways. As in the mother, these hormones lower the baby's ability to digest, grow, and fight infection. In particular they cause food to be broken down faster and less efficiently, preventing calories from being converted to weight gain.

Prolonged levels of stress hormones in utero are also believed to affect the baby's autonomic nervous system, conditioning it to respond to stress in a specific manner. It is thought that such conditioning may lead to increased irritability, restlessness, crying, and digestive disturbances in the newborn. A few researchers speculate that continuous high levels of stress hormones may even affect the development of the brain and central nervous system. Constantly bathing the growing nerve cells with epinephrine causes fundamental changes in the way nerve impulses are transmitted. Research like this leads some scientists to believe that such stress tuning in utero may have lifelong effects, not only on stress-response patterns but on stress-related illnesses that people develop in adulthood.

Life Events and the Perception of Stress

In the broadest sense, stress is anything in people's social-emotional world that causes them to feel distress or unease. People describe such situations as "difficulties," "hardships," or "problems," and they describe their resulting feelings as "anxious," "upset," "threatening," or "unsatisfied." Thus stress not only relates to outside events but, more important, to the way in which a person internally *perceives* those events. While most people would view loss of a job as a stressful event, only some people would view writing a report as stressful.

What is important is not only people's perception of an event but their ability to deal with it. According to this definition, even so-called positive events can be anxiety-producing for some people. For example, holidays and vacations are sometimes unsatisfying or upsetting because they require adaptation or change from normal routines. Also, people sometimes fear that they will have difficulty handling a particular situation or expect too much of themselves.

One of the greatest contributions to stress research was made by Seattle psychiatrists Thomas Holmes and Richard Rahe. They set up a scale that ranked a variety of life events in terms of the amount of

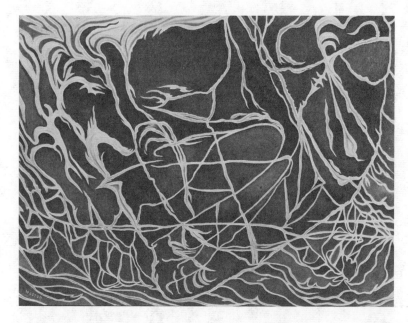

Stress *is defined as "anything in a person's world that causes him or her to feel distress or unease"; lack of stress causes a person to feel calm and peaceful.*

Tensions, *Harold Weston, 1960. Collection of Whitney Museum of American Art, New York. Gift of the National Council on the Arts and Government and the Friends of the Whitney Museum of American Art.*

Ocean Image, *Vija Celmins, 1970. Graphite and acrylic spray, 12¾" x 17½". Collection, The Museum of Modern Art, New York. Mrs. Florene M. Schoenborn Fund.*

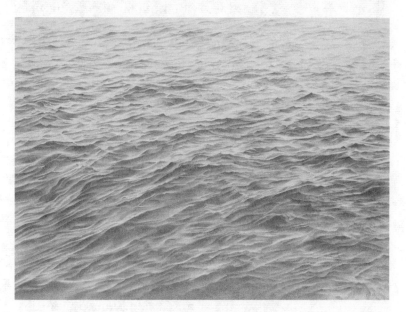

stress they produced and the amount of coping they required. Holmes and Rahe asked a broad cross-section of people, including psychologists, teachers, and doctors, to rate many universal events such as getting married, getting divorced, having a baby, changing jobs, moving, and so on. Holmes and Rahe used marriage as a reference point and assigned it an arbitrary value of 50 on a scale of 1 (low stress) to 100 (high stress). They found a remarkable uniformity among the responses. A subsequent survey clearly demonstrated that the onset of illness is often correlated with stressful life changes. People who had a high number of points based on recent life experiences had five times as great a chance of developing health problems.

Stress scale for pregnant women

STRESSFUL EVENT	STRESS IN A FIRST PREGNANCY	STRESS IN A SUBSEQUENT PREGNANCY
A baby or child of yours died	—	9.6
Your husband/partner died	—	9.5
You were told by your husband/partner that you were no longer loved	9.5	9.1
You separated from your husband/partner	9.1	9.1
Your baby was abnormal	—	8.3
You were in contact with someone who had an infectious disease, like German measles, which might affect your baby	8.9	8.1
Your husband/partner was unfaithful	8.8	9.0
Increasingly serious arguments developed with your husband/partner	8.8	8.6
You were the cause of a traffic accident in which someone was badly injured	8.6	8.7
Someone close to you (in the family or outside) died	8.5	9.0
You almost miscarried *after* 3 months	8.1	7.5
You heard that something you took (medication, alcohol, cigarettes) during pregnancy might be harmful to the baby	7.9	7.8
You were seriously ill during pregnancy	7.9	7.5
Your husband/partner became unemployed	7.8	7.1
Your baby needed some special treatment after the birth	7.6	7.6
You almost miscarried *before* 3 months	7.5	6.6
You had a pregnancy terminated (during the past 12 months)	7.5	7.1
Increasingly serious arguments developed with your mother	7.5	7.7
Someone close to you (in the family or outside) developed a serious illness	7.5	7.9
Medical complications arose during the delivery	7.3	7.1
Your husband's/partner's business failed	7.3	7.1
A major financial crisis arose	7.3	7.5
You were pregnant and your husband/partner did not want you to be	7.1	5.7

STRESSFUL EVENT	STRESS IN A FIRST PREGNANCY	STRESS IN A SUBSEQUENT PREGNANCY
You had difficulty in arranging for someone to look after your family while in hospital	—	6.6
You miscarried during the past 12 months	6.9	6.3
You were involved in a legal action which could have damaged your reputation	6.8	7.1
Your husband/partner was not present at the delivery	6.6	5.3
You had to have an anesthetic during the delivery and were not awake when your baby arrived	6.6	5.4
The labor/delivery was very painful	6.5	6.3
You were separated from your family or a close friend	6.0	6.7
You had an X-ray during the pregnancy	6.0	5.4
Increasingly serious arguments developed with your in-laws	5.6	5.7
You had a serious illness or were badly injured and had to be off work and/or in hospital for at least a month	5.5	7.1
You had blood pressure trouble	5.5	5.6
Your obstetrician was unable to be present at the delivery of your baby	5.5	3.5
You had a cesarean operation	5.4	5.2
There were problems in the sexual relationship during the pregnancy	5.1	4.9
You had recurrent urinary tract infections	5.1	5.1
You found out you were pregnant and did not want to be	—	4.3
A new person came to live in your household (not baby)	5.0	4.3
You had to have stitches and were uncomfortable for a long time after the delivery	4.7	4.0
Your baby had a birthmark or something similar spoiling his/her appearance	4.7	4.3
You developed varicose veins	4.6	4.6
You were severely constipated	4.5	3.7
You had severe vomiting/morning sickness	4.4	3.4
Your baby was very small at birth	4.0	4.0

(continued)

STRESSFUL EVENT	STRESS IN A FIRST PREGNANCY	STRESS IN A SUBSEQUENT PREGNANCY
The labor/delivery had to be induced	4.0	3.5
Your doctor told you you were going to have twins	3.8	4.5
You had an amniocentesis investigation during the pregnancy	3.4	4.1
Your baby arrived after the expected date	3.2	3.4
You moved to a new house	2.9	2.7
You stopped work	1.9	1.5
Your baby arrived before the expected date	1.9	2.3
You had an ultrasound investigation during the pregnancy	1.6	2.2
Your baby was not the sex you hoped for	1.0	2.1

Used by permission. Barnett, B., et al., *Journal of Psychosomatic Research*, 27:4, p. 316.

Effects of Support

A number of other studies that were landmarks in stress research dealt with the effect *support* had on people under stress. Support is a relatively new term in the health-care field, and can broadly be defined as anything that makes a person feel good, function more effectively, or be more optimistic. Support leads people to feel loved, nourished, and satisfied; it raises their self-esteem and makes them feel part of something larger than themselves. Support can come from close relationships with family and friends, from jobs or hobbies that give people positive feedback, and from systems of belief that give meaning to their life.

The studies on stress and support showed that people did not tend to become ill in the face of many life changes or major life events if they had strong support systems. Support tends to counteract stress and protect people from the health-related effects of stress. In other words, support is the functional opposite of stress.

One theoretical model of stress, designed by Irwin Sarason, is of particular relevance to pregnant women. It holds that stressful situations result in or involve a "call to action." This call to action causes people to "appraise the situation" at hand in terms of their ability to handle it successfully. Such an appraisal is based on past life events but is evaluated in the context of present social support. Depending on how people evaluate themselves, they will react with self-preoccupying thoughts or task-oriented thoughts: they will become anxious and worry, or they will try to make constructive plans.

Support, Stress, and Pregnancy Complications

Most stress researchers consider pregnancy to be a stressful experience. As nursing professor Jane Norbeck states, "Pregnancy is an event with demands, constraints, opportunities, and an uncertain outcome . . . [But] it is not uniformly stressful among women or for the same woman at different times in her life. Instead, the context of other life events and the availability of social support were regarded as the variables of central importance to the appraisal" of the expectant woman.[1]

Stress researchers have noted that pregnancy is generally a time of emotional disequilibrium, which includes mood fluctuations, anxiety, and ambivalence. This characteristic disequilibrium is likely to be of greatest consequence among women who are under stress apart from their pregnancy. One study found that only 25 percent of expectant mothers who were not rated as under *prior* stress found their emotional disequilibrium to be severe, as opposed to 81 percent of those mothers who were considered to be under stress prior to becoming pregnant.

Over the last twenty years there have been many studies examining the relationship between stress on the pregnant woman and the physical complications of pregnancy, labor, and delivery. These studies are useful to the pregnant woman because they point up the extent to which dealing with stress can reduce the likelihood of problems for her or her baby.

The earliest such studies simply dealt with whether the mother felt stressed or anxious during her pregnancy and studied the responses in relation to one complication or another. Separate studies had similar findings: women who had high levels of anxiety did indeed have more complications, including nausea and vomiting, spontaneous abortions, longer labor times, labors that did not progress, postpartum complications, low-birth-weight and premature babies, and newborns in fetal distress or below-average condition. Another study specifically found that stress was as important a factor in complications as were known medical indicators of potential pregnancy problems such as maternal illness.

Whereas the initial studies simply dealt with feelings of anxiety or stress and one particular pregnancy complication, later studies took a number of complications into account simultaneously. Toxemia, premature labor, prolonged labor, cesarean section, low-birth-weight babies, and babies who required special medical attention after birth were all grouped together in a category called complications of preg-

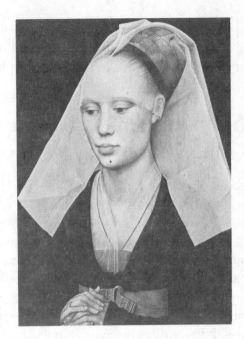

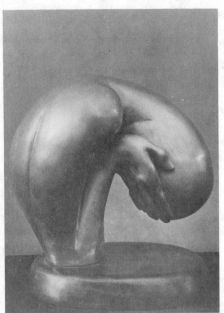

nancy. Mothers who had high levels of anxiety were found to have much higher incidences of these complications than mothers who had low anxiety.

Once there was sufficient evidence that stress was a significant factor in pregnancy complications, researchers undertook more sophisticated studies designed to determine what the stress consisted of. It was found that family conflicts, numerous life-change events, and high anxiety correlated with pregnancy complications, as did job, economic, and interpersonal problems. One study showed a significant relationship between high anxiety and pregnancy complications in the first trimester. Complications in the second and third trimesters correlated with a high level of life changes.

In 1972 Katherine Nuckolls of Yale Nursing School did a landmark study of several hundred pregnant women in terms of stress and social support. Nuckolls found that women who had a number of life changes during their pregnancy and the preceding two years, but who also had strong support systems, had one-third as many complications as a matched group of women who had a number of changes but didn't have strong support. Nuckolls concluded that stress by itself is not the cause of problems; rather, a combination of social factors act together to increase a woman's "susceptibility" to problems. It is this susceptibility, combined with genetic and environmental factors that leads to complications in pregnancy.

Norbeck later refined Nuckolls' study in an effort to clarify the role support plays in preventing the complications of pregnancy. Norbeck's goal was to determine the importance of support, as opposed to the mothers' own ego strengths and attitudes toward the pregnancy. In

Do you have enough support?

Do you confide in someone each day, once a week, less than once a week, never?

Do you feel secure in your environment each day, once a week, less than once a week, never?

Do you feel that you have some control over your environment each day, once a week, less than once a week, never?

Do you feel that people approve of you each day, once a week, less than once a week, never?

Do you have an intimate relationship with someone each day, once a week, less than once a week, never?

Does your support come from family, friends, community?

Do you feel you have enough money? Usually? Sometimes? Never?

Do you have a strong set of personal beliefs? A strong religious affiliation?

addition to using a broad support questionnaire, Norbeck specifically asked her subjects how much *tangible support* they could count on in the event that they needed a ride to the clinic, needed to borrow money, or needed help because they were sick in bed. The study showed that complications correlated with maternal depression and lack of self-esteem as well as with stress and high amounts of life change.

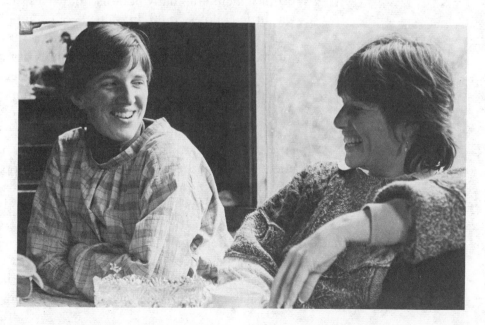

Support *is the functional opposite of* stress. *A mother with support feels loved, nourished, and satisfied. Photo by Michael Samuels.*

Norbeck found that social support played a buffering role, with tangible support being the most important factor in terms of preventing complications. Norbeck's study showed that high stress and low support increased the chances of a pregnant woman having severe emotional disequilibrium. High stress tended to be associated with complications during pregnancy, whereas high emotional disequilibrium tended to be associated with problems with the newborn. Norbeck believes that the stress model is more complicated than researchers have thought up to now. She feels that stress not only involves many factors, but that these factors do not operate independently. Rather, they interact and affect other self-care behaviors such as nutrition, smoking, and exercise.

A study by Thomas Picone tends to verify the concept that a pregnant woman's diet, for example, is affected by stress. He found that mothers under stress did not gain as much weight and had a higher incidence of low-birth-weight babies than did mothers who took in the same amount of calories but were not under stress. He speculates that stress causes hormonal and metabolic changes that lower the body's ability to use the calories it is getting (see p. 140).

Gabriel Smilkstein has developed a test for *family function* that measures how well a pregnant woman's family works together. His findings showed that family function was a better predictor of pregnancy complications than life events or previous obstetrical history. He also found that poor family function correlated strongly with mothers' complications after delivery.

Not only do these studies help to clarify what is important for the developing infant, they give an indication of what parents can do to improve their pregnancies and lower the possibility of complications for both mother and baby. Until such studies were undertaken, most people, including many doctors, midwives, and nurses, thought there was little couples could do, outside of good prenatal care and nutrition, to affect the outcome of pregnancy. Yet the complexity and interrelatedness of factors causing complications point to the fact that there are numerous small ways in which expectant mothers and fathers can improve the course of a mother's pregnancy. Anything parents can do to lower stress, cope with it more effectively, improve their family functioning, or strengthen support lines will act as preventive medicine. In this regard the father's behavior can have almost as great an effect as the mother's obviously does. His support and understanding, as well as his knowledge of what is important in the expectant mother's life-style, can have a beneficial effect on the outcome of the woman's pregnancy.

It's important that expectant parents realize that stress, like other circumstances that influence pregnancy, is only a *risk factor*. That is, stress is a contributing agent rather than the sole cause of pregnancy problems. Further, not every pregnant woman experiencing

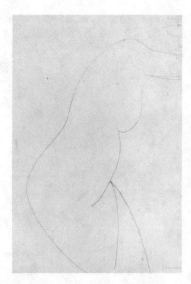

Relaxation techniques are at the heart of all the methods of prepared childbirth. Nude, *Constantin Brancusi, 1920. Solomon R. Guggenheim Museum, New York.*

significant stress will develop complications; rather, these women's *chances* for complications are statistically somewhat higher. Women with highly stressful lives and low support systems should not be disheartened by what they have read. The stress material should be viewed as information that can help them reduce the *possibility* of complications.

RELAXATION AND SUPPORT

The two broad methods for counteracting stress are *relaxation* and *support*. Relaxation techniques are widely taught during pregnancy and are at the heart of all methods of prepared childbirth. The goal of these techniques has always been to relieve pain and anxiety during labor and birth, but they also work to relieve stress. Indeed, they relieve stress during pregnancy and after delivery just as effectively as they do during childbirth.

Several aspects of current obstetrical care help to enhance the mother's sense of support during pregnancy and delivery as well as afterward. By meeting regularly with a childbirth educator, obstetrician, and/or midwife, the expectant mother forms a special relationship with that person and sets up a medical support system. Joining other expectant mothers and fathers in prenatal classes helps to create a support group of lay people who are sharing similar experiences. And the information on pregnancy and childbirth that is learned in these classes helps expectant parents bring to labor and delivery a sense of confidence and understanding. All these factors create a unique situation in medicine. Although there is detailed information on the way stress, relaxation, and support affect a wide variety of medical situations, obstetrics is the only medical specialty that has so broad-based and well-worked-out a system for teaching relaxation techniques and providing support.

The relaxation and support that expectant parents acquire during the prenatal period have broader application and greater significance than most people realize. As their primary goals, most childbirth classes work toward making the mother as comfortable as possible and enabling her to minimize the use of drugs for pain control during labor, delivery, and the first postpartum days. We believe that the skills the classes develop can also be used as powerful tools in both the treatment and prevention of illness. Such learning can positively affect the health of mother and baby throughout their lives.

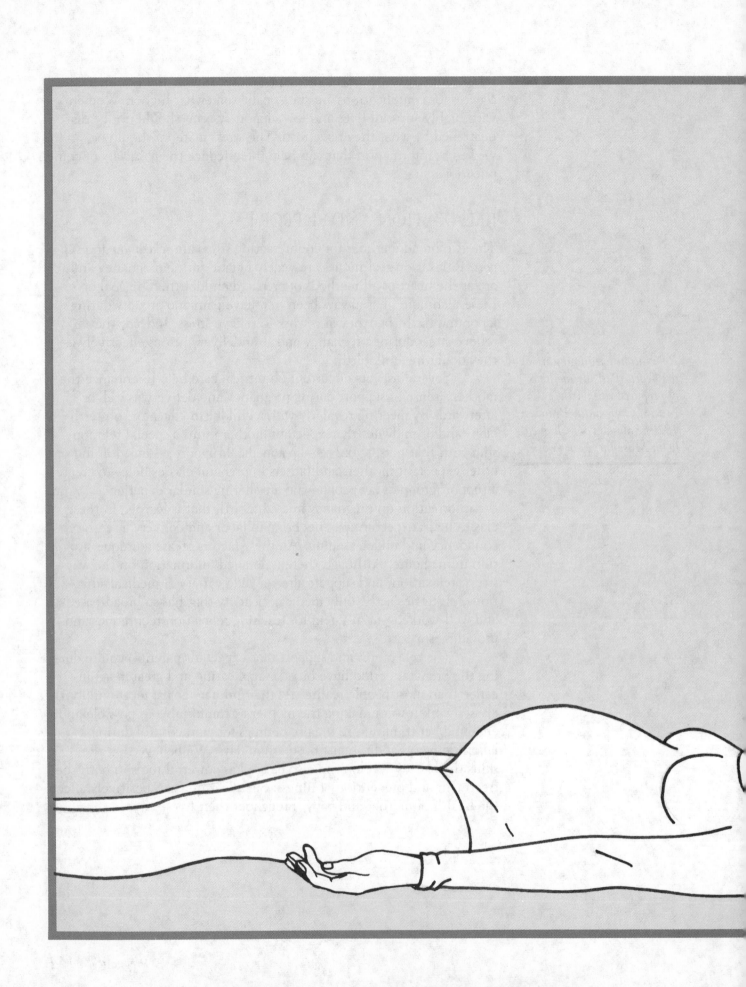

Relaxation and Prepared Childbirth Techniques

The Rationale for Prepared Childbirth

During the last fifty years a wide variety of childbirth preparation techniques have become an increasingly important part of the practice of both obstetrics and midwifery. The reasons for this trend are twofold. First, many expectant mothers have sought doctors and midwives who practice prepared childbirth because they want to participate actively in delivery and make it as positive and fulfilling an experience as possible.

The second reason for the growth in popularity of prepared childbirth has had to do with birth attendants themselves. Initially doctors and midwives wanted to take the fear out of childbirth, make it a joyful experience, and make the mother as comfortable as possible throughout her labor and delivery. But by the 1950s doctors had also begun to realize that obstetrical anesthesia, especially general anesthesia, not only altered the mother's delivery experience, it had potentially serious consequences for her and the newborn as well. As a result, the use of general anesthesia has been largely eliminated, and other types of anesthesia are used with more caution in childbirth.

During the time when mothers were given large amounts of sedatives in labor, many babies were born *anoxic*, that is, limp and bluish because of lack of oxygen. Often such babies did not begin to breathe on their own and needed to be resuscitated. Recognizing that

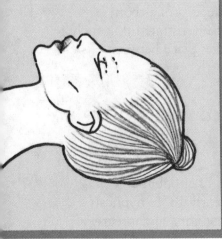

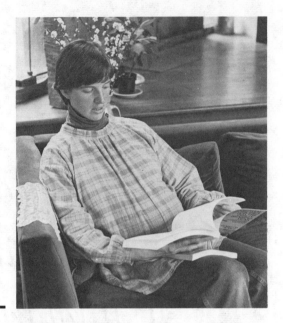

The expectant mother has a wide variety of prepared childbirth techniques to choose from. Photo by Michael Samuels.

these newborns' condition at birth was compromised by drugs and that the babies felt the effects of the drugs for the first four to seven days, doctors began to be concerned that anoxia might be a significant factor in brain damage and other long-term neurological problems as well.

Since the 1960s there has been a great deal of research into how even the smallest amount of drugs and anesthesia affect the baby. Several newborn behavior evaluation scales have been developed, the most famous of which is the Brazelton scale. These scales demonstrate the subtle but definite effects of many drugs that had been thought to be safe. For instance, Brazelton found that babies whose mothers were given high doses of barbiturates such as secobarbital or pentobarbital (150 mg. or more) had a delayed weight gain and an impaired ability to nurse. These babies showed significantly lower muscle tone and muscle strength scores on the Brazelton test. Effects such as this are significant enough that the Committee on Drugs of the American Academy of Pediatrics has recommended that doctors use only those drugs that have been shown to have the least effects on newborn behavior. Since the late 1970s it has also been demonstrated that such drugs interfere with the bonding process that takes place between mother and baby in the first hour or two after birth.

Historical Roots of Prepared Childbirth

HYPNOSIS

One of the earliest attempts to affect the quality of childbirth by psychological means was through hypnosis. In the early 1800s hypnosis was first used to produce anesthesia in surgical patients, and as early as

1837 it was used in France for women giving birth. Proponents believed that *suggestion* or *suggestive therapy,* as it was then called, worked by getting a woman to concentrate on an idea other than pain. In addition to talking to the mother, the obstetrician often massaged her and encouraged her to breathe in a certain way. Studies of suggestion showed good results with 70 percent of mothers.

Suggestive therapy was very popular in France and Germany around the 1880s and on into the early 1900s, but by the 1920s the focus of large-scale application of hypnosis as an obstetrical tool had switched to Russia. Based on Pavlov's *psychological conditioning,* the Russians developed their own theory of how hypnosis worked. They believed that hypnosis altered *conditioned* or *learned reflexes,* so that a negative reflex that was perceived as painful could be supplanted by a positive reflex that was perceived as a "sensation" (see p. 157). By the 1960s the Russians had used hypnosis in hundreds of thousands of births.

NATURAL CHILDBIRTH

Meanwhile a new system of prepared childbirth called *Childbirth Without Fear* or *Natural Childbirth* was developed by an English obstetrician named Grantley Dick-Read. Read's method stemmed from an incident in which he delivered a woman who felt no pain during the birth of her baby. Based on this experience, he developed a theory that pain was not a necessary or inevitable part of labor, rather, that it was caused by images of fear that women had been taught by their culture. He believed that such images created muscle tension in the uterus, cervix, and abdomen, which caused real pain. Out of this theory came Read's famous triad: "Fear, tension, pain."

The method of prepared childbirth that Dick-Read developed involved three aspects. First, it explained the anatomy and physiology of childbirth to mothers. Second, it taught them physical relaxation. Third, it stressed the therapeutic relationship between the pregnant woman and her doctor.

Anatomy and physiology were taught in a series of eight classes, using models and drawings as visual aids. The early classes were designed to dispel the notion that childbirth must be painful. The rest of the classes described normal labor and delivery. Throughout the description the word *pain* was never used, because it was felt that the contractions of labor were not comparable to other kinds of pain. It was also felt that the use of the word *pain* would contribute to producing fear and tension.

Following each lecture, the mothers were taught relaxation, physical conditioning, and breathing exercises. Dick-Read based his relaxation exercises on the technique of *progressive relaxation* taught by the muscle physiologist Edmund Jacobson. That technique involved contracting different muscle groups individually, becoming aware of the feeling of tension that was produced, and then letting go. Dick-Read advised expectant mothers to practice tensing and relaxing muscles throughout the last two trimesters, and to use relaxation between contractions when they were in labor.

Dick-Read's work was joined and endorsed by an English physiotherapist named Helen Heardman, who believed that "women should train themselves for the *physical exertion* of labor in much the same fashion that an athlete should train . . . for an athletic event."[1] In addition to sound sleep and a balanced diet, she encouraged women to engage in such athletic pursuits as cross-country walking, climbing, swimming, skiing, skating, riding, and handling boats, as well as team games, athletics, and gymnastics.

Heardman made a famous analogy between the experience of labor and mountain climbing. In this regard she wrote that after climbing awhile,

> the legs, due to an accumulation of fatigue products, ache almost beyond bearing; but a brief rest, sitting on a stone or lying down, rapidly removes the waste products of combustion and with them this feeling. The sight of the mountain crest spurs the individual and he toils on. The muscular sensation can certainly be called discomfort, but no mountaineer would seek an analgesic during his ascent, however toilsome, or an anesthetic while he attained the triumph of the summit. This explains why so many women, while admitting to discomfort [in labor], refuse relief. Loss of self-control and missing the "summit" would spell failure to them (and control becomes increasingly difficult with increased administration of drugs). Encouragement, companionship, reassurance, and praise help far more to build up to the climax, and encourage pride of achievement. The women are experiencing the need for the very qualities of patience, self-control, and concentrated hard-work which they possess and can use, and the goal is in front of them, just within reach, after nine months of waiting.[2]

Recent research indicates that Heardman's analogy to strenuous exercise is remarkably apt. During labor, just as during heavy exercise, chemicals called *endorphins* are released in the brain. These chemicals are a natural narcotic that relieves pain and elevates mood.

The final component of Dick-Read's program involved the relationship between the expectant mother and the doctor. Read pointed out that this relationship can be "the greatest and most harmless anesthetizing agent." The woman's faith in the doctor and the reassurance provided by the doctor's presence serve to prevent the mother from becoming afraid and creating tension in her body. Read felt that the doctor's presence was most important during *transition*, the active stage of labor just before dilation of the cervix is complete. This is the time when the mother is most likely to feel discomfort, without yet having her goal in sight. By 1950, due to Dick-Read's and Heardman's charismatic personalities and their wide success, Natural Childbirth had become the dominant method in England. In subsequent years variations of the method spread throughout the United States.

PSYCHOPROPHYLAXIS

By the late 1940s a new method that stemmed from the old technique of hypnosis was gaining popularity in Russia. Three doctors, Platonov, Velvovsky, and Nicolaiev, developed a system they called *psychoprophylaxis.* It held that childbirth could be completely painless, since pain was a conditioned or learned reflex. This idea was based on studies that showed that if an animal was given a *positive reinforcement,* such as food, along with a painful stimulus, such as a shock, the animal would eventually salivate rather than pull away, having learned to associate the shock with the positive reinforcement rather than the pain. Thus Russian researchers believed that women could be reeducated not to focus on discomfort during labor and delivery. The idea wasn't to *relieve* pain but to *prevent* the possibility of pain. As the method evolved, the focus shifted from totally painless childbirth to concentrating on making the mother as comfortable as possible.

Psychoprophylaxis was taught in six sessions. In the introductory session mothers were interviewed to see if they had fears or negative attitudes toward pregnancy and childbirth, and these were "corrected." In subsequent classes the women were taught anatomy and physiology to show them why childbirth would be painless. In the final classes the mothers were taught specific types of breathing, massage movements, pushing techniques, comfort positions, and relaxation to be used in labor and delivery. The method became

What is important is not which method of prepared childbirth a woman chooses but whether she looks forward to the birth of her baby joyfully. Reclining Nude, Pierre Auguste Renoir, 1902. Oil on canvas, 26½" x 60⅝". Collection, The Museum of Modern Art, New York. Gift of Mr. and Mrs. Paul Rosenberg.

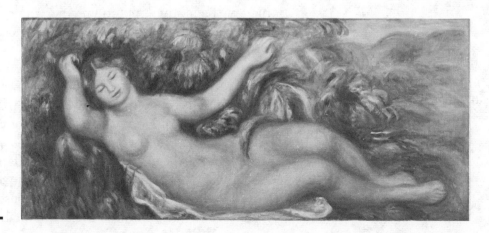

spectacularly successful in Russia. By 1953 it had been used by over 300,000 women.

LAMAZE

The French obstetrician Ferdinand Lamaze learned of *psychoprophylaxis* during a trip to Russia and returned home determined to popularize the method in France. Like the Russians, Lamaze called the method Painless Childbirth, but he changed it to fit the French rather than the Russian viewpoint, adopting more Dick-Read-like relaxation exercises and adding a new *pant-blow* breathing technique to control pushing in the final stages of labor. In addition, Lamaze taught a much more detailed anatomy and physiology course. Six to nine classes were held, each one being followed by a period of breathing, relaxation, and delivery exercises.

The first session dealt with conception and the early physiology of pregnancy; the second with fetal development and the latter part of pregnancy. The third session went to the heart of the Lamaze method, showing how conditioned reflexes could enable a woman to replace pain and fear with joyful expectation, redefining contractions as *sensations* rather than birth pains. In the fourth session expectant mothers were taught breathing exercises; in the fifth, relaxation. The last two sessions focused on the various positions and breathing techniques a woman could use during different stages of labor. Within a few years Lamaze's method had spread to a number of countries around the world, including the United States.

In the last thirty years there has been a proliferation of prepared childbirth methods, most of which have incorporated the best elements of Dick-Read or Lamaze and added components of their own design. For instance, Bradley emphasizes the father's role as labor coach, and Kitzinger stresses imagery in her *Psycho-Sexual Method.* But all the methods offer some degree of education, relaxation and breathing exercises, and support, which seem to be at the heart of their success. Each of these aspects can have powerful effects on the functioning of the mother's autonomic nervous system, endocrine glands, blood flow, and perception of pain.

The well-known childbirth educator and author Elizabeth Noble observes that as birth education has come of age, there has been a good deal of reevaluation. The trend is away from rigid rules and toward emphasis on the mother's own internal cues. For example, Noble and others question the technique of rapid, high-chest breathing to prevent the mother from pushing too soon or too hard. This breathing method can result in hyperventilation and make the mother feel lightheaded or faint. There is also a movement away from having mothers hold their breath when they are pushing in the second stage of labor (see p. 328), because the abdominal pressure that is built up decreases the amount of oxygen reaching the baby. Noble concludes by saying:

> Childbirth education should be kept simple, with emphasis on natural events and normal physiology, not on contrived techniques. If a couple and their attendants can learn to view childbirth as an involuntary process, one that need only be allowed to happen rather than be controlled, the laboring woman will be better able to direct her energy within, instead of dissipating it by attempting to put her mind outside her body. Women need to gain trust in their bodies which is difficult with the extreme medicalization of health care, especially birth, that has occurred in our society.[3]

More important than which of the methods a woman chooses or has available to her is whether or not it enables her to look forward eagerly to the birth of her baby. An attitude of joyful anticipation can incorporate the Dick-Read idea of replacing culturally acquired fears with positive images, the Lamaze idea of altering the pain threshold by creating new circuits in the brain through understanding of anatomy and physiology, and the Bradley idea of having a trusted person to offer support and coaching. From our point of view, an expectant mother should concentrate on allaying any fears she might have, developing the ability to relax her body deeply, and learning enough to understand what is happening in labor and have a clear image of the outcome. Finally, an expectant mother should focus on setting up her pregnancy and delivery in a positive environment with supportive people. The exact manner in which any mother will work this out will vary from taking a specific course to reading widely on her own, to finding a doctor or midwife she totally trusts and following her or his instructions.

Relaxation Techniques

Although relaxation seems like a deceptively simple process, it has profound psychological and physiological effects on the body. Psychologically, relaxation reduces fear and anxiety and replaces them with a sense of calmness and well-being. Relaxation also lessens a person's response to stressful stimuli. Physiologically, relaxation causes slower breathing, slower heartbeat, lower blood pressure, and altered adrenal hormone levels.

Specifically in regard to pregnancy, relaxation maximizes blood flow to the uterus, placenta, and fetus. During labor and delivery, relaxation continues to optimize blood flow to these organs, but in addition, it makes uterine contractions more effective. Tensed muscles and high levels of stress hormones both tend to produce irregular, ineffective, and painful contractions. When a mother is relaxed, her contractions tend to take place in a vigorous, steady manner that she is likely to perceive as strong sensations similar to hard work, rather than as pain.

Relaxation is characterized by turning inward—by concentrating on one's own body and mind rather than on external events. Inherent in the relaxed state is a certain feeling of detachment; that is, a lack of concern for how one is doing. Dr. Wolfgang Luthe, one of the originators of *Autogenic Training*, a German system that includes a very popular method of prepared childbirth, has described the relaxed state as "a casual, relaxed attitude involving minimal or no goal-directed voluntaristic efforts in the sense of energetic striving, and

Relaxation, like meditation, is characterized by turning inward and viewing events with a feeling of detachment.

Jizo-Bosatso, Hanabusa Itachō, 17th century Japanese. The Metropolitan Museum of Art. Rogers Fund. Purchase, 1936.

Kuan Yin, Chinese, 17th century. *The Metropolitan Museum of Art. Fletcher Fund.*

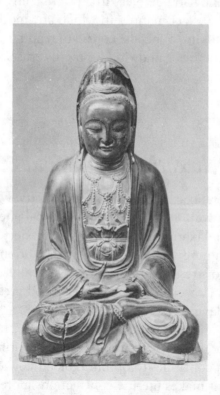
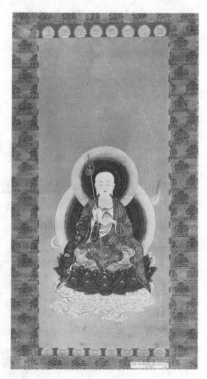

Everyone has certain areas or muscles that get tense when they are nervous or under pressure. Here are the most common areas to check for tension:

Eyes

Jaw

Neck and shoulders

Lower back and pelvis

apprehensive tension-producing control of functions leading to the desired result."[4] Thus people do not so much "do" relaxation as permit it to happen. They merely let go and allow relaxation to take place.

Interestingly, people are often confused as to how to identify feelings of relaxation. One of the best ways to differentiate between feelings of muscle tension and relaxation was taught by physiologist Edmund Jacobson in his method called *Progressive Relaxation.* This is the technique on which Dick-Read and most other prepared childbirth programs based the relaxation component of their courses. Jacobson instructed people to contract a single muscle or group of muscles by making a specific movement and holding it for a given period of time. When they let go after several moments, they would experience the feeling of relaxation in that muscle group. The contrast between the two feelings heightened people's awareness of the sensation of relaxation. By methodically going through each of the muscle groups, people learned to distinguish between relaxation and even small amounts of tension in various parts of their bodies.

Often people hold their muscles in a slightly contracted state without noticing it. The more nervous and tense people tend to be, the more likely they are to be unaware of constant, low-level tension because they have come to accept it as normal. Most people find they are least aware of slight tension in the muscles around the eyes, jaw, neck, and shoulders, or around the pelvis and lower back. Few childbirth educators teach Jacobson's method in its entirety anymore, because it is very time-consuming, but parents who are interested can easily teach themselves from Jacobson's book *How to Relax and Have Your Baby,* which is still available.

Our own health-care philosophy was profoundly influenced by the experience of learning Jacobson's relaxation techniques in preparation for the birth of our first child. Michael had had previous training in hypnosis, meditation, and visualization, and he had already started using an autosuggestion method of stress reduction. But he had never achieved levels of relaxation as deep as those he learned from the childbirth classes that he attended with Nancy. And it was there that he realized for the first time the importance of relaxation in preventive

When to briefly relax

During stressful times in the household (before dinner, before bed).
After stressful times (after the kids go to school, after a family fight).
During planned rest times (coffee break, lunch hour).
More often during high-stress periods.
More often when you feel as if you might be getting sick.

medicine. For Nancy, the relaxation classes and her two wonderful deliveries convinced her of the powerful control she had over her own body, not only during birth but whenever she felt under stress.

Recent research shows that the maximum effects of relaxation can be achieved with only four to eight hours of instruction and twenty minutes of practice a day. There are almost as many methods for learning to relax as there are instructors, and no one method has proved superior to the others. In fact, all the methods have great similarities. The common aspects that seem the most important are (1) a set of clear instructions that one trusts, (2) a comfortable position in which one's muscles can relax, (3) a passive attitude of allowing relaxation to take place, (4) a quiet place in which one won't be disturbed, and (5) a deep, regular rate of breathing.

Autosuggestion, which can be taught in a short time, is one of the most popular methods for teaching relaxation today. In auto-suggestion, the teacher initially recites the directions to the class slowly. Then, after a mother has become familiar with the exercise, she can give herself the instructions mentally. In using any of our relaxation exercises, a woman can have someone slowly read the directions out loud, tape record the exercise herself and play it back,

By raising her hand slightly at the wrist, a woman can feel when the muscles in her forearm contract gently; by dropping her hand, she can become aware of the feeling of relaxation in those same muscles.

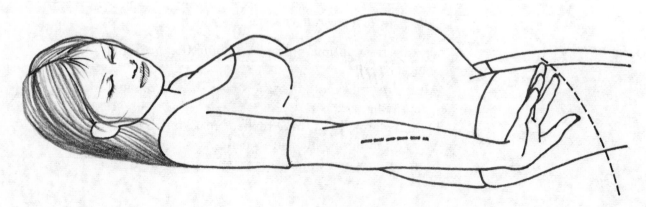

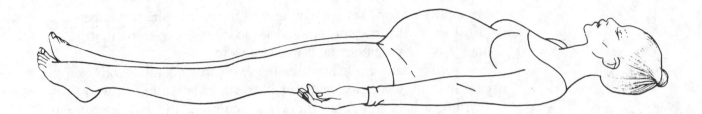

Learning to relax muscles consciously is an important preparation for labor and delivery. The more profoundly a woman can learn to relax her body at will, the more comfortable she can make herself during contractions.

An exercise for relaxation

Find a tranquil place where you won't be disturbed. Sit with your legs uncrossed and your arms at your sides. Close your eyes; inhale slowly and deeply. Pause a moment. Then exhale slowly and completely. Allow your abdomen to rise and fall as you breathe. Do this several times. You now feel calm, comfortable, and more relaxed. As you relax, your breathing will become slow and even. Mentally repeat to yourself, "My feet are relaxing. They are becoming more and more relaxed. My feet feel heavy." Rest for a moment. Repeat the same suggestions for your ankles. Rest again. In the same way, relax your lower legs, then your thighs, pausing to feel the sensations of relaxation in your muscles. Relax your pelvis. Rest. Relax your abdomen. Rest. Relax the muscles of your back. Rest. Relax your chest. Rest. Relax your fingers. Relax your hands. Rest. Relax your forearms, your upper arms, your shoulders. Rest. Relax your neck. Rest. Relax your jaw, allowing it to drop. Relax your tongue. Relax your cheeks. Relax your eyes. Rest. Relax your forehead and the top of your head. Now just rest and allow your whole body to relax.

You are in a calm, relaxed state of being. You can *deepen* this state by counting backward. Breathe in; as you exhale slowly, say to yourself, "Ten. I am feeling very relaxed. . . ." Inhale again, and as you exhale, repeat mentally, "Nine. I am feeling more relaxed. . . ." Breathe. "Eight. I am feeling even more relaxed. . . ." Seven. "Deeper and more relaxed. . . ." Six. "Even more. . . ." Five (pause). Four (pause). Three (pause). Two (pause). One (pause). Zero (pause).

You are now at a deeper and more relaxed level of awareness, a level at which your body feels healthy, your mind feels peaceful and open. (It is a level at which you can experience images in your mind more clearly and vividly than ever before.) You can stay in this relaxed state as long as you like. To return to your ordinary consciousness, mentally say, "I am now going to move. When I count to three, I will raise my left hand and stretch my fingers. I will then feel relaxed, happy, and strong, ready to continue my everyday activities."

or simply read the exercise over several times until she remembers the instructions. It is the concept and sequence of the exercise that is important, not memorizing it word for word.

Expectant mothers and fathers who are unfamiliar with exercises like autosuggestion may feel a little awkward at first or wonder if anything is happening, but they should continue the exercise without worrying. Doctors have found that there is a measurable drop in muscle tension the first time people consciously try to relax. As they practice more and more, people become aware of changes in sensation that they describe as feelings of heaviness, lightness, numbness, tingling, floating, or even absence of feeling. Others describe warmth, coolness, or a radiating or pulsing sensation. The more people practice conscious relaxation, the better they will become at it and the deeper the levels they will achieve. Like learning to ski or ride a bike, relaxation becomes a habit ingrained in neuromuscular pathways.

The sooner a pregnant woman begins to set aside time for relaxation, the better. First, relaxation will help her relieve fatigue, worry, and discomfort while she is pregnant. This is important for the baby as well as herself. Second, the more time an expectant mother spends relaxing, the better prepared she will be for labor. Because labor tends to be a long process, we feel it is important for a woman to be able to remain in a relaxed state for 45 to 60 minutes without falling asleep. And while frequent practice sessions are very good, we feel it is more useful to practice two or three times a week for an hour than to practice every day for only 15 minutes. Long sessions, in which deep, sustained levels of relaxation can be achieved, are particularly valuable during the last six to eight weeks of pregnancy.

When to use relaxation during pregnancy

Use the exercise just described to relax your whole body, including the uterine muscles and the baby.
Relax your body and mind in order to relieve worries.
Relax your body and mind when you are upset, angry, or unhappy.
Relax your body when you are fatigued.
Relax your body and mind before going to sleep.
Relax your body and mind at particular stress points during the day.
Relax your body when you feel sick or physically uncomfortable.
Relax a part of your body to anesthetize it if it hurts.
Relax your body completely at the first sign of any illness, to help prevent or heal disease.

Visualization Techniques

Visualization, or picturing images in the mind, is now an important technique used in medicine as well as some methods of prepared childbirth. Actually, people visualize all the time without realizing it: they see events from the past in their mind's eye, envision plans and goals for the future, and picture solutions to problems they are working on. Despite the fact that most people visualize constantly, they do not make conscious use of this skill.

Although visualization is an age-old tool of medicine and religion, it is only recently that visualization exercises have been applied to childbirth. Interestingly, prepared-childbirth pioneer Grantley Dick-Read wrote at length on the importance of mental imagery in childbirth. He believed that it was the mental images instilled in a woman by her culture that were responsible for the fear and tension at the root of the pain sometimes felt in childbirth. Dick-Read believed that by changing a woman's mental imagery, one could decrease her fear and pain. He wrote, "Is it unreasonable that we should pause to consider the mental image of labor within the mind of the woman? Is it not essential that we should create by education and instruction the true and natural happiness of motherhood within the vision of her mind? The mental picture of her anticipated experience should be the image of all that is beautiful in the fulfillment of her love."[5]

Researchers have found that visualization works best when people are relaxed. Relaxation not only helps people clear their minds, it lowers the level of anxiety they feel about fearful and negative images. The same nerve and muscle pathways that are involved in a "real" action are also involved when people picture that activity in their mind. The more vividly people can picture a scene in their imagination, the more the body reacts as if the experience is actually taking place. Researchers have recorded changes in almost every physiological system in response to visualization. When a woman pictures running to catch a bus, her heartbeat and respiration actually rise, and small electrical impulses are detectable in her running muscles. Similarly, when a woman pictures herself in a relaxing activity, such as lying on a beach, her breathing, heart rate, and muscle tension decrease.

We separate visualization techniques into two basic categories: receptive and programmed. *Receptive visualization* involves clearing the mind and letting images arise spontaneously. It is one of the fundamental tools of psychiatry, providing access to inner feelings and ideas. Through receptive visualization the expectant mother and father can get in touch with both the positive and the negative feelings they have about pregnancy, childbirth, and parenting. This will help them to deal with their fears and anxieties, as well as make them more aware of their positive feelings. *(text continues on page 168)*

Feelings aroused by the prospect of parenthood

PLEASURABLE	FEARFUL
Parenting instinct; oceanic feelings of wanting a baby, stimulated by daydreams or sight of a positive parent-child experience	Fear of being tied down to responsibility; fear of being an inadequate parent or disliking the task
Pride in conceiving a child—female fertility, male potency	Fear of not being able to conceive
Earthy feeling of fullness, verdancy; harmony with natural rhythms	

FEELINGS ABOUT PREGNANCY ITSELF

Female feeling of being healthy, big, slow-moving, relaxed	Female fear of being fat, ungainly, physically uncomfortable
Male feeling that the expectant mother looks soft, happy, glowing	Male fear of wife looking big and unappealing
	Fear of woman being sick
	Dislike of having to give up activities and habits, change life-style

FEELINGS ABOUT CARING FOR AN INFANT

Joy in touching, picking up, cuddling baby	Fear of picking up the baby: won't do it right; baby will cry
Contentment with rocking baby, watching baby sleep	Worry that baby is fragile, can easily be hurt
Pleasure at breast-feeding baby	Disgust at having to change dirty, smelly diapers
Delight in taking baby to beach, hiking, picnicking with family and friends	Resentment at not being able to do things because of the baby; at baby crying
Happiness at thought of staying home, taking care of baby	Male resentment at woman not working, bringing in extra money

PLEASURABLE	FEARFUL
	Female resentment at being stuck at home
	Fear of not having enough money to raise a child and having to give up own pleasures
	Fear of being left alone with baby, having to support the baby alone
	Feeling jealous of all the attention the baby gets, requires
Enjoyment of image of a healthy, strong baby	Fear of illness in the baby
	Fear of not being a good parent
Increased interest in sex; lack of concern over birth control	Decreased interest in sex; fear of somehow hurting the baby through lovemaking
	Fear of miscarrying
	Female fear that father will suddenly leave during pregnancy

FEELINGS ABOUT CHILDBIRTH

PLEASURABLE	FEARFUL
Excitement and joy at new life, at witnessing a profound, primeval event	Fear of participating in such a personal, physical event
Female pride in doing well	Female fear of pain, of not being able to deliver the baby without anesthetics
Male pride at helping mother, being needed	Male fear of not knowing what to do or not wanting to be there, of not loving the mother during labor
Feeling proud of and loving the baby	
Knowing instinctively how to care for baby	
Feeling that family is made richer by the birth of the baby	

(continued)

Programmed visualization involves choosing and holding particular images rather than letting images arise spontaneously. Like receptive visualization, programmed visualization has specific effects on people's mental and physical states and on their lives. Programmed visualization is useful in helping to achieve goals and make changes. For pregnant women, concentrating on positive images of birth can help to strengthen their confidence, increase their peace of mind, and enhance their joyful anticipation.

Relaxation and visualization techniques are of general use long after the actual hours of labor and delivery. As wonderful and significant an event as birth is, it constitutes a relatively small percentage of the time the parents spend nurturing their baby. This nurturing begins

Visualizing peaceful scenes causes a pregnant mother and her baby to become relaxed.

Girl In A Boat With Geese, *Berthe Morisot, 1889. National Gallery of Art, Washington, D.C. Ailsa Mellon Bruce Collection.*

The Seine At Giverny, *Claude Monet. National Gallery of Art, Washington, D.C. Chester Dale Collection.*

How to use receptive visualization to get in touch with inner feelings

Visualize how you'd like to spend your time at work, at home.

Visualize how you'd like family relationships to be—how you'd like your children and mate to treat you, how you'd like to treat them.

Visualize what would be the most pleasurable family vacation or weekend you can imagine.

Visualize things you could do to improve problem areas in your personal life, your family life.

Visualize which situations make you or your family members sick or healthy.

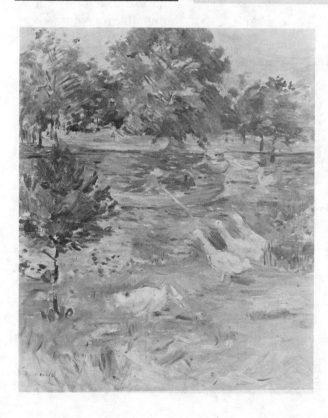

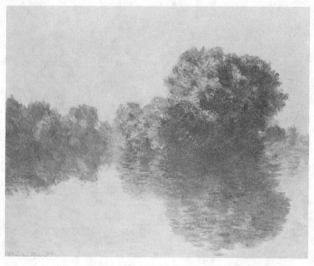

Using programmed visualization before the baby is born

VISUALIZE	IN ORDER	FOR EXAMPLE, IMAGINE
Yourself in enjoyable scenes with a small baby	To maximize your positive expectations about becoming a parent	A family picnic in a meadow, taking a walk with the baby, or showing the baby to relatives and friends
Yourself having fun taking care of a small baby	To strengthen your confidence about being a parent	Playing with the baby during its bath, feeding the baby, tickling the baby as you change its diaper
Yourself being pregnant and feeling radiant and healthy	To increase feelings of well-being and create good health during pregnancy	Walking exuberantly down the street in maternity clothes, feeling good when you wake up in the morning, happily eating all kinds of good foods
Yourself doing well during labor and delivery	To build up your confidence and relieve inevitable anxiety about the birth process	Being relaxed and focused during labor, joyful during the hard work of delivery, calm and rested after delivery
A strong, healthy baby	To feel glad about the baby and relieve inevitable momentary concerns about the baby's health	A radiant, beautiful baby
Positive energy flowing into you and your unborn baby	To make yourself and the baby strong	Yourself and the baby bathed in warm sunlight

at conception and continues until the child is fully grown. Viewed from this perspective, pregnancy is simply the beginning, and birth an early landmark along the parenting continuum. Thus deliberate use of relaxation and strengthening one's own support networks during pregnancy become an early part of parenting. And they contribute as much to the baby's health as they do to the mother's.

Using receptive visualization before the baby is born

SUBJECTS TO THINK ABOUT	SPECIFIC QUESTIONS AND CONCERNS	TYPICAL POSITIVE OR NEGATIVE IMAGES
Nutrition	What foods does my body crave?	Milk, leafy green salads, lean meats, and seafood
	What foods don't interest me now?	Alcohol, pasta, hot chili
Exercise	What kind of exercise appeals to me now?	Walking, swimming
	Am I getting enough exercise?	I feel energetic, draggy
Sleep	Am I getting enough sleep?	I feel tired in the morning
	Do I need naps?	I feel sleepy in the afternoon
Sex of the baby	What sex will the baby be?	Image of a girl; image of a boy
Kind of delivery	What kind of delivery would be ideal for me?	A natural delivery with no drugs; a delivery that uses some kind of anesthesia so I don't feel the contractions
Method of feeding the baby	What method of feeding the baby makes me feel the happiest?	Nursing the baby; feeding the baby with a bottle only; nursing and occasionally using formula to give me time off
Preparations for the baby	What things do I feel are important to do before the baby is born?	Get a special cradle? Buy a dresser? Set up a whole room? Buy new clothes? Borrow well-loved baby articles from friends?

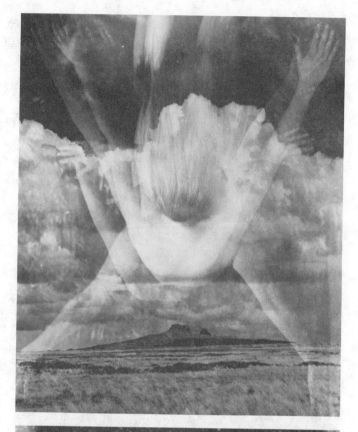

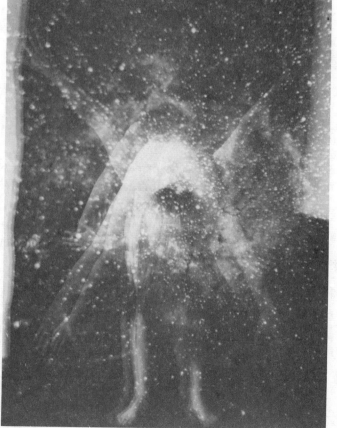

Through visualization, we can soar and go beyond the boundaries of our bodies. Soaring (top) and Grounding (bottom). Photos by Michael Samuels.

Relaxation and visualization during labor and delivery

Relaxation is a key technique for labor and delivery, and most natural childbirth systems make use of it. The more a woman practices deep body relaxation before labor begins, the more effectively she'll be able to use it during labor. Initially she should follow complete instructions for relaxation (see p. 163), but as she becomes familiar with the sensation of relaxing, she can simply concentrate on remaining deeply relaxed for longer and longer periods. Labor and delivery vary greatly in length, but most likely they will last a number of hours. Thus it is good if a woman learns to stay relaxed and focused for an hour or more. When the muscles around the uterus are relaxed, the woman is not fighting or struggling with the contractions. If she is *mentally* relaxed and tranquil as well, her perception of the experience is profoundly altered and she can work with her contractions. Images that a woman holds in mind while relaxed can greatly increase her ability to remain calm and tranquil. Like relaxation, visualization is a skill that improves and becomes easier with use. Together, relaxation and visualization can make a woman more comfortable during labor and delivery and can help to make childbirth a tremendously rewarding and exhilarating experience.

IMAGES FOR CHILDBIRTH

I am calm and relaxed.
The baby feels my calmness and shares it.
The baby and I are rested and ready for the work we will do.
The baby is naturally doing just what it should.
My uterus is contracting by itself.
With each contraction my cervix is dilating a little more.
The contractions of my uterus are massaging the baby.
My belly feels as if it is suspended in warm water, floating lightly.
My abdomen feels almost as if it were separate from the rest of my body. I can watch the contractions come and go as if they were slow waves breaking on shore.
My breathing is slow and even.
My legs, hands, and jaw are loose. My belly and bottom are loose.
The baby and I rest deeply in between one contraction and the next.
In a while the baby will be here. The baby and I are doing beautifully. The baby will be beautiful.

IMAGES FOR CHILDBIRTH

The baby is descending naturally. With each contraction the
  baby descends a little more.
The baby's head fits perfectly in my pelvis.
My hand against my back equalizes the pressure of the baby's head
  against my back.
Soon the baby will be here.
The baby and I are doing beautifully.
It feels good to push now. It is wonderful, exhilarating work.
The baby and I can still rest between contractions.
The baby is almost here.
My vagina stretches tight as the baby's head crowns, then
  emerges. I think of coolness, coolness.
I can see my baby's head.
Now the baby is here. The baby is beautiful. What a sense of
  completion.

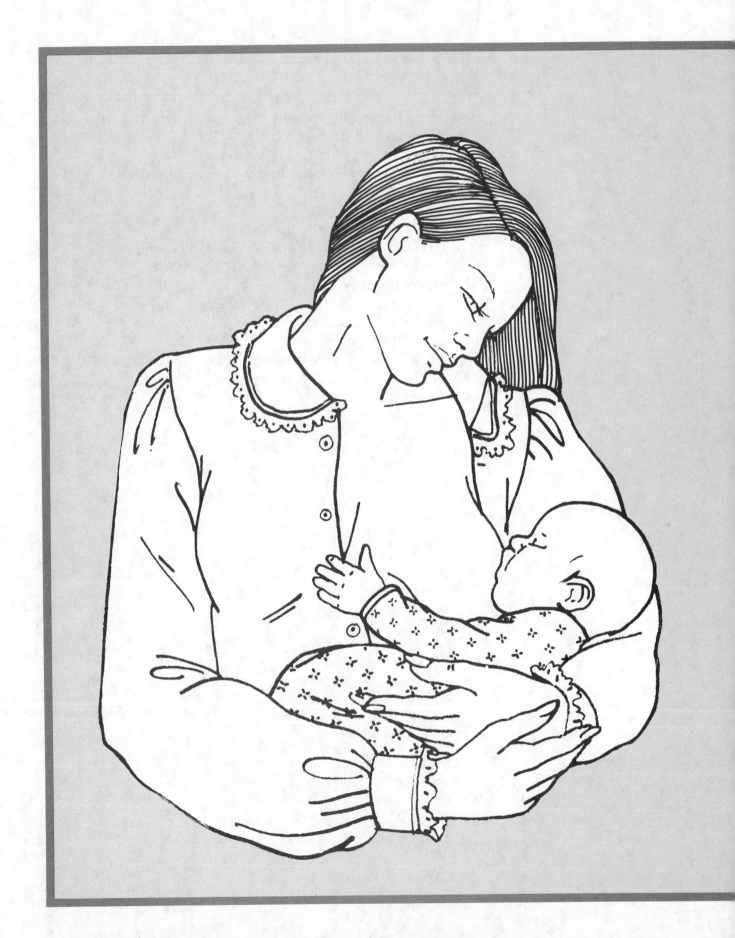

Preparing to Breast-feed

What Doctors Recommend

Just as the mother's body has an incredibly complex and beautiful system for feeding the baby in the uterus, it has one for feeding the baby after it is born. For hundreds of thousands of years the human species has nurtured its infants by breast-feeding. Indeed, it has only been within the last hundred years or so that mothers have had any alternative. But while a baby can grow and become healthy on formula, scientists have discovered that nursing has numerous medical and psychological advantages for the baby. Moreover, studies show that nursing has positive effects on the mother as well.

As a result of recent scientific findings, the American Academy of Pediatrics has made a strong and sweeping recommendation that full-term newborn infants be breast-fed: "Ideally, breast milk should be practically the only source of nutrients for the first four to six months for most infants."[1] The same committee has recommended that pregnant women study information on both the theoretical and the practical aspects of breast-feeding so that they will understand the importance of it and make preparations should they decide to nurse. The committee went so far as to suggest that laws be passed enabling women to take off from work the first three or four months after birth and/or that nurseries adjacent to the mother's work space be provided in order to promote nursing.

Unfortunately, studies over the last few decades have shown that the number of mothers who were breast-feeding when they were discharged from the hospital has dropped progressively. Whereas in 1946, 65 percent of mothers in the United States were breast-feeding at approximately one week, in 1956 that figure had dropped to 37 percent, and by 1966 it had reached a low of 27 percent. More recent studies have shown a general leveling off, with a significant increase among married women and women with at least a high school education. As of 1972, only half of the 28 percent of mothers that began breast-feeding were still nursing their babies two months later, and only 6 percent were still nursing at six months.

Every species produces milk that is specifically adapted to its infants' life-style as well as its physiological needs and capacities. The milks of individual species differ in the kind and quantity of protein (amino acids), fats, minerals, vitamins, and trace elements they contain, as well as in immunological composition. Thus even when cow's milk is diluted, altered, and modified in modern-day prepared formulas, it neither matches human milk nor provides many of its advantages. Without question, human milk is best suited to the nutritional needs of human babies.

The prominent breast-feeding expert Dr. Derrick Jelliffe tells the following story to illustrate how the milk of different mammals is evolutionarily adapted to each species' needs. The blue whale gives birth to enormous newborns that have tremendous calorie needs. But

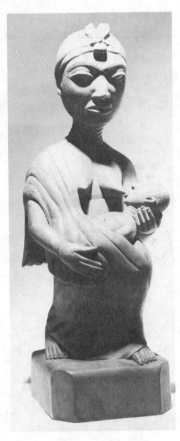

For hundreds of thousands of years the human species has nurtured its infants by breast-feeding. Ashanti mother and child, Ghana. Lowie Museum of Anthropology, University of California, Berkeley.

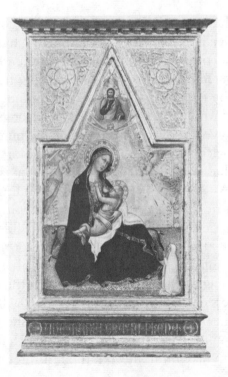

Quite simply, human milk is best suited to the nutritional needs of human babies. Madonna and Child, *Andrea di Bartolo. National Gallery of Art, Washington, D.C. Samuel H. Kress Collection.*

the newborn whale cannot hold its breath for long while it is nursing underwater. Thus the female blue whale has evolved a milk that is as rich as cream (over 50 percent fat), and has developed a very powerful letdown reflex that literally pumps milk into the baby's mouth in brief, enormous squirts. Neither this type of milk nor this type of mechanism would be suitable for most other mammals.

Nutritional Differences Among Milks

Human milk is especially rich in nutrients needed for brain development: lactose, cholesterol, and specific amino and fatty acids. Babies absorb *lipids*, basic elements in fats and cholesterol, more easily from human milk than from cow's milk because of their structure and composition. In fact, at present most formulas remove butterfat from cow's milk and replace it with vegetable oil, which is more readily absorbed by human babies. Unfortunately, vegetable oils have almost no cholesterol, an important substance needed for nerve development and brain growth. Newborns can synthesize cholesterol to some extent, but it is not yet known if their ability is adequate in this case. Also, vegetable oils are two or three times higher in polyunsaturated fats than is human milk. The implications of this for full-term babies are not known, but in premature babies it can cause a vitamin E deficiency and a kind of anemia.

It is very interesting to note that adults who were breast-fed for several months as infants show lower cholesterol levels than adults who were formula-fed. And there is some evidence that adolescents who had been breast-fed as babies for even a short time had less cholesterol buildup in the arteries of their hearts than did those who had been exclusively bottle-fed. Scientists speculate that ingestion of cholesterol in human milk may aid babies' bodies in learning how to man-

Advantages of breast-feeding

- Human milk is rich in nutrients needed for brain development.
- Human lipids are easier to absorb than those in cow's milk.
- Human milk has antibodies to protect the baby from gastrointestinal and respiratory diseases.
- Human milk promotes healthy lactobaccillus growth in the baby's intestinal tract (cow's milk promotes the growth of other bacteria).
- Breast-feeding avoids potential allergic reactions to cow's milk.
- Breast-feeding promotes bonding and encourages a warm relationship, based on touch, between mother and baby.

ufacture enzymes that digest cholesterol and prevent heart attacks in later life.

Human infants have a tremendous need for amino acids, the units from which proteins are built. It has been found that some of the amino acids present in cow's milk are difficult for the newborn's liver to use in manufacturing important proteins. This difficulty is even more pronounced in premature babies, whose blood actually shows different amounts of certain amino acids when they are fed cow's milk. In comparison with human milk, cow's milk has generally higher levels of protein and may overload infants who are routinely fed formula. But cow's milk has a very low amount of a specific protein building block called *nucleotides*, which is thought to play an important role in protein production and growth. A quarter of breast milk's building blocks are nucleotides, as compared to only 6 percent of cow's milk.

Iron, an important mineral derived from food sources, is primarily used in the human body to bind oxygen to red blood cells. Babies are born with abundant stores of iron in their red blood cells, liver, and spleen, which their body has accumulated during pregnancy. In fact, humans have more iron stores as newborns than at any other time in their lives. These stores are enough to last until a baby has tripled its birth weight, provided that it is breast-fed.

All mammalian milks tend to be low in iron, but recently scientists have found that the amount of iron in human milk is ideal for enabling two special proteins to work in the baby's digestive system at optimum capacity. Remarkably, these proteins, *transferrin* and *lactoferrin*, have the ability to kill *E. coli*, a common but potentially harmful intestinal bacteria. However they can only work if they are not overloaded with iron. In view of the baby's high stores at birth, pediatricians no longer recommend giving breast-fed babies supplemental iron before they are six to nine months old.

Cow's milk formulas, on the other hand, are less than ideal in terms of iron. First, processing totally destroys the transferrin and lactoferrin proteins in formula. Second, the form of iron naturally present in cow's milk is not well absorbed by the baby's digestive system, although present formulas are better than those of ten years ago.

Another important mineral that babies need is zinc, which is necessary for enzymes that are part of the energy production cycle. Zinc is present in very high levels in *colostrum*, the starter milk that the mother produces for the first several days after the baby is born. It is present in low amounts in regular breast milk, as it is in formula, but it is much better absorbed from human milk.

The amounts and ratios of calcium, phosphorus, magnesium, and sodium, as well as zinc, are very different in cow's milk than in human milk. Elevated levels of certain minerals and proteins in cow's milk pose a potential strain on the newborn's kidneys, which are still immature. Finally, the amounts of different minerals also vary between colostrum and mature human milk, indicating that in some way not yet fully understood these constituents in breast milk are specially regulated to meet the newborn's needs at various stages of development.

Immunological Differences Among Milks

One of the prime factors in breast milk that *is not* and *can not* be duplicated in formulas is the presence of a large number of maternal *antibodies,* complicated substances that help to fight infection. This is very important, because the newborn's immune system is not fully functional: it still cannot effectively make antibodies, and it has only had a chance to develop antibodies to infections that the mother has had during pregnancy.

There are three major kinds of human antibodies: IgG, IgM, and IgA. Babies are born with high levels of IgG, which has come across the placenta from the mother, but they have very low levels of IgM and IgA. Babies' immune systems do not become capable of making these antibodies at adult levels for varying periods of time: IgM levels develop by one year and IgG by four years, but IgA does not reach adult levels until adolescence. Mature human milk and colostrum, especially, have all three kinds of antibodies, but are highest in IgA.

IgA protects against infections of the lungs and gastrointestinal system. This has been important historically, and continues to be even now in third world countries, where pneumonia and diarrhea are among the major causes of serious illness and death in newborns and young children. The mechanism by which breast milk comes to contain high levels of IgA is quite remarkable. IgA, like all antibodies, is made by white blood cells called *lymphocytes.* Lymphocytes live all over the body, but special groups live in the walls of the intestine, where they learn to recognize and make antibodies against common local intestinal germs. During the last trimester of pregnancy, a number of these lymphocytes in the mother's intestines are somehow signaled and actually migrate to her breasts. By the time the baby is born, some of these relocated cells have begun to produce IgA that goes directly into the milk. Breast milk also contains an enzyme without which IgA cannot break up harmful bacteria. This particular enzyme is found in much greater quantities in human milk than in cow's milk.

Not only does breast milk contain antibodies against intestinal infections, it also has specific antibodies against meningitis, polio, influenza, tetanus, strep, staph, and a variety of other viruses and bacteria. Thus it is not surprising that all over the world breast-fed babies have been found to have lower incidences of intestinal, respiratory, and ear infections. Such statistics are most pronounced in third-world

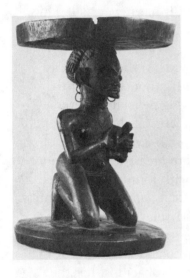

The presence of large numbers of antibodies in breast milk cannot be duplicated by formulas. These antibodies aid the newborn's immature immune system. African stool, Angola, 19th–20th century. The Metropolitan Museum of Art. The Michael C. Rockefeller Memorial Collection. Purchase, Nelson A. Rockefeller gift, 1971.

countries where infection rates are generally higher because sanitation and refrigeration are often inadequate. Breast-fed babies in these countries actually have much better rates of survival in the first year, which is why the World Health Organization strongly recommends breast-feeding. It is significant to note that even in the United States, babies who are given manufactured formula and who have the benefits of good sanitation, refrigeration, and antibiotics have over *twice* the illness rate and *three* times the hospital admission rate of breast-fed babies. These figures are based on studies made as recently as 1979 and 1980 and include illnesses such as ear infections, pneumonia, bronchitis, vomiting, and diarrhea.

The initial human milk, colostrum, contains high levels of white blood cells. In fact, there are over 2 million white blood cells per cubic centimeter in colostrum. Most of these are *macrophages*, giant cells that manufacture the digestive enzymes *lysozyme* and *lactoferrin*, which explode and kill bacteria. The rest of the white blood cells in colostrum are *lymphocytes* that can make antibodies against illnesses the mother has had. While they last, these cells enable the baby to make antibodies against illnesses that it has never had. Thus breast-fed babies acquire from their mothers a kind of *temporary immunity* to many diseases.

Babies are born with no bacteria growing in their intestines because the mother's uterus is sterile, but within hours after birth babies acquire bacteria through eating. These beneficial bacteria quickly multiply and become permanent residents of the digestive tract, helping to break down food, make vitamin K, and dispose of harmful bacteria. Interestingly, babies who are breast-fed have very different intestinal bacteria than babies fed with formula: breast-fed babies have an almost pure culture of *lactobacillus bifidus* in their intestinal tract, while bottle-fed babies have mostly putrefactive bacteria such as *E. coli*. This is what accounts for the stronger smell of bottle-fed babies' stools. Manufacturers have begun to add lactose sugar to formula in order to encourage the growth of lactobacillus, but they have not been able to add a special substance in breast milk that promotes the growth of lactobacillus. Although scientists don't understand how a pure lactobacillus culture is maintained in breast-fed babies, they feel it helps to protect babies against harmful intestinal infections.

Preventing Allergies

Very recently doctors have come to believe that breast-feeding has advantages for babies in terms of allergies. Since 1976 several studies have demonstrated that breast-fed babies have much lower incidences of all kinds of allergies, including skin rashes, food allergies, and breathing difficulties. This advantage particularly applies to babies with a strong family history of allergies as well as to babies who have no history of allergic illness among their parents and siblings.

Researchers have discovered the mechanism by which babies become sensitized to various *allergens,* or allergy-causing substances. The newborn's intestine, unlike the adult's, cannot stop large molecules from passing through its wall into the bloodstream. Thus cow's milk proteins, which are actually foreign to the baby, enter its bloodstream. White blood cells identify them as foreign substances and then make antibodies against them.

Scientists don't know why some babies become allergic and others do not, but it is probably due in large part to genetic background. In babies who become allergic, numerous antibodies are made, priming the whole immune system and resulting in the symptoms of allergy. Within six days after birth bottle-fed babies show measurable levels of antibodies to cow's milk in their blood. They also have much higher levels of IgE, the antibody associated with allergies, than do breast-fed babies. Babies who are allergic to cow's milk or who "tolerate it poorly" have many more digestive problems than breast-fed babies, including more frequent spitting up, more bouts of diarrhea, and more colic.

In an effort to prevent allergies, many pediatricians now recommend that babies *only* be breast-fed, or that they be given cow's-milk-free formulas. If there is a strong allergic history pediatricians may even recommend that a nursing mother refrain from ingesting cow's milk products herself, since the molecules can actually come through to the baby in her milk.

Breast-fed babies are protected against foreign molecules in a special way. IgA, the major one of the three types of antibodies that pass in the mother's milk, and the last one that the baby learns to make by itself, coats the baby's intestine and prevents foreign molecules from getting through. This protection is most important in the first two to three months. During this time the baby is colonizing its own intestine with small patches of the white blood cells so that it can begin to make IgA by itself.

Preventing Obesity

In addition to adult heart disease and adult allergies, obesity is another long-range problem that may be associated with bottle-feeding. Obesity is more than a social concern; it is a medical matter that affects life expectancy. It is estimated that one-quarter to one-third of all adults in our culture are obese, though it is not known to what extent these weight problems are related to infant obesity. But infant obesity is common, and it is frequently associated with bottle-feeding. During the first few years of life the baby makes most of its fat cells and sets up patterns for regulating its energy intake. At the same time the baby is developing habits about how much seems to be a satisfying amount of food. Because of this pediatricians advise against excessive weight gain in the first few years.

Bottle-feeding is more typically associated with overeating than is breast-feeding. The reasons for this are quite complicated and have to do with the inherent nature of these two very different ways of nourishing a baby. First, studies have shown that mothers who bottle-feed tend to encourage a baby to take all of the bottle, but no more. This means the baby tends to eat the same amount regardless of its size or how hungry it is. Second, studies show that mothers who bottle-feed their babies tend to introduce solid foods much earlier, thereby greatly increasing the baby's caloric intake at a young age. Finally, it's known that the composition of breast milk changes during the course of a feeding (see p. 415). Toward the end of the feeding the milk is much richer in fat and protein. Some doctors have theorized that this richness tends to fill the baby up and becomes associated with the cessation of hunger at the end of feeding, whereas a bottle-fed baby has no taste associations with the end of the feeding because the milk composition remains the same.

Breast-feeding and Bonding

Not surprisingly, nursing tends to promote long-term bonding between mother and baby (see p. 348). Studies have shown that within the first few days after delivery, mothers who have prolonged "skin-to-skin" contact with their babies during nursing develop different mothering patterns as the baby grows. Nursing mothers tend to engage in more soothing behavior and more eye-to-eye contact, and they are less likely to leave their baby with others. The act of nursing is a pleasurable, sensual one for both mother and baby, which tends to develop communication between them. It is a "dyadic" process, that is, both mother and baby learn together.

Cross-cultural studies show that a nursing baby tends to remain closer to its mother and sleeps with the mother more frequently. These studies also show that the mother gives precedence to the nursing baby and reacts more strongly to its crying, and is more likely to swaddle and rock the baby. Nursing mothers also tend to touch their baby more and spend more time with it. Babies who breast-feed tend to keep the nipple in their mouth for longer periods of time than do bottle-fed babies. This longer feeding time for the nursing mother correlates with more time communicating with the baby.

Mothers who nurse their babies speak of the great emotional satisfaction they derive from breast-feeding. Although some mothers

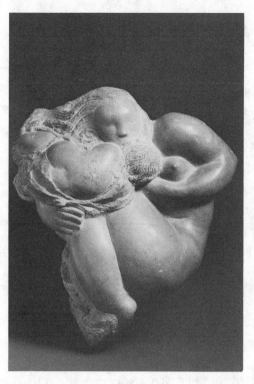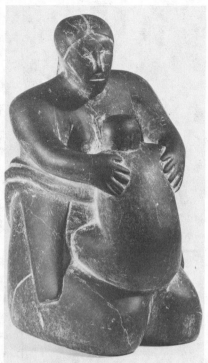

Nursing tends to promote long-term bonding between mother and baby.

The Cloud, *Jose de Creeft, 1939. Collection of Whitney Museum of American Art, New York.*

Seated mother and child, Eskimo, 20th century. The Metropolitan Museum of Art. Harris Brisbane Dick Fund and Houghton Foundation, Inc.

have problems in the first few weeks of nursing, the great majority of women who breast-feed say that it has given them many of the most ecstatic moments they have ever experienced. Breast-feeding seems to touch some of the same deep emotional sensations and feelings that mothers experience when they are giving birth. In fact, a number of doctors believe that nursing is the natural step that follows birth in a normal maturational sequence of maternal development. Certainly in biological terms nursing is intimately tied to birth and the postpartum process, since milk production occurs automatically, and the baby's sucking stimulates the mother to release a hormone that causes her uterus to clamp down, which stops bleeding and helps return the uterus to its normal size (see p. 352).

Evolutionary biologists believe that the profound satisfaction mothers get from nursing is no accident; rather, it is the result of ancient, inborn *bioprograms* that are built in to the species. These programs have developed over hundreds of thousands of years to give the species an evolutionary advantage. Bioprograms help to give a mother a strong sense of what to do with her baby even if she has never seen a newborn before. Like instincts in primates and other animals, these programs are the foundation upon which parenting is built, and they yield immense satisfaction if they are played out in a natural way. But bioprograms are more complex and subtle than instincts and can be elicited at different times, by different factors. Ideally, bioprograms are combined with social support factors and

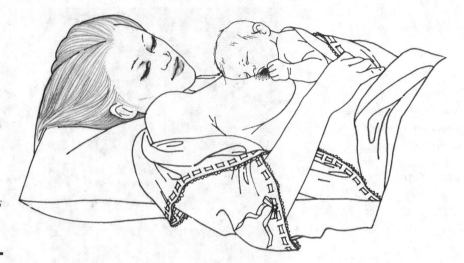

Nursing is a wonderful sensual experience that promotes long-term bonding between mother and baby.

knowledge acquired from experienced women, medical personnel, courses, and books.

For mothers, nursing offers a close, intimate time with the baby. Physiological factors almost ensure that the nursing session be peaceful and relaxed; a mother who is agitated will not be able to initiate the reflex that squeezes the milk down from the breast sinuses. Perhaps even more than pregnancy breast-feeding is an act of love, an act of giving generously of oneself. In return, the mother is rewarded by the baby's immense satisfaction when its hunger is assuaged and by the baby's growing understanding of the mother as the source of so much pleasure and contentment.

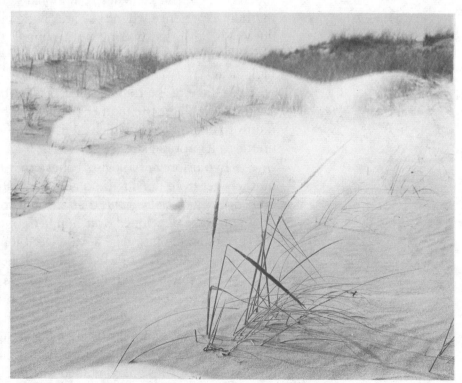

A woman's desire to nurse and the satisfaction she receives from it are the result of ancient inborn bioprograms. Earth Mother, *photo by Michael Samuels.*

The Decision to Breast-feed

A woman can make the choice to breast-feed at any time from prior to pregnancy to several days after the birth of her baby. But generally, for the mother's own ease, the earlier she decides to breast-feed, the better. If she makes the decision early in pregnancy, she will have ample time to prepare herself physically as well as mentally.

The more motivated a mother is to nurse, the more likely she is to succeed. Her desire to nurse will help her learn a new skill and conquer any of the problems that sometimes arise in the first week or two. If a mother is not very motivated, such problems, though they are temporary, may cause her to give up breast-feeding before she and the baby have had a chance to establish a mutually satisfactory routine. Obstetricians and midwives have also observed that mothers who belatedly make the choice to breast-feed often have a more difficult time establishing good nursing.

Before making a choice, it's important that a pregnant woman acquaint herself with the physical facts of nursing and with the advantages for the baby. If she has particular fears or concerns, as many women do, she needs to discuss them and lay them to rest. To get a real sense of the rewards she'll experience with nursing, she can talk to mothers who are nursing or have nursed their babies happily.

Unfortunately, for many pregnant women, especially first-time mothers, the reality of pregnancy and the impending birth are so overwhelming that the thought of nursing the baby, as well as bathing and diapering it, remains vague and rather distant right up to the end of pregnancy. From a rational perspective this doesn't make any sense, yet almost all mothers can remember and sympathize with such feelings. Expectant mothers should be reassured that a lack of intense interest in nursing and nursing preparation is very common and doesn't reflect on their future success at breast-feeding. If a pregnant woman has any thought of nursing at all, she should prepare to do so as early as possible in order to minimize problems and make nursing easier for herself and the baby. Even if a mother is uneasy about breast-feeding, she is urged to go over the advantages it offers the baby and to consider nursing for at least the first few weeks.

Concerns About Nursing

There are several factors that explain why women are sometimes hesitant about breast-feeding. Often they have conscious or unconscious worries about nursing that are based on misinformation or lack of information. Also many pregnant women, especially first-time mothers, have little experience with friends or acquaintances who have nursed. Unfortunately there is little general support for nursing in this

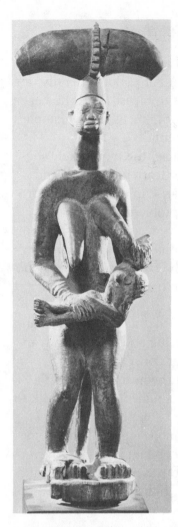

Some women fear that nursing will cause their breasts to sag. Actually, normal enlargement and lack of support during pregnancy are what cause breast ligaments to stretch. Mother and child, Yoruba, 19th–20th century. The Metropolitan Museum of Art. Michael C. Rockefeller Memorial Collection, bequest of Nelson A. Rockefeller, 1979.

country, whereas in Europe and many third-world countries, nursing is expected and accepted more matter-of-factly. Finally, working mothers sometimes feel there may be insurmountable conflicts between their work and breast-feeding.

Many women have physical concerns as to whether nursing will make their breasts sag. Although pendulous breasts are considered a sign of maturity and beauty in many tribal cultures, they are not in our culture, with its emphasis on youth and fitness. Doctors have found that breast sagging has to do with pregnancy, not nursing. During late pregnancy the breasts enlarge due to the growth of ducts and the increasing number of alveoli (see p. 30). If pregnant women gain a great deal of weight, their breasts may enlarge even more than otherwise. These changes in breast size take place whether a mother intends to nurse or not. The increased weight of the breasts tends to stretch the *ligaments of Cooper,* the tough, fibrous bands that support the muscles that underly the breasts. The most effective way to prevent these ligaments from stretching is to provide strong support with a well-fitted maternity or nursing bra that is replaced whenever the elastic wears out. Of course, nursing causes some physical changes to take place in the breasts. Often the nipples protrude more, and the breasts may increase or decrease somewhat in size, although this is generally the result of weight gain or loss after pregnancy.

Some women simply feel uncomfortable or embarrassed at the thought of nursing. Talking to mothers who have enjoyed breast-feeding may help to allay their anxieties. Also, a mother should realize that she need never nurse publicly if she does not want to. In fact, many new mothers find that nursing in company is too distracting and they need to be alone or just with the family so that they can pay attention to how the baby is doing. If a woman is motivated, but she can't resolve her feelings of discomfort, counseling during pregnancy may be helpful. If after serious consideration a woman finds that she still feels very uncomfortable with the idea of nursing, it may be better for her relationship with the baby to bottle-feed.

A few women, especially those with small breasts, are concerned that they may not have enough milk to meet the baby's needs. Actually there is no correlation between breast size and milk production. The size of the breasts is determined by the amount of fat, muscle, and connective tissue in them; milk is produced by alveoli (see p. 30), which make up a relatively small amount of the breast mass. Ultimately the amount of milk a mother produces depends on how much the baby sucks, the amount of prolactin her pituitary gland produces in response to the sucking, and her willingness to let the baby nurse on demand. This is why mothers can automatically meet the needs of a growing baby, and mothers of twins can usually supply all of both babies' needs.

A dramatic example, often quoted by obstetricians, demonstrates the natural capacity of women to succeed at breast-feeding. In the 1930s in France, only 38 percent of women nursed successfully. During World War II formula became unavailable, and even cow's milk was scarce. Over 90 percent of mothers were able to nurse during the war years, even under very stressful conditions.

Another concern that many women have is that they will be "tied down" by nursing; this is especially likely if a mother has to or wants to return to work quickly. It is true that a nursing mother needs to be more available to her baby than a mother who bottle-feeds, and some women do chafe at this constant demand for their time and attention. However, most mothers who nurse find the experience so rewarding that they are willing to adjust their schedule to meet the baby's needs. Even a mother who bottle-feeds has to spend time preparing the bottles and feeding the baby. Indeed, many nursing mothers feel that they have more time to themselves, and that the time they spend with the baby is more pleasurably spent if they nurse, especially at night when they can simply bring the baby into bed with them.

Most working mothers take a six- to eight-week leave after a birth. Even if a mother ceases to nurse at this point, she should realize that her breast-feeding has been of tremendous value to the baby. Of course, the more time the mother takes off after the birth, the less scheduling problems she is likely to have, because the frequency of feedings drops steadily over the first few weeks and months. After they return to work, many mothers are able to make arrangements to have their baby at work, or they pump and store their milk for future feedings. If a mother does not want to go to the trouble of expressing her milk at work, by the second month or so she will find that her milk supply can adjust so that she can nurse when she is at home and simply have the baby fed formula during work hours. In this case most pediatricians would recommend a *non-cow's-milk* formula to lessen the baby's chances of developing allergies.

Preparing to Breast-feed

Many women engage in no special preparations for breast-feeding and have little or no trouble establishing good nursing. However, there are several things that generally make the beginning of nursing easier. Also, certain physical characteristics have been found to correlate with initial ease or difficulty of nursing.

First, pregnant women should not use anything that tends to make their nipples dry, cracked, or sore. Expectant mothers should avoid using soap, alcohol, benzoin, or any drying creams or lotions on their nipples throughout pregnancy, but especially during the last trimester. Usually, this is not a problem, though women sometimes forget and use soap on their nipples when bathing. Soap removes the normal moistening oils that are produced around the nipples.

Most women's nipples are overprotected by clothing. When the nipples receive very little friction, they don't tend to build up a thick layer of epithelial cells. There are several techniques that help to toughen the nipples in preparation for nursing. Women with small breasts can go without a bra. Women with large breasts who are concerned about sagging can cut holes out of the center of their bra cups, which will allow their nipples to rub against the fabric of their clothes. Mothers should also expose their nipples to air and sunlight as much as possible in the last few months before delivery. Touching the nipples, either in lovemaking or in exercises (see following), also gets the nipples used to friction and helps to prepare them for the extensive manipulation they will receive during breast-feeding. Although some doctors and midwives no longer emphasize nipple-toughening exercises, it's only common sense that rubbing will thicken the skin of the nipples, just as going barefoot builds up calluses on the soles of the feet. Toughening the nipples is important because nipple soreness is one of the most common complaints in the early days of nursing.

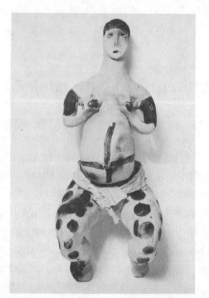

Doctors and midwives feel that good prenatal preparation makes the beginning of nursing easier. Pregnant woman, Caraja Indians, Brazil. Photograph courtesy of The Museum of the American Indian, Heye Foundation.

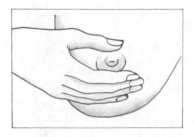

From week 36 on most doctors and midwives recommend that the mother manually express colostrum from her nipples in preparation for nursing. Manual expression clears the breast sinuses, stimulates the muscles around the breast ducts, and helps a mother become familiar with handling her breasts.

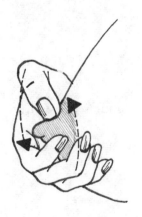

Many doctors and midwives believe that nipple rolling exercises help to break fibrous bands around the nipples, making it easier for them to become erect. Nipple rolling is not recommended until after week 36, because it can stimulate uterine contractions.

Nipples that protrude require little preparation for nursing other than general toughening to help make them impervious to the constant friction of nursing. If the mother's nipples don't protrude, it can be difficult for the baby to "get on" when it nurses. This can be very frustrating for the baby, as well as upsetting and demoralizing for the mother. Also, the baby's repeated attempts to get the nipple in its mouth are one of the causes of sore nipples for the mother.

In the correct nursing position, the baby draws the mother's nipple deeply into its mouth so that its tongue can press the nipple against the roof of its mouth. This is much easier if the mother's nipples stand out from the surrounding areola when they have been stimulated. By the seventh or eighth month of pregnancy, two-thirds of all mothers will find that their nipples stand up, while about one-third will find that they have *flat nipples* that invert when stimulated. Many mothers who have flat nipples in early pregnancy will notice that hormonal changes will cause their nipples to become erect by the middle of pregnancy. There is a very small number of women who have truly *inverted nipples*, which never protrude with or without stimulation.

Most doctors and midwives believe that there is much a mother can do during pregnancy to make her nipples stand out and to prevent the baby from having problems getting on. Some doctors believe that flat nipples are firmly anchored to underlying breast tissue with fibrous bands, whereas nipples that protrude are only loosely attached to the breast tissue underneath. Other people feel that it is simply a matter of strengthening the erector muscles that cause the nipple to protrude. Whatever the cause of flat nipples, most doctors and midwives recommend nipple pulling or rolling exercises (see chart on p. 192).

In addition, many doctors advise that mothers begin breast massage and manual expression of colostrum after week 36 of pregnancy. Massage and expression are not recommended before that time because they cause the release of the hormone *oxytocin* (see p. 248), and there is concern that this might cause premature labor in a few women. These exercises are thought to clear the breast sinuses and ducts of early thick colostrum, establishing a free and easy flow. Expressing colostrum stimulates the tiny muscles around the ducts that squeeze the milk down, and stretches the ducts themselves so that they can hold more milk.

Like nipple rolling, manual expression helps to make flat nipples stand out. Some people believe that it also helps to establish special neuro-hormonal circuits that will condition the letdown reflex (see p. 414). It does get the mother used to touching her breasts and caring for them in a natural, relaxed way. No matter how motivated mothers are to nurse, few of them handle their breasts and nipples to the same degree or with the same lack of self-consciousness that they need to in nursing. This is true even for mothers who have nursed before, because they frequently get out of practice between babies.

Breast massage

- Place hands palm down at top of one breast.
- While keeping thumbs in place, firmly rub the fingers of each hand down the sides of the breast and around the bottom, without touching the nipples.
- Bring thumbs and other fingers together, firmly squeezing the breast tissue, and then slide the fingers off breast.
- Repeat these motions 10 to 15 times with each breast.
- Lubricate hands with oil or cocoa butter if desired.

Manual expression of colostrum or breast milk

- Use one hand to support the breast.
- Use thumb and index or middle finger of other hand to express milk, placing fingers opposite each other on the outer edge of the areola.
- Press fingers back into breast; at the same time, spread fingers apart, then bring them back together, squeezing the areola gently but firmly.
- Move fingers around areola in a circle, pressing at each location until the flow stops. This empties all sinuses around the nipple.
- Begin this exercise at 36 weeks.

Nipple rolling

- Place thumb and forefinger on sides of nipple and areola, without touching end of nipple.
- Holding thumb and forefinger steady, turn the hand gently in either direction, twisting nipple.
- Practice several times on each nipple.
- Begin this exercise after 36 weeks to prepare for nursing.

Finally, the ability to express milk manually can be of great use throughout the nursing period. In particular, it can be invaluable when the mother's breasts become swollen and overly full with milk in the early days of nursing. Later, if a mother wishes to leave her baby to go to work or go out, manual expression will enable her to store her milk so that it can be fed to her baby while she is away.

If an expectant mother wants to practice nursing techniques, she should refer to the chapter on nursing to learn about the various positions. Some doctors even recommend that the mother hold a pillow or doll in the crook of her arm and practice grasping her breast with the "steering hand" and "rooting" her nipple against the pillow or doll. In this way she can attempt to make some of the nursing actions second nature. Another way a woman can familiarize herself with nursing is to seek out experienced nursing mothers and observe them when they feed their babies. Whereas it may make a new mother nervous or uncomfortable to be observed, most experienced mothers do not mind at all and, in fact, will be happy to demonstrate and share what they know.

More than ever, doctors acknowledge the health benefits of breast-feeding for the newborn. Not only is breast milk nutritionally superior to other milks, but it helps to prevent infections, allergies, and obesity. In addition, it promotes bonding between mother and baby and adds to the warmth and poignancy of their relationship, providing great pleasure and satisfaction for both of them.

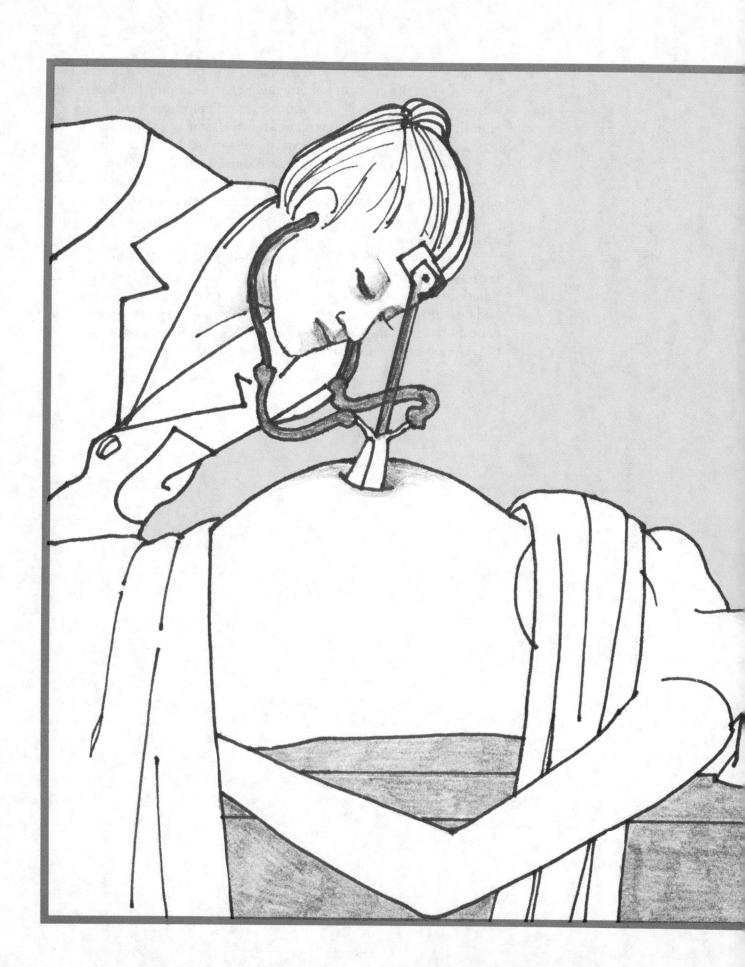

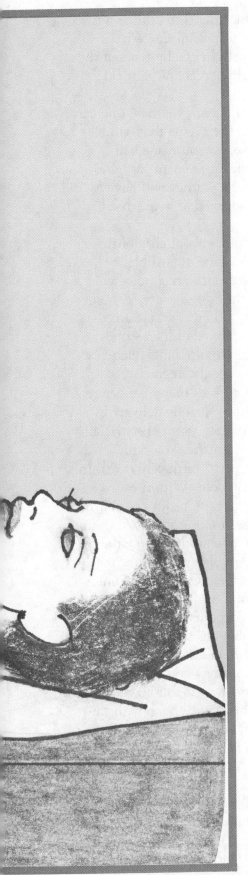

CHAPTER 11

Choices for Childbirth

Choosing the Doctor or Midwife

The relationship that a pregnant woman and her husband have with their doctor or midwife is a very intimate and important one. Not only will this person assist the mother during labor and delivery and advise the parents of what is best for the baby, he or she will also affect the way the mother perceives the whole experience of being pregnant and giving birth. The mother's view of the birth process is a significant factor in determining what happens to her during delivery and in determining how she deals with her experience.

As much as a mother tries to visualize and influence what will happen to her during birth, she cannot fully control the process or its outcome. Birth is one of the great experiences in life, requiring the participants to give up specific expectations and views and accept whatever unfolds. The trust that the mother and father have in the doctor or midwife becomes a very important part of this process.

For a woman birth requires letting go and relying on her body. To do this effectively the mother must be in an environment in which she feels comfortable and has confidence in the people who are assisting her. The environment and the people who can best help a mother achieve these feelings will vary greatly from one woman to another.

Every birth is unique, so it's not useful for the parents to outline a rigid step-by-step plan of how they want the birth to take place. What's important is that each mother get in touch with her feelings about the kind of environment and people that will help her feel most at ease (see p. 168).

We have said that birth is a journey. Like any journey, one can plan the destination, but one cannot plan all the events that will take place along the way, or even necessarily the exact route one will travel. Often the most meaningful and significant moments are the ones that are unexpected. And memories of the journey will have as much to do with how one *dealt* with what happened as with what actually took place.

Currently there are two basic philosophies about childbirth. One group wants to make the experience as natural as possible. Another group advocates the general use of advanced technological procedures in the belief that they maximize the baby's safety. A home delivery is the epitome of the first philosophy, whereas an electronically monitored delivery in a hospital is the epitome of the second. This dichotomy in obstetrical philosophies has resulted in a quandary for many pregnant women and for many obstetrical caregivers.

Women today face greater childbirth choices than ever before. In most parts of the country a mother can choose among delivery by a lay midwife, a nurse-midwife, a family practitioner, or an obstetrician. She can choose to give birth either at home, in a "free-standing" birth center separate from a hospital, in an "alternative" birth center within a hospital, or in a traditional hospital delivery room. Within each of these settings a mother has some option about positions for childbirth, use of an episiotomy, and availability of drugs or monitoring.

Before interviewing doctors or midwives a mother and father should develop a general concept of the kind of birth they'd like to have. Most expectant mothers have intuitive feelings and ideas which will give a sense of the mother's attitude toward birth, her hopes and fears, and what she feels will make it a joyful experience. But these feelings must be meshed with the realities of having a baby. To accomplish this a woman needs to talk to other mothers about their birth experiences and begin to read about pregnancy and childbirth. After she has gained some background information, it will be valuable for her to use visualization exercises to help her get in touch with the kind of birth situation that will make her feel most comfortable. From all her talking, reading, and thinking can come a list of preferences that she should discuss when she interviews doctors and midwives.

The choice of a particular doctor or midwife is critical in determining many of the alternatives in the birth situation. Each practitioner has his or her own set of beliefs and training that condition or create the kind of medicine they practice. For example, a midwife may have been trained to walk a woman who is experiencing a slow first

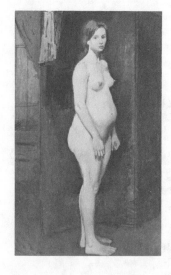

The relationship a pregnant woman develops with her doctor or midwife is very significant; to a great extent it will influence how she perceives the experience of being pregnant and giving birth. Nude, *Raphael Soyer, 1952. Collection of Whitney Museum of American Art, New York.*

Questions to ask a prospective obstetrician or midwife

- Do you practice in a group, and will I have a choice of practitioners? Do the others have similar philosophies on how to manage labor?
- Do you plan to be away for any period of time around my due date?
- Do you deliver at home? In a particular hospital? In a birth center?
- Do you view birth as a natural physiological process, and what is your policy on routine intervention?
- Do you practice natural childbirth? How many of your mothers deliver without medication?
- Do you use a particular method of natural childbirth, for example Bradley, Lamaze, or a combination?
- Do you or does someone you recommend teach childbirth education classes? What do they cover?
- Do you recommend amniocentesis or ultrasound? Under what conditions?
- Do you explain to a mother what is going on in labor and allow her some choice and involvement in making decisions?
- Do you remain with a mother continuously during labor, or do you have a nurse or labor coach do so?
- Who can be present during labor and delivery—father, friends, siblings, birth coach?
- Do you allow visitors not approved by the mother? Will you allow a mother to restrict observers other than her family or friends?
- Do you allow a mother to deliver in her own clothes?
- Do you require any prep before birth, such as a shave or an enema?
- What is your policy about fetal monitoring? Do you use a fetoscope, Doptone, or a continuous external or internal monitor?
- Do you routinely use an IV?
- What is the labor room like? Do you allow or encourage a mother to walk around, move, and change position in labor? Eat or drink in labor?
- Do you have time limits for the different stages of labor?
- How many of your patients receive pitocin to stimulate labor?
- Do you rupture the membranes routinely?
- If labor begins with the spontaneous rupture of membranes, do you set a time limit for when the baby must be born? If so, how long is it?
- How long do you allow a mother to be overdue before intervening? Then what do you do?

Questions to ask a prospective obstetrician or midwife

- What is your cesarean rate? Your group's rate? The hospital's rate?
- If a mother requires medication for pain, what type do you recommend?
- If you work at a hospital, can a mother deliver in the labor room provided it is an uncomplicated delivery?
- Do you allow the lights to be dim during an uncomplicated delivery if the mother requests it?
- Do you allow the mother to view the birth in a mirror if she cannot see it in the position she is in?
- What type of birth table or bed do you use? What positions do you allow a mother to deliver in?
- Do you encourage pushing in the second stage of labor? What positions do you allow a mother to push in?
- How many of your patients do you deliver with forceps or a vacuum extractor?
- Do you use massage, oil, and/or heat on the perineum to avoid an episiotomy? How often do you use an episiotomy?
- Do you allow the mother to touch the baby as it's being delivered?
- Do you allow the placenta to deliver naturally?
- When do you cut the umbilical cord?
- Do you routinely do a manual exploration of the uterus after delivery?
- Do you encourage bonding? Is the mother allowed to hold and nurse the baby immediately? For how long?
- What medical procedures are routinely performed on the baby?
- If the baby is healthy, can procedures like eyedrops and weighing be delayed?
- How soon will you discharge a mother after delivery?
- Does the hospital have complete rooming-in? If not, when must the baby be in the nursery?
- What are the visiting hours for the father?
- Can siblings visit?
- What is your policy on circumcision?
- How do you handle common complications of labor, such as unusual presentations or failure of labor to progress?
- How do you handle breech deliveries? Do you try to turn the baby manually? Are you experienced at delivering breech babies vaginally? Do you routinely do a cesarean for breeches?
- Do you do vaginal births after cesareans (VBACs)?
- Who can be present at a cesarean? Father or friend?
- What anesthesia do you use for a cesarean?

labor, whereas a doctor may have been trained to administer a drug to speed up contractions. The obstetrical style of a particular doctor or midwife consists of his or her normal routines and responses to both variations and complications in labor and delivery. Whereas a woman cannot determine everything that happens during childbirth, she can choose the style and philosophy of the person who delivers her baby.

A woman generally selects a doctor or midwife very early in pregnancy, sometimes before even becoming pregnant. An expectant mother's decision may be made on the basis of the medical insurance she has, by remaining with her previous gynecologist or midwife, through the recommendation of other mothers, by contacting professional organizations and support groups (see chart), or by obtaining a referral from another doctor the mother has seen. In order to make her choice on the basis of obstetrical style, a mother has to learn how the doctor or midwife handles specific situations, either by talking with other patients or, better still, by talking at length with the doctor or midwife.

In speaking with a practitioner, the mother and father should ask how he or she handles both normal deliveries and cesareans and should bring up any specific concerns or requests they might have. While it will be impossible to find out exactly how a practitioner will deal with every situation, the prospective parents will be able to get a feeling for his or her obstetrical style and personality and whether or not their attitudes toward birth are similar. If there seems to be a serious disagreement over philosophy or one important issue, the parents should interview other practitioners.

For many women the process of selecting a doctor or midwife is neither quick nor easy. First, a mother has to educate herself enough to decide what questions to ask. Then she has to obtain the names of

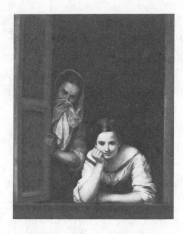

Many doctors and midwives now believe that a woman should have a supportive person who remains with her continuously during labor and delivery. A Girl And Her Duenna, *Bartolome Esteban Murillo, c. 1670. National Gallery of Art, Washington, D.C. Widener Collection.*

people whose philosophy and style are likely to match hers. Finally, if she is not lucky enough to feel confident about the first person she sees, she may need to interview several people. This in itself can be time-consuming, costly, and sometimes disconcerting.

The emphasis on choosing the right person to deliver the baby may seem overstated during the first part of pregnancy, but it's valuable to make the choice early because it enables the expectant mother to build a relationship with the doctor or midwife. Also, if a woman is to make a switch, it is easier to do so early in pregnancy. As pregnancy progresses most women become attached to the practitioner they have been seeing and find it harder and harder to make a break with the person. But ultimately it is worth all the effort for a mother and father to find a doctor or midwife they trust and feel comfortable with.

The Importance of Constant Companionship

In addition to picking a doctor, some women pick a labor coach or experienced woman friend to remain with them throughout labor and delivery. Many midwives and doctors have observed that women who are constantly attended during labor seem to be less anxious and to deal better with contractions. In 1974 Marshall Klaus and John Kennell, the neonatologists who were instrumental in developing the concept of mother-infant bonding, did bonding studies in Guatemala. In the course of these studies they noted a dramatic difference between unattended mothers and mothers who were continuously attended by a woman who had experience with childbirth but was not a midwife. This difference prompted Klaus and Kennell to do a study on the effect of a supportive companion during labor and delivery. They note that out of 150 cultures studied by anthropologists, a family member or friend remained with the mother continuously in all but one. In many cultures the midwife, grandmother, and husband all remained with the woman. Klaus and Kennell refer to a supportive lay woman by the term *doula.*

In their Guatemalan doula study Klaus and Kennell randomly divided first-time mothers into two groups. The first group was assisted by a lay woman, previously unknown to the mothers, who rubbed their backs, talked to them, and stayed with them throughout labor. In addition, this group was periodically checked by a nurse. The second group was simply visited by the nurse for checks. The findings of the study were remarkable. In the doula group the average labor was significantly shorter (9 hours versus 19 hours), and there were significantly fewer labor complications and problems with the newborn. Mothers in the doula group had a 12 percent cesarean rate, as opposed to a 19 percent rate in the other group, and required drugs or forceps only 7 percent of the time as opposed to 21 percent. Babies in the doula group had less incidence of fetal distress as evidenced by meconium staining (see p. 129) and by difficulty in breathing after birth. Mothers in this group also exhibited different behavior during bonding with their baby. Following the birth these mothers tended to remain awake longer, and they stroked, smiled at, and talked to their babies more. Often they had milk dripping from their nipples as soon as their baby was handed to them.

Klaus and Kennell theorize that these rather noteworthy differences are due to the fact that mothers in the doula group produced lower levels of stress hormones during childbirth because they were less anxious. They conclude that it is almost inevitable that a woman who is left alone in labor will become anxious and produce higher levels of stress hormones, interfering with uterine contractions and slowing down blood flow to the baby (see p. 140 and p. 276).

According to Klaus and Kennell, the concept of a constantly attended labor and delivery may be as important as the concept of bonding, and they strongly suggest that mothers have a supportive companion who remains with them continuously. They believe that family members may be more effective as doulas than people who are unknown to the mother, and that the father can function as a doula if he remains with the mother consistently. Many researchers agree with Klaus and Kennell's concept of constantly attended labor. The idea of the father staying with the mother during labor is not entirely new. Over the past ten to twenty years many United States hospitals have allowed the father to stay with the mother. What has not always been stressed is the value of the father's *continuous* presence.

Some researchers feel that it is important to have a female attendant and/or an experienced person present in addition to the father. They feel that another woman is more likely to have an intuitive grasp of the mother's feelings, that a woman is more likely to be sympathetic and attentive to the mother and less likely to become impatient with her or be influenced by a male obstetrician. A woman who is experienced in *managing* labor, as many midwives and mothers will attest, often has very specific nonmedical means for reassuring a mother and increasing her comfort during labor.

If an obstetrician is not able to provide continuous support, which is usually the case, and if the mother feels she would be helped by the presence of someone other than the father, she should decide if she wishes to be accompanied by a friend or labor coach. And then she should make arrangements with the practitioner and the hospital well ahead of her expected delivery date. Not all hospitals allow companions other than the father, and some obstetricians actually will not work with a labor coach. In either case, the mother needs to learn this early in case she then wishes to change her birth plans.

From our personal experience and research, it seems that the

(text continues on page 205)

Alternatives for childbirth

NONINTERVENTIONIST OBSTETRICS

- Mother allowed to move about freely in labor and delivery and pick her own positions.
- No medicines or medical procedures are routinely used.
- Birth is allowed to proceed in an instinctual, natural manner that is thought to optimize innate hormonal patterns that speed labor and produce natural opiates (endorphins) that make labor more comfortable, even ecstatic.
- Mother-baby bonding emphasized and baby is not separated from the mother.
- Not all mothers want or feel comfortable with this approach or have an uncomplicated labor or delivery.
- Many doctors believe such an approach puts some babies at greater risk, although a number of studies indicate that it is just as safe.
- Truly noninterventionist obstetrics is most readily available in the United States in home deliveries or alternative birth centers, although a number of obstetricians who deliver in hospitals generally agree with this philosophy.

INTERVENTIONIST OR TECHNICAL OBSTETRICS

- Uses routine medical procedures such as monitoring in an attempt to optimize the health of all newborns.
- Generally restricts mother's movements during labor and delivery.
- Does not always emphasize mother's participation, choice, or sense of intimacy.
- Definitely has a higher cesarean section rate.
- Techniques are thought by noninterventionists to slow labor and sometimes actually to cause labor and delivery complications.
- Thought by proponents to be the safest system in terms of infant health statistics.
- Currently most births in the United States tend toward the technical, although many obstetricians have personal philosophies that are relatively noninterventionist.

PREPARED CHILDBIRTH

- Mother participates fully in labor and delivery. She works hard, feels all sensations, is often uncomfortable at certain points, but generally has profound feelings of joy and accomplishment.

Alternatives for childbirth

- Mother and baby have no side effects from drugs that may complicate bonding or early nursing.
- Many methods are taught, including Lamaze, Bradley, Jacobson, Kitzinger, or individual systems. The trend is away from dogmatic systems (especially breathing techniques) and toward systems that allow the mother to follow her own body's signals.

MEDICATED CHILDBIRTH

- At present, anesthetics handled by skilled personnel have minimal side effects on the baby.
- Barbiturates and demerol given in low doses in early labor can help a mother who is very uncomfortable.
- A continuous epidural (anesthesia injected around the spinal cord) stops all sensation below the waist, allows the mother to move her legs and push, has minimal effects on the baby, and can be given during the entire latter part of labor. It is generally considered the best anesthesia for the latter part of labor, but may not be available in small hospitals without anesthesiologists.
- A spinal (a single shot of anesthesia injected *into* the spinal canal) not only stops all sensation below the waist, it prevents the mother from pushing and means the baby must be delivered with forceps or a vacuum extractor. It is not given until late in labor because it doesn't last long.
- Certain medications or some given in high doses depress the mother and baby. These include large amounts of Demerol or barbiturates, local nerve blocks like paracervicals, and general anesthesia.
- Noninterventionists believe that all medications alter the natural process of labor and delivery and may slow labor.

PRESENT AT LABOR AND DELIVERY

- Husband or father: familiar, loving, involved person who can be continuously present; may or may not be trained to coach mother in labor and won't be trained to deal with specific complications; occasionally may make mother anxious.
- Nurse: training, interest in, and motivation for prepared childbirth can vary widely; must follow hospital rules; not present continuously; goes off at end of shift regardless of mother's stage of labor; generally unknown to mother and not chosen by mother.
- Labor coach or doula: assists mother continuously throughout labor and delivery; may be prepared childbirth instructor, mid-

Alternatives for childbirth

wife, experienced friend, or, occasionally, the doctor; varies in experience with dealing with labor complications; sometimes not allowed by hospital rules; considered by many to be one of the most important aspects of birth care; some birth experts feel the doula must be a woman.

- Family members, friends, or siblings: reassure mother by promoting a nonmedical, intimate atmosphere, or may make mother more anxious (particularly children); often not allowed because of hospital rules.
- Others, including residents, medical students, or hospital observers: may decrease personal or sexual atmosphere of birth; may make mother anxious and slow labor; but are essential in training future doctors, labor coaches, and midwives.

LABOR PROCEDURES

- Noninterventionist approach involves no routine shave or enema, allows the mother to wear her own clothes, does a minimum of internal exams to see how labor is progressing, monitors the fetal heartbeat intermittently, and encourages mother to move about freely during labor and drink juice or tea.
- Interventionist approach may routinely use medical procedures such as IV, continuous fetal monitoring, artificial rupture of the membranes, and drugs to stimulate labor or ease discomfort.

DELIVERY PROCEDURES

- Noninterventionist approach allows a woman to choose her position for delivery; may use oil or massage to relax the perineum and avoid an episiotomy; dims lights to shield the baby's eyes; delays cutting of the cord until baby has received placental blood; allows the placenta to deliver naturally; only does cesareans for rare presentations or emergencies.
- Interventionist approach uses a delivery table with stirrups and surgical lights; does routine episiotomies to prevent perineal tearing; may use forceps or a vacuum extractor to deliver the baby; uses drugs or manually extracts the placenta; routinely does cesareans for dystocia (failure of labor to progress), as well as for emergencies, breech, and other presentations.

PROCEDURES THAT AFFECT BONDING

- Noninterventionists encourage bonding by placing the baby directly on the mother and allowing it to nurse and remain with the mother and father for at least an hour, often in private; by delaying weighing the baby and putting drops in its eyes, and in some cases by not routinely suctioning out the baby's nose and throat.

- Interventionists may briefly take the baby to weigh, measure, examine, suction out its nose and throat, and give a vitamin K shot and eyedrops.

- Some hospitals may routinely separate the newborn from its mother and place it in a nursery for variable amounts of time. This procedure does not allow bonding to take place in the critical period of the first hour after birth.

- In hospitals with full rooming-in the baby remains with the mother continuously and she has primary responsibility for it. Bonding researchers feel this situation optimizes bonding, lessens the chances of postpartum depression, and eases the mother's transition to caring for the baby at home.

- Hospitals and doctors vary in terms of when they routinely send mother and baby home. Some mothers are uncomfortable with hospitals and do better at home; other mothers feel more comfortable and get more rest if they remain in the hospital for several days.

importance of constant companionship cannot be overestimated and will be a growing trend in this country. However, whether the doula must be a woman is open to question. The answer depends in part on how comfortable the father feels in supporting the mother and how comfortable the mother feels with the father's support. The choice of a labor companion also depends on whether the mother happens to know a woman who she feels would be calm and supportive during her labor and delivery. This is not a situation of judgment but of personality—the mother's, the father's, and the doula's. In deciding who will attend her in labor, the mother is urged to follow her deepest intuitive feelings.

Whether an experienced labor coach is necessary or useful is a related question. The answer depends in part on how the mother's labor progresses and on whether there are complications, such as a breech presentation, that are beyond a mother's control. However, the events of labor are not generally predictable, and most midwives and labor coaches acknowledge that it is much more difficult to help a mother when they are called in late in labor. For these reasons we believe it is preferable for a mother to have an experienced labor coach or midwife attending her during labor and delivery, particularly with first deliveries.

Resource groups and organizations

American Academy of Husband Coached Childbirth
P.O. Box 5224
Sherman Oaks, Calif. 91413
(Teaches the Bradley method and has lists of local chapters.)

American Academy of Pediatrics
P.O. Box 1034
Evanston, Ill. 60204
(Has literature for parents and families.)

The American College of Home Obstetrics
664 North Michigan Avenue, Suite 600
Chicago, Ill. 60611

The American College of Nurse Midwives
1522 K Street, N.W., Suite 1120
Washington, D.C. 20005

American College of Obstetricians and Gynecologists
Suite 2700, Resource Center
1 East Wacker Drive
Chicago, Ill. 60601
(Has resource publication.)

American Foundation for Maternal and Child Health
30 Beekman Place
New York, N.Y. 10022

American Society for Psychoprophylaxis in Obstetrics (ASPO)
1840 Wilson Blvd.
Suite 204
Arlington, VA 22201
(Teaches Lamaze technique, offers literature, and has lists of local chapters.)
Association for Childbirth at Home, International
Box 1219
Cerritos, Calif. 90701

Cesarean/Support, Education, and Concern
22 Forest Road
Framingham, Mass. 01701

Cooperative Birth Center Network (CBCN)
Box 1, Route 1
Perkiomenville, Pa. 18074

Coping with the Overall Pregnancy Experience (COPE)
37 Clarendon Street
Boston, Mass. 02116

The Farm
156 Drakes Lane
Summertown, Tenn. 39483

Frontier Nursing Service
Wendover, Ky. 41775

Holistic Childbirth Institute
1627 10th Avenue
San Francisco, Calif. 94122

Home-Oriented Maternity Experience (HOME)
511 New York Avenue
Tacoma Park
Washington, D.C. 20010

Informed Home Birth, Inc.
P.O. Box 788
Boulder, Colo. 80306

International Childbirth Education Association (ICEA)
Box 20048
Minneapolis, Minn. 55420

La Leche League International, Inc.
9616 Minneapolis Avenue
Franklin Park, Ill. 60131
(Provides support for nursing mothers, list of local chapters, and a pattern for making a baby-carrier.)

MANA (Midwives' Alliance of North America)
% Concord Midwifery Service
30 So. Main St.
Concord, N.H. 03301

Maternity Center Association, Inc.
48 East 92nd Street
New York, N.Y. 10028
(Brochure on free publications.)

National Association of Parents and Professionals for Safe Alternatives in Childbirth (NAPSAC)
P.O. Box 267
Marble Hill, Mo. 63764
(Extensive directory of home-birth organizations throughout the world.)

U.S. Government Printing Office
Washington, D.C. 20402
(Information and publications on pregnancy.)

Yearly obstetrical report for a small general hospital

	TOTAL	VAGINAL	PRIMARY CESAREAN	REPEAT CESAREAN
Dr. A	112	93	21	8
Dr. B	75	53	18	4
Dr. C	44	39	5	–
Dr. D	77	52	12	13
Dr. E	85	54	21	10
Dr. F	77	60	12	5
Dr. G	149	95	43	11
Dr. H	84	65	14	5
Dr. I	32	27	4	1
Dr. J	74	60	10	4
Dr. K	73	54	14	5
Dr. L	38	27	8	3
Dr. M	43	32	9	2
Dr. N	31	25	3	3
Dr. O	51	40	6	5
Dr. P	102	79	18	5
Dr. Q	95	62	28	5
Dr. R*	25	25	0	0
Dr. S*	4	4	0	0
TOTAL	1295	952	253	91

* Cesareans performed by other doctors.

Primips (1st baby)	656	**TYPE OF DELIVERY**
Multips (2nd or 3rd baby, etc.)	629	Spontaneous	816
# babies delivered	1300	Low forceps	93
Males	646	Mid forceps	38
Females	654	VBAC's
Live births	1294	attempted	10
Stillborns	6	completed	15
Infant deaths (1 twin)	8	
Twins	13	**BREECHES**
Triplets	1	Primip cesarean	40
Under 2500 gms.	82	Multip cesarean	24
		Vaginal primip	3
		Vaginal multip	9
		Transverse lie	4

PLANNED HOME DELIVERY (IN HOSPITAL)		ANESTHESIA (continued)	
Vaginal	10	Pudendal	32
Cesarean	1	Local	678
		None	125

HOME DELIVERIES		INTRAPARIUM	
Drs. R & S	26	Episiotomy	572
Midwives	13		

ANESTHESIA		MONITORING	
Spinal vaginal	1	Fetal monitor used	1321
Spinal cesarean	9	External monitor	727
General vaginal	3	Internal electrode	449
General cesarean	24	Internal pressure	21
Epidural vaginal	101	pH scalp sampling	12
Epidural cesarean	311	OCT (stress test)	71
Caudal	1	Nonstress test	416
		Ritodrine (stop premature labor)	21

The Place of Birth

Just as a mother has a choice of *who* will deliver her baby, she also has some choice of *where* to deliver her baby. As in choosing a doctor or midwife, choosing the delivery site is a matter of personal style and obstetrical philosophy. One of the most important aspects of this decision is the degree of intervention inherent in the four most common birth settings: home, free-standing alternative birth center, alternative birth center within a hospital, and hospital delivery room.

By far the most common delivery site in this country is the hospital delivery room. The overwhelming majority of doctors who practice at hospitals or medical centers feel that a hospital is the safest place to deliver a baby because of its technical support system. At the same time, in recent years home birth has gained considerably in popularity, after dropping to very low levels in the United States during the 1950s and 1960s.

Options other than the hospital delivery room and the home have arisen recently, largely in an attempt to bridge the gap between the two extremes. The development of hospital- and non-hospital-related birth centers is attributable to a number of cultural factors. As

(text continues on page 212)

Place of birth

ADVANTAGES

- Widely available, traditional, accepted.
- Well-staffed by qualified doctors.
- ACOG regards hospitals as safest because of availability of surgical and emergency equipment and personnel.
- Equipped to handle high-risk patients and complicated labor and deliveries with fetal monitoring, sonograms, laboratory tests, anesthetics, blood transfusion, and cesarean sectioning.
- Resuscitation and infant intensive care available for newborns that are premature or ill.
- Technical, medical outlook during labor, delivery, and after birth reassures some mothers and makes them feel confident and comfortable.
- Hospital staff to care for mother and baby after birth can give mother physical help, rest, and support.
- Visiting hours, when limited, may keep new mother from becoming overtired.
- Presence of other new mothers and their infants may provide a special social experience.

DISADVANTAGES

- Greatest likelihood of routine use of medical interventionist techniques such as prepping, fetal monitoring, IV, induced labor, drugs, anesthetics, episiotomy.
- Greatest likelihood of medically caused complications or illness such as long or disturbed labor, baby depressed due to anesthetics, birth injuries due to forceps, mother tearing, or infections.
- Mother has least control over environment and is most subject to rules and procedures—during labor, delivery, and after birth.
- Hospital environment and procedures can be frightening, frustrating, insulting, or degrading.
- Hospital is generally an unfamiliar place with little privacy.
- Unlikely that mother will know her labor attendants, have them with her continuously, or have the same one throughout the whole labor.
- Mother most likely will have to remain in bed throughout labor and use a delivery table.
- Hospital rules often minimize mother's (and family's) early contact with the newborn.

- Most hospitals require the baby to be in the nursery for some period every day.
- Hospital births tend to be expensive.

BIRTH ROOMS AND BIRTH CENTERS

ADVANTAGES

- Combine availability of technical medical services with warmth of nonmedical atmosphere.
- More likely to be staffed by nurse-midwives.
- Physicians and nurses staffing birth rooms tend to be less interventionist than those in technical hospital settings.
- Support natural childbirth and bonding.
- Hospital rules are minimized.
- Mother can have family members, labor coach, and friends present for labor and delivery.
- Mother does not have to move from room to room during labor and delivery.
- Mother can often go home soon after birth.
- Generally less expensive than a regular hospital delivery.
- Increasingly available.

DISADVANTAGES

- Birth centers not close to a hospital have less immediate access to some medical equipment.
- Still may involve a fair amount of medical rules and intervention—for example, some birth rooms routinely require monitoring, others won't admit mothers over 35.
- Still an unfamiliar environment that a mother must go to.

HOME DELIVERIES

ADVANTAGES

- Mother is in a familiar, supportive place—does not have to be moved, and has the most control over her environment.
- Mother avoids unfamiliar and/or unsupportive attendants.
- Nurse-midwife is present for the whole labor.
- Family and friends can be present at any point and for any amount of time.
- Least chance of medical intervention and possible ensuing problems.
- Best environment for bonding; baby need never be separated from mother.
- Least expensive.

HOME DELIVERIES *cont.*

DISADVANTAGES

- Many women are consciously or unconsciously apprehensive about the unconventionality of home deliveries and their possible dangers.
- Technical and emergency training of medical staff may vary (especially in infant resuscitation) and be difficult to assess.
- Medical procedures and extra personnel not available (*see Hospital advantages*).
- If problems arise, mother must be transported to the hospital in active labor or after the baby is born.
- Considered less safe than a hospital birth by ACOG (although a number of studies indicate home delivery is as safe).
- Not widely available.

prepared childbirth became popular in the United States in the 1950s and 1960s, mothers came to view birth as a natural event in which they could actively participate rather than as an illness that required medical procedures. The increasing adoption of prepared childbirth by obstetricians also made women aware of the influence that consumer pressure could have on the medical profession. The women's movement lent further support to the idea of women being responsible for their own bodies and taking control of their own lives. Finally, the rise in popularity of holistic medicine in the 1970s emphasized health, rather than illness, as a reference point. And it made people aware of the negative effects sometimes wrought by medical intervention and drugs, as opposed to more natural remedies.

Hospital births of the 1960s not only tended to make birth a technical medical procedure, they almost always separated the mother and baby for a significant period of time soon after birth. Such rigid, rule-oriented circumstances further increased mothers' dissatisfactions with hospital births in those years. Fortunately, the studies of Klaus and Kennell showing the positive effects of mother-infant bonding (see p. 467), combined with consumer pressure, have resulted in sweeping changes in birth and newborn nursery procedures.

Studies showing that mothers who had home births were more relaxed and had less complications with labor and delivery convinced many birth experts that home birth had some compelling features. Ultimately this led doctors to incorporate some of the positive aspects of home birth into special hospital environments such as alternative birth centers and even into normal hospital rules and regulations. However, medical developments simultaneously caused obstetrics to become more technical and more interventionist, as shown by the recent rise in fetal monitoring, cesarean sections, and amniocentesis.

HOME BIRTHS

Generally the least technical, least interventionist birth takes place when the mother delivers at home, attended by a well-trained midwife or doctor. Because home births are the most natural and take place in quiet, familiar, private circumstances, the mothers tend to be more relaxed and less frightened. The mother is free to move around and free to choose who is with her at various stages, including any older children. The home delivery mother is never left alone and is never

Common criteria for home delivery

INITIAL SCREENING

- Maternal age between 18 and 35 for a first baby, between 18 and 40 for subsequent births
- Less than 20 minutes travel time to the backup hospital
- Healthy mother with no preexisting chronic diseases
- Normal obstetrical history with no previous pregnancy complications for mother or baby
- No previous cesarean section (generally)

REASONS FOR RULING OUT HOME DELIVERY

- Development of a medical problem such as high blood pressure, excess amniotic fluid, herpes (within 6 weeks of delivery), intrauterine growth retardation, placenta previa, or abruptio placenta
- Determination of inadequate pelvis for this particular baby
- Breech presentation or twins (generally)

CAUSES FOR TRANSFER TO HOSPITAL

- Premature labor
- Premature rupture of membranes (sometimes)
- Inaccessibility of hospital due to weather conditions
- Failure of labor to progress
- Meconium staining of the amniotic fluid
- Fetal distress during labor
- Excessive maternal bleeding
- Retained placenta or deep tear requiring surgery
- Poor condition of baby, including low birth weight, respiratory distress, low Apgar score, or development of neonatal jaundice

separated from her baby or members of her family. Studies have shown that these mothers are often in a state of ecstasy after they give birth. Klaus and Kennell have called this exuberance after a home birth *ekstasis,* and they have found that observers at the birth were also elated. They note that there is invariably tremendous support and attention directed toward the mother both during and after the birth.

Several studies have shown that home deliveries are as safe as hospital deliveries. The researcher Tew found that the shift from home birth to hospital birth that took place in England between 1965 and 1974 did not result in improved newborn health statistics. In the Netherlands the Dutch home birth expert Kloosterman found that there was no difference in infant mortality statistics between cities that had 50 percent home births and cities that had 100 percent hospital births. In the United States a study by Estes on 418 planned home births, of which 289 were completed, showed that the infant mortality rate among babies delivered at home was lower than that of babies delivered in the hospital.

In the United States Mehl matched 1,046 women who planned a home delivery (all but 12 of whom eventually delivered at home) with an equal number of women who planned a hospital birth. He found no difference between the two groups in terms of infant mortality or neurological problems. Moreover, he found that the women who delivered in the hospital had much higher rates of all manner of obstetrical interventions, including drugs to promote labor, episiotomy, forceps, c-sections, and anesthesia. Mehl also found that hospital mothers had greater rates of complications, including tears, fetal distress, failure of labor to progress, birth injuries, and newborn infection. Only one large study, done in Oregon in 1977, found that home birth was less safe for babies. Out of 200,000 hospital births and 3,000 home births, it was found that the neonatal death rate was twice as great among babies born at home. Both Mehl's study and the Oregon study have been called into question for their scientific methods. Mehl's study was criticized because the sample was too small and the groups were not well matched. The Oregon study was criticized because the two groups were not matched in any way and the home group included many unattended births, as well as miscarriages and unplanned premature deliveries. Definitive studies of the relative safety of home birth versus hospital birth are still to come.

Most reputable physicians and midwives who deliver at home believe that home delivery is a safe alternative for a well-screened low-risk population, that is, for mothers who are healthy, have careful prenatal care, and have a pregnancy with no medical complications. But even among a well-screened population, Kloosterman estimates that there is a real but very small risk of less than 1 per 1000 that a complication will arise in which the transit time to a hospital would be a serious disadvantage to the mother or baby.[1] He suggests that parents

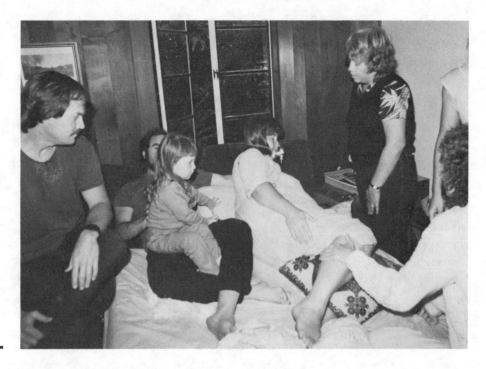

A home delivery allows a woman to give birth in familiar surroundings with a minimum of medical intervention. Photo by Linda O'Neil.

must weigh this risk against the atmosphere of a hospital birth and the problems sometimes caused by hospital procedures.

The home birth movement has contributed greatly to current obstetrical thought and practice, affecting the experience of even those mothers who give birth in hospitals. Many leading birth experts believe that home birth is probably the ideal situation for delivery and bonding. Sheila Kitzinger, the British childbirth educator, has said, "The birth of a child is a family event and as such should, ideally, take place at home as a normal part of life."[2] On the other hand, the highly respected Harvard pediatrician T. Berry Brazelton has said, "I am not entirely in favor of home births, although I see their value at the present time—as a way for a mother to establish herself as being in control of this important event in her life. . . . I would much prefer that hospitals or hospices make such an attractive, homelike, family situation available that there was no need to push for home births. In other words, if home births are on the rise, the medical system has no one to blame but itself."[3]

ALTERNATIVE BIRTH CENTERS

Alternative birth centers, whether within or separate from a hospital, are intended to bridge the gap between home birth and a hospital delivery room. Alternative birth centers have a more informal, home-like, nonmedical atmosphere with easy chairs, plants, and stereos. More important, the nurses and doctors who work there generally have a noninterventionist philosophy toward birth. When a mother gives birth in such a center, she is much less likely to have medication

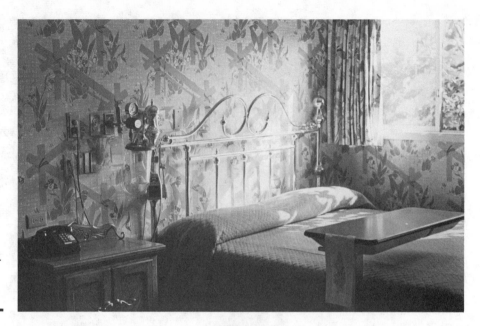

An alternative birth center gives a mother a mixture of the advantages of a home delivery and a hospital delivery. Photo by Michael Samuels.

or medical procedures. Although there is tremendous variation in whether or not the same person remains with the mother continuously, most birth centers are staffed by practitioners, labor coaches, and nurses who have extensive experience with natural childbirth. Many centers also routinely allow friends and siblings to be present at the birth. Finally, most birth centers have an excellent atmosphere for bonding and their rules are structured to promote it.

Freestanding alternative birth centers (not within a hospital) such as the Maternity Center in New York City, generally, have the most informative educational programs, allow the mother the most control, and are the least interventionist. But many doctors are not in favor of freestanding centers because they involve transportation to a hospital in case of an emergency.

Birth rooms, alternative birth centers located within hospitals, have proximity to emergency medical care. For this reason they are more often staffed and controlled by doctors and hospital nurses; in many cases midwives are not allowed to practice at hospital birth rooms. As opposed to freestanding birth centers, birth rooms may vary widely in how noninterventionist they are. The associated hospital's rules and the doctor's philosophy will both affect this. Many hospitals have rather strict protocol for their birth centers. For example, women over the age of thirty-five may be excluded simply because of their age, no matter what their health status. But it has become increasingly possible for a mother to find a doctor or midwife who will deliver her in a birth room with the same lack of intervention as characterizes home births or alternative birth centers.

One of the most famous birth centers in the world is run by Dr. Michel Odent at the public hospital in Pithiviers, France. Instead of a delivery table or bed, the birth room in Pithiviers simply has a low

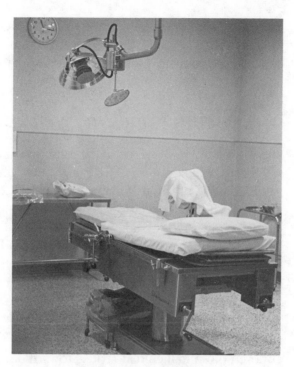

A hospital delivery provides access to the most up-to-date technology. Photo by Michael Samuels.

platform covered with mats and cushions, to encourage the mother to choose her own position throughout labor and delivery. In an adjacent room there is a low hot tub, which is sometimes used to help a woman relax during early labor. Odent believes in providing mothers with a calm, intimate, private setting in which their instinctive knowledge of birth can be their guide. Most women at Pithiviers deliver in a supported squatting position without intervention. Medical authorities such as Marshall Klaus, Sheila Kitzinger, and Elizabeth Noble believe that Pithiviers is a model hospital birth center and that many of its practices point to the future of obstetrics.

THE HOSPITAL DELIVERY ROOM

The hospital delivery room is still the site of the great majority of births in this country. Although a delivery room birth is likely to be medical in nature, it can vary greatly in how interventionist it is, depending on the philosophy of the doctor and on the rules of the hospital. Even in the least interventionist centers, the delivery room has a medical atmosphere, and hospital rules tend to take control of the birth away from the mother.

Most practicing obstetricians in the United States feel that in terms of infant mortality, the hospital is statistically the safest site for delivery, particularly for mothers whose pregnancy or labor has been associated with any risk factors. In a hospital delivery the mother and baby have all the advantages of the most up-to-date technology, along with the possible psychological and medical disadvantages that can accompany medical procedures. But even in hospital delivery rooms there is a trend toward a more natural delivery and increased control for the mother. Again, the degree to which this is true varies greatly depending upon the doctor and the hospital.

Siblings and the New Baby

Having a baby is an event that profoundly affects the whole family, siblings as well as parents. No matter how much siblings look forward to the coming of the new baby, they cannot help being affected by variations in family relationships, routines, and living arrangements. These changes require adaptation on the part of all family members. This adaptation needn't be stressful or negative; it can be a source of excitement and stimulation for growth and development. But too many changes at once, even good ones, can be overwhelming, especially for children.

Psychologists have identified a number of characteristics common to children after the birth of a sibling. On the positive side, children often make great strides toward developmental landmarks and become more independent in response to the presence of a new baby. On the negative side, older siblings tend to go through a period of attention-getting and regression. Children of all ages frequently become hostile or aggressive with the new baby, their mother, or playmates. Studies have shown that 90 percent of children under the age of three, particularly boys, have distinctly negative reactions to the birth of a sib. Studies also show that young children temporarily have a significant increase in problems with their daily routines. For unknown reasons, both boys and girls seem to react more negatively to the birth of a brother than a sister. As the new baby gets older and

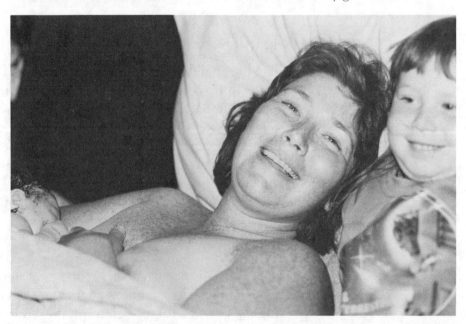

Young children should be given special preparation if they are to witness the birth of a sibling. Photo by Linda O'Neil.

begins to move about, the problems between the siblings are likely to be accentuated rather than to drop off.

Psychologists believe that at least some of the problems encountered among older siblings are due to their being separated from the mother at the time of the birth. Much of this separation is caused by hospital rules and regulations. Studies have shown that when older sibs can visit the mother—even once—during her hospital stay, much of the disturbance caused by the separation is eased.

In addition to separation from the mother, there are a number of other changes that immediately take place in the sibs' lives. For instance, many families make changes in their living space, either moving or reorganizing. In either case, siblings often end up in a new bedroom. This can be particularly upsetting for very young sibs who were sleeping with the parents and are now displaced by the new baby. Most psychologists agree that all such moves are less traumatic if they are made well in advance of the baby's arrival.

Recently there has been a trend toward having siblings present at deliveries, most commonly with ones at home or in alternative birth centers. It is thought by some birth educators that including siblings at the birth will minimize their separation anxiety and lessen future sibling rivalry. Thus far, there are no studies of the long-term effects on siblings who attend a birth, but there are studies on how siblings behave during a birth. Typically, in the first part of labor sibs interact with their mother, but as labor progresses and she becomes more self-involved, they tend to draw back and observe her. After the delivery they become involved with the new baby, looking at it and touching it. Although none of the children became terribly upset by the birth, some did seem to be upset with certain aspects of labor and delivery. Six- to ten-year-olds in particular found the blood to be upsetting, but most children ignore the surgical aspects or only watch intermittently during these parts. Two studies of home births found the experience to be positive for most children. An Australian study showed no difference two months after the birth between sibs who had been present at the delivery and those who had not.

Because of the current lack of data concerning long-term effects on siblings who attend a birth, many researchers in the field, including Marshall Klaus and John Kennell, question the practice. Leonard, who has done several sibling studies, suggests that children under four not be present unless there are older siblings who can participate with them. The English sib experts the Robertsons advise against having young sibs present because they cannot adequately verbalize fears that are aroused and thus be reassured about them. The pioneering French obstetrician Michel Odent also questions whether the presence of siblings may not adversely affect the mother, preventing her from following her most instinctive feelings. However, other researchers point to the positive responses of some children who

Helping sibs deal with birth of a new baby

BEFORE THE BIRTH

- Make sleeping, school and day-care changes far in advance.
- Explain to the child about the new baby and encourage questions.
- Involve the child in preparing for the new baby and in making arrangements for housekeeping after the baby is born, for example, washing baby clothes or freezing meals.
- If planning a hospital birth, show pictures of the hospital room or take the child for a visit if possible; also have the child practice talking to the mother on the phone.
- Discuss with the child where he or she will be during the birth and who will be with him or her. Solicit ideas and feelings, and try to pick the most supportive plan—having a close friend or relative come to the home *or* taking the child to the home of a close friend or relative.
- If children are to be present at the birth, prepare them in advance through discussion and pictures that demonstrate how much blood there is and how the baby, umbilical cord, and placenta will look.

DURING BIRTH

- If the child is not present at the birth and labor is slow, call the child occasionally to let him or her know how the mother is progressing.
- If the child is present at the birth, make sure one person takes care of him or her, explains what is happening, and sees that the child gets to eat or sleep when necessary; the child should be encouraged to come and go from the room at will.

AFTER THE BIRTH

- After a hospital birth, the mother should go home as soon as she feels able to, in order to minimize separation from other children.
- Daily sibling visits to see the mother (especially) and the baby in the hospital should be strongly encouraged at times when the children are not hungry or sleepy.
- If the children were present at the birth, they should be encouraged to talk about their impressions of it.
- If the mother is breast-feeding, she should not be surprised if a younger child wants to try nursing again; if the mother is not comfortable with this, she can simply express some milk for the child to taste.

attend a birth and to the absence of short-term ill effects as support for the idea of having children share the birth experience.

Thus parents must make their own decision as to whether they wish to have siblings present. Much of the choice is determined by where the mother gives birth, because very few hospitals in the United States allow sibs to be present. Ultimately what matters is the way the parents, and in particular the mother, feel about having the children present. If the parents feel at ease and excited about the prospect, they'll be encouraging and supportive of the children. But if the mother or father feels ambivalent or uncomfortable, he or she may communicate these feelings to the children, which could make the situation more difficult for the mother. At least two birth centers have found that a large number of parents who initially show interest in having sibs witness the birth do not bring their children along when the mother goes into labor.

Not only should the parents consider how they feel about having the children present, they need to consult with the children about *their* feelings. If a decision is made to have the children present, they should be prepared in advance. The parents should discuss with the children on a number of occasions how labor and delivery proceed, how the mother will feel, the noises she will make from work or discomfort, and what they will see. In particular, they should explain why there is blood when the baby is born, how the baby will appear, and what the placenta will look like. Some childbirth educators advise parents to show the child colored pictures, slides, or movies. Many parents who have had their children present at a birth advise that one adult should be there just to take care of the sibs, talk to them, feed them, and take them out of the room whenever they or the mother wish it. If possible, the children should be given some choice in who takes care of them.

The choices a woman makes about childbirth will radically affect her satisfaction with the experience. The decisions about who will deliver her, where she will give birth, and who will be present to help her should be made after careful thought and discussion. Often these decisions are particularly difficult for the first-time mother to make because she lacks either experience or knowledge. We hope that by emphasizing these choices and providing detailed information about them we will help each woman to pick the alternatives that will make the birth experience most positive for her and her baby.

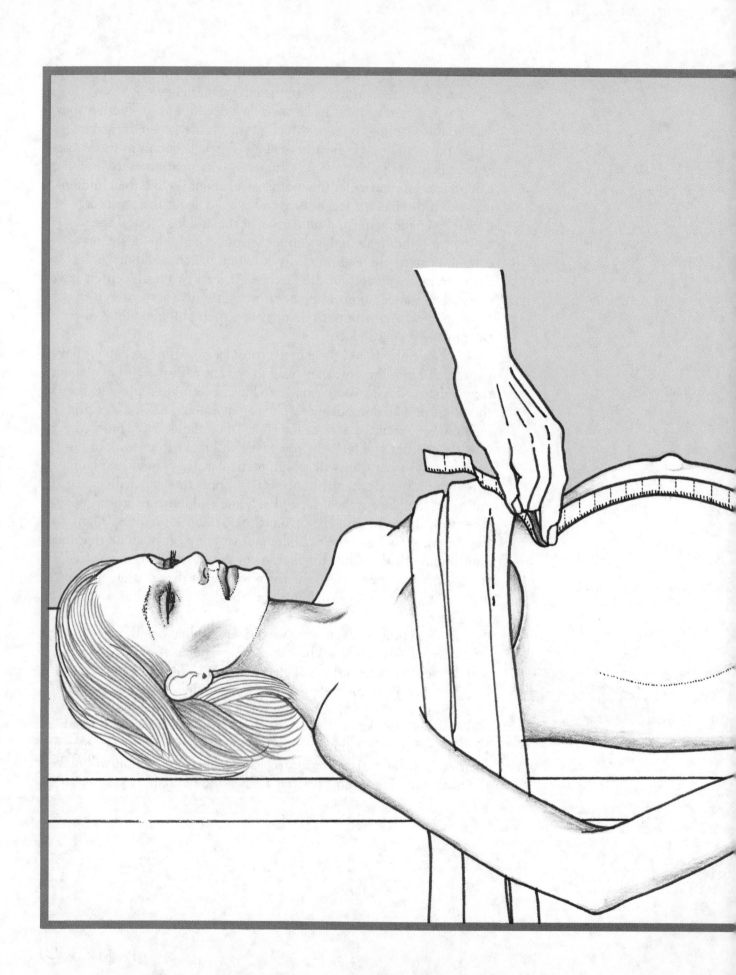

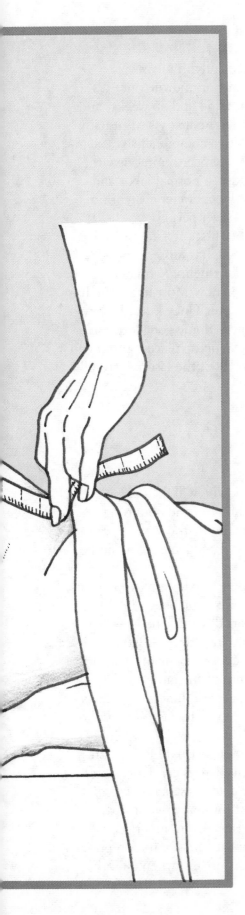

Prenatal Care and Medical Concerns

Prenatal Care

Good prenatal care is essential for optimizing the health of mother and infant. Prenatal care is true preventive medicine. It has emotional and educational aspects that are the primary considerations for the great majority of women who have healthy, uncomplicated pregnancies. The expectant mother's routine appointments allow her to become familiar with the person or persons who will assist her in delivering the baby. During her prenatal visits the mother can establish a relationship with the doctor or midwife based on trust and understanding, and the practitioner likewise has a chance to get to know the mother. At each stage of her pregnancy the mother has a chance to talk about the medical, emotional, and practical concerns that she has. Finally, she becomes used to dealing intimately with her body in the presence of medical people. Often this takes some time, particularly for women who have not been pregnant before and are not used to going to doctors.

The majority of women routinely go through their prenatal visits without any problems, but regular visits to the doctor or midwife can help to pick up potential problems. Early detection and treatment of such uncommon problems as high blood pressure, gestational diabetes, small-for-date babies, or twins or breech presentations increase the chances of making sure the baby will be healthy.

In the United States prenatal care typically involves six to twelve hours total. The mother sees the doctor or midwife once a month until she is 32 weeks pregnant, again at 34 and 36 weeks, and then weekly thereafter until the baby is born. The first visit is usually a long one, in which the doctor or midwife does a comprehensive examination, and the mother (and father) have a chance to interview the practitioner and find out how he or she handles a normal labor and delivery (see p. 199). Subsequent visits involve a briefer evaluation, some routine lab tests, and a question-and-answer period.

Generally, by the time she goes for her first prenatal visit, a woman already knows that she is pregnant. She has missed a period, and she may have noticed breast tenderness or tingling, and perhaps nausea, fatigue, constipation, or urinary frequency. Most likely she has confirmed her pregnancy either with a home pregnancy kit or by having a lab do a urine or blood test for human chorionic gonadotropin (HCG). HCG is a hormone made by the developing placenta that can be detected as early as 42 days after the *first* day of the last menstrual period.

THE INITIAL VISIT

The History

During the first visit the doctor or midwife will do a complete physical exam, including performing some lab tests and obtaining a full history. Although some women don't realize it, the history provides the doctor with information that is just as valuable as the findings from the physical exam and the tests.

First the mother's general health will be reviewed to find out if she has or has ever had illnesses that might affect the baby's health, such as high blood pressure, diabetes, or heart disease. Then she will be questioned about her reproductive history, including previous pregnancies, miscarriages, abortions, stillbirths, congenital malformations, or cesareans. Next, her family history and that of the father will be taken, concentrating on multiple births and genetic illnesses, such as chromosomal abnormalities, mental retardation, Tay-Sachs disease, or sickle-cell anemia.

The doctor or midwife will also take a menstrual history, stressing the date of the last menstrual period. This date is crucial to determining the baby's *gestational age* and the *due date* or *estimated date of confinement*. The gestational age is important for many reasons, the main one being that the doctor or midwife uses this information in assessing the baby's growth each time the mother comes in for a prenatal visit. Gestational age becomes of prime concern when a mother goes into labor prematurely, since the more premature a baby is, the more likely it is to have medical problems.

In calculating the actual date of conception, the doctor or midwife will question the mother closely about the length of her last menstrual period and the amount of flow. About 20 percent of the time mothers actually experience spotting at the time of implantation (see p. 58), which roughly corresponds with the time of the first missed period in women who have a 28-day cycle. Occasionally a mother spots during the first month and doesn't realize that she is pregnant, which can throw off the due date by a month.

The due date is calculated according to *Knaegele's rule:* 7 days are added to the first day of the last *true* menstrual period, and then three months are subtracted. Technical as this formula sounds, it is at best a guess, particularly if a mother has irregular periods. There are several other fairly accurate ways that gestational age can be estimated or confirmed at a later time. For example, the menstrual information can be compared with the mother's first awareness of *fetal movement.* This normally takes place at 18 to 20 weeks with a first pregnancy and at 16 to 18 weeks with subsequent pregnancies. Another basis for confirmation is *fetal heart sounds,* which are normally first heard at 16 to 20 weeks with an obstetrical stethoscope called a *fetoscope,* or between 12 to 20 weeks with an ultrasound device called a *Doptone.* Some practitioners prefer to use a fetoscope in initial prenatal visits so that the baby is not unnecessarily exposed to ultrasound in the early developmental stages. The doctor or midwife can also confirm the due date by the size of the enlarging uterus, as routinely determined by physical examination. In certain circumstances an *ultrasound examination* may also be used to visualize the baby's size and corroborate its gestational age.

In calculating the due date it's important to keep in mind that few babies are actually born on the calculated due date, which is just an estimate based on the average length of pregnancy. In fact, most babies are born sometime within two weeks before or after their due date. This is useful for parents to keep in mind, so that they don't fix their minds on a particular day. When parents do this, they can find themselves shocked if the baby comes earlier than expected or frustrated if the baby is later.

The Physical Exam

The second part of the initial visit involves a complete physical and an extended gynecological exam. Generally a nurse will record the mother's weight and height as a baseline for comparison throughout the pregnancy and as a context for nutritional counseling. The nurse will also take the mother's blood pressure to make sure it is within satisfactory limits. This figure too will be used as a baseline for comparison throughout pregnancy.

The doctor or midwife will then proceed with a regular physical exam, first checking the mother's general appearance to assess her overall health, energy level, and emotional state. Next the practitioner will check the skin for pallor or rashes, the eyes for signs of high blood pressure, and the ears, gums, and throat for signs of infection. Then he or she will feel the mother's neck and throat to check on the size of her thyroid, listen to her heart and lungs to rule out respiratory or cardiac problems, and examine her back, muscles, and joints to check for strength and alignment.

The last part of the physical exam involves three purely obstetrical aspects. First, the doctor or midwife will examine the mother's abdomen, feel her uterus, and measure the height of her uterus from the *fundus* or top to the pubic bone. There is a direct correlation between the height of the fundus and the age of the baby. Up to 12 weeks, the fundus is equal to or below the pubic bone. Thereafter, the height of the fundus increases in a regular progression (see p. 230). In examining the abdomen, the practitioner will also look for stretch marks or scars from abdominal surgery, as well as check the muscles in the middle of the abdomen to see if they have become separated during a previous pregnancy (see p. 102–03). Depending upon the timing of the initial visit, the doctor or midwife may also feel for fetal movements, listen for fetal heartbeat (see p. 225), and in the later months of pregnancy will determine what position the baby is in (see following).

The second part of the reproductive exam is a standard vaginal checkup. As in any pelvic exam, the doctor or midwife will look for rashes or a discharge that would indicate a vaginal infection, or any tenderness. Then the practitioner will insert a *speculum* into the vagina, look at the cervix, take a Pap smear, and do a gonorrhea culture. Next is a *bi-manual exam* in which the woman's uterus and ovaries are felt with one hand on the abdomen and the other in the vagina. This reveals the tilt of the uterus, and its softness and mobility. At the end of the bi-manual exam, the doctor or midwife will insert one finger into the mother's rectum. This enables the practitioner to feel the uterus and ovaries from the back and from an inch further up than the vagina allows.

The third part of the reproductive exam involves determining the size and shape of the mother's pelvis to make sure that it is adequate for the baby's head to pass through during delivery. Few women have a pelvis that is too small for a vaginal delivery; the human female pelvis has evolved over millions of years to fulfill just this need. During the vaginal exam the doctor or midwife will feel the woman's pubic bones in front, the symphysis where the pubic bones meet, the side-

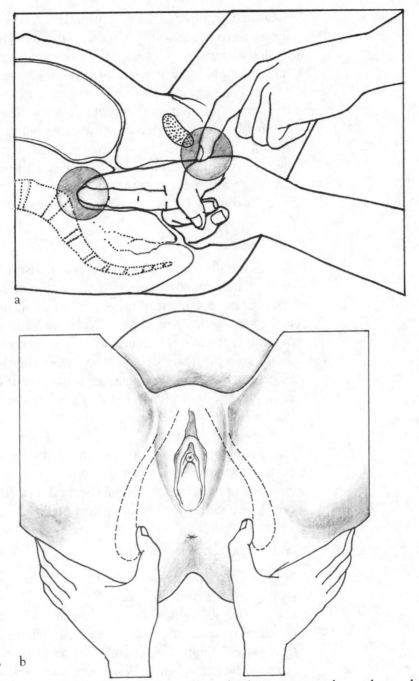

a

During the initial pregnancy exam the doctor or midwife will determine the size and shape of the mother's pelvis to make certain it is adequate for the baby to pass through. The doctor measures both the inlet, *the distance from the sacral promontory to the pubic bone (a), and the out-let,* the distance between the ischial spines (b).

b

walls of the pelvic basket, the ischial spines on either side, and the sacrum and coccyx at the back (see p. 28).

To measure from the back to the front of the pelvis, the practitioner inserts the index and middle fingers into the vagina until they touch a bump at the bottom of the sacrum called the *sacral promontory,* and then tilts these fingers up until the side of the index finger hits the pubic bone in the front (see illustration). The other hand is used to mark where the pubic bone hits, and the span is measured on a ruler. This distance, which is referred to as the *diagonal conjugate,* is the only way that the *inlet,* the top of the pelvic basket (see p. 29), can be measured on physical examination. It is one of the most important measures in determining whether a mother's pelvis is large enough for a vaginal delivery. Occasionally women find this part of the exam uncomfortable, but it does not take long.

Next the doctor or midwife measures the diameter of the *outlet*, the bottom of the pelvic basket. This measurement gauges the distance from one side of the pelvis to the other between bumps called the ischial tuberosities. The distance is judged externally, using either calipers or the practitioner's hand. The practitioner locates the bumps by pressing against the mother's buttocks while she has her legs in stirrups or pulls them back.

Lab Tests

Finally, during the first prenatal visit certain routine laboratory work is done on the mother. Blood is drawn from her arm for several tests: a *hemoglobin test* to make certain she is not anemic, a *VDRL* to make sure she does not have *syphilis,* and a *rubella antibody titer* to determine if she has immunity to German measles. This sample is also used to establish what blood type the mother has and whether her blood is Rh positive or negative. In the event that the mother is Rh negative, she is often given a *RhoGam* shot at 28 weeks to prevent her from making antibodies against the baby's blood type which used to be the cause of "blue babies" (see p. 48). A urine sample is taken to do a routine *glucose test* to make sure the mother is not developing *gestational diabetes* (see pp. 47–48), a *protein test* to make sure she is not developing proteinuria (see p. 48), and a culture to make sure she does not have a kidney or bladder infection.

SUBSEQUENT VISITS

Subsequent visits are generally much briefer, although a number of matters are regularly checked. First the doctor or midwife will talk to the mother about how she is feeling and whether or not she has any problems or concerns such as morning sickness, backache, constipation, or leg cramps (see chart). The practitioner will also ask about symptoms such as headaches, visual problems, dizziness, or swelling of the ankles, face, or hands that might indicate a complicated condition called *preeclampsia* (see p. 265). Finally, he or she will also check to make sure that the mother does not have any signs such as abdominal pain or vaginal bleeding that might indicate premature labor or placental problems.

At each prenatal visit the mother's blood pressure is routinely checked and a urine sample is taken to make certain that she is not spilling protein or glucose. She will also be weighed, and the increase will be compared with the normal range of weight gain for the baby's gestational age (see p. 92). The mother's weight gain gives a good indication of her nutritional status and some indication of how the baby is growing. Current expectations are that the mother will gain an average of 10 pounds in the first 20 weeks and 15 pounds in the second half of pregnancy.

During routine visits the doctor or midwife will do a brief phys-

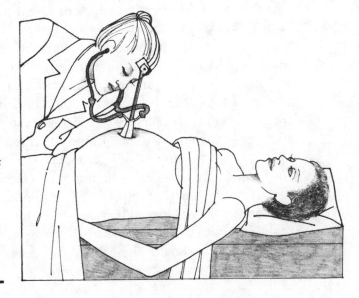

At each visit the doctor or midwife listens for the fetal heartbeat with a fetoscope (as shown) or a Doptone. The first fetal heart sounds are generally heard at 16 to 20 weeks with a fetoscope, and as early as 12 weeks with a Doptone.

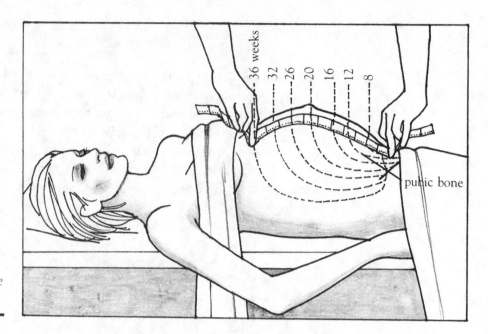

36 weeks
32
26
20
16
12
8

pubic bone

At each prenatal visit the doctor or midwife measures the distance from the pubic bone to the fundus, *the top of the uterus. This measure gives a very good indication of the rate at which the baby is growing. Between 18 and 30 weeks the height of the fundus in centimeters approximately equals the age of the baby in weeks.*

ical exam, measuring the height of the mother's fundus and comparing it with previous measurements. Along with the mother's weight gain, the height of the fundus gives a good indication of the baby's rate of growth. As mentioned earlier, the height of the fundus is equal to or below the pubic bone during the first 12 weeks of pregnancy. At 16 weeks the fundus is about halfway between the pubis and the navel. Between 18 and 30 weeks of pregnancy the height of the fundus in centimeters should equal the age of the baby in weeks.

   In the brief physical exam the doctor or midwife will check the mother's ankles for swelling and question her as to whether she feels fetal movements, and if so, how frequent they are. The practitioner will also listen to the mother's abdomen with a fetoscope or Doptone to check for fetal heartbeat. With the Doptone, the practitioner can hear the fetal heartbeat and demonstrate it to the mother between 9 and 12 weeks, long before she can even feel fetal movements.

   During the latter part of pregnancy, as part of the physical exam, the doctor or midwife will routinely feel the mother's abdomen to check what position the baby is in. This is traditionally done using the *maneuvers of Leopold,* a set of four classic hand positions. First the practitioner gently palpates or touches the top of the abdomen with the tips of the fingers to determine whether the baby's head or rump is at the top of the uterus: the head feels hard and round and moves in response to a gentle push; the rump feels larger, bulkier, bumpier, and doesn't move much in response to pressure. In the second maneuver the practitioner palpates the sides of the mother's abdomen with the palms in order to see which way the baby is facing: the baby's back feels smooth and hard; the baby's front has both soft and hard bumps that may move in response to pressure.

Generally the third and fourth maneuvers simply confirm the information yielded by the first two. In the third maneuver the doctor or midwife takes the thumb and opposing fingers of one hand and presses just above the mother's pubic bone. This maneuver verifies whether the head or rump is at the bottom, as determined by the first maneuver. Often the practitioner can feel the baby's brow if the head is down, thereby confirming which way the baby is facing as established by the second maneuver.

In the fourth maneuver the doctor or midwife places hands on the sides of the mother's abdomen, facing her legs. The hands are slid down around the baby to reconfirm whether it is up or down and which way it is facing. During the last several weeks of pregnancy this maneuver will also allow the practitioner to determine if the head or presenting part is *engaged,* that is, if it has dropped down into the pelvic canal. Once this occurs the head will not be movable. With a first pregnancy, engagement, or *lightening,* takes place in the last few weeks before delivery; with subsequent pregnancies, engagement takes place during labor. When the baby is head down but not engaged—the most common position during prenatal checkups—the practitioner's hand will stop when it bumps the baby's brow, while the other hand will continue to slide down the mother's abdomen unhindered. This maneuver tells the doctor or midwife the angle of the baby's head as well as whether it is engaged.

Taken together, the four maneuvers give extensive and valuable information on the baby's position. For this reason they are also used when the mother goes into labor. During this part of the exam a

(text continues on page 235)

a

b

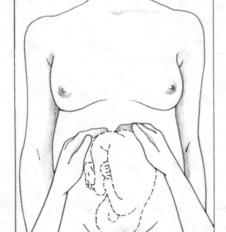
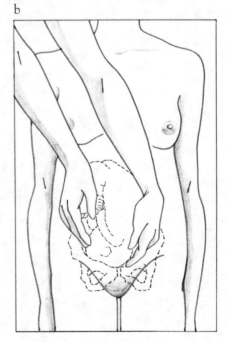

At each visit in the latter part of pregnancy the doctor or midwife will check the baby's position or lie, with a series of four hand maneuvers. The first maneuver determines if the baby's rump or head is at the top of the uterus (a). The second maneuver tells which way the baby is facing (b).

Common concerns of pregnant women

Nutrition (see pp. 75–93)
- Get a balanced diet to meet increased nutritional needs, paying particular attention to extra protein and calories.
- Gain an average of 25 to 30 pounds: approximately 10 pounds by 20 weeks, and another 15 pounds in the remaining 20 weeks.
- Take iron, folic acid, and vitamin C supplements in the second and third trimesters.
- Eat a high-fiber diet with lots of fruits and vegetables to avoid common problems with constipation and hemorrhoids.

Exercise (see pp. 95–109)
- Do pelvic and abdominal exercises throughout pregnancy.
- Avoid straight sit-ups, weight lifting, or other exercise that involves holding the breath which elevates intra-abdominal pressure.
- Do aerobic exercises at a conversational pace.
- Precede exercise with a slow warm-up and follow with a slow stretch-out.
- Work to maintain good posture: keep pelvis and shoulders back, chin up.
- Lift from a squatting position to prevent back strain.

Sex (see pp. 110–15)
- There is no medical reason to limit sexual intercourse or orgasm during pregnancy *unless* there is a specific threat of abortion or premature labor.
- Vary lovemaking positions to accommodate the woman's changing size and shape.
- Use techniques other than intercourse to achieve sexual satisfaction, based on the needs and feelings of both the mother and father.

Chemicals and drugs (see pp. 117–35)
- STOP SMOKING.
- Stop drinking (although an occasional drink is probably not a risk).
- Limit caffeine in coffee and soda to less than 2 to 4 cups a day.
- Do not use cocaine (which may cause birth defects) and avoid marijuana (which may cause fetal distress).

- Do not take any prescription or over-the-counter medication without consulting your doctor or midwife.
- Do not expose yourself to solvents or other dangerous chemicals at home or in the workplace.

Stress (see pp. 137–51)
- Pregnancy and birth are natural phenomena but they require change and adaptation.
- Use relaxation techniques to deal with stress.
- Pamper yourself with daily activities that are enjoyable.
- Share concerns with relatives and friends in frequent, intimate conversations.
- Attend a prenatal group for support as well as for information.
- Set aside quiet times with the father to discuss concerns, points of conflict, and plans for the pregnancy, birth, and newborn period.
- Rapidly seek reassurance for questions and worries either from the doctor or midwife, or from experienced mothers.

Immunizations
- Do not be vaccinated for rubella or mumps during pregnancy.
- Avoid flu or polio shots unless there is a serious epidemic.
- Avoid a tetanus-diphtheria shot unless the mother has never been vaccinated or has not been vaccinated within 10 years.
- The following vaccines are acceptable if necessary to meet travel requirements: typhoid, yellow fever, cholera, and hepatitis A.
- Rabies immunization is acceptable if necessary.

Personal hygiene and bathing
- Brush and floss teeth regularly to prevent cavities and gum disease.
- Avoid putting soap or drying agents on the nipples or areola in preparation for nursing; creams or lanolin are all right.
- There is no medical reason to limit tub bathing or swimming, since water does not enter the vagina except under pressure (but be careful of slipping in the tub).
- Do not douche without instructions from your practitioner.
- To prevent toxoplasmosis, wash hands after handling red meat and have someone else change kitty litter or use rubber gloves.

Clothing
- Wear loose, comfortable clothing; avoid clothes or stockings that are tight and may restrict circulation.

(continued)

Common concerns of pregnant women

Clothing (cont.)

- Choose clothing that can adjust as size and shape change; maternity clothes are generally not needed until the fourth or fifth month, although they may be more comfortable.
- A well-fitted maternity or nursing bra provides support and relieves or prevents breast discomfort, upper backache, and breast sagging (see p. 188); nursing bras open to allow the nipples to rub freely in preparation for nursing. Breast size generally does not change after the fourth month of pregnancy.
- Wear low-heeled, comfortable shoes that help to maintain good posture, prevent backache and leg cramps, and avoid falls due to changes in balance.
- A maternity girdle will provide abdominal support and help to prevent backaches if a woman has loose abdominal muscles, is obese, or has had a number of previous pregnancies.
- Support hose or tights will help women with leg swelling, varicose veins, or leg cramps.
- Cotton underpants lessen the chances of rashes or vaginitis.

Employment

- There is no medical reason for a woman not to work during pregnancy, provided she remains healthy.
- Women should avoid sitting or standing in one position for long intervals; women in sedentary jobs should get up and walk at frequent intervals.
- It is advisable for a pregnant woman to rest during lunch and morning and afternoon breaks.
- It is important that a pregnant woman's work not cause her to strain physically or become too fatigued.
- Women should feel free to stop work or cut back if they become chronically fatigued or feel themselves under constant emotional stress.
- A woman's work should not expose her to dangerous chemicals or physical hazards such as radiation or microwaves.

Travel

- Provided a woman is healthy, there is no medical reason to restrict travel, including airplane travel, during pregnancy.
- The mother should wear seat belts in cars, placing the lap strap below her abdomen and the shoulder strap above it.
- A woman should be sure to move about every several hours when traveling to promote circulation and prevent leg swelling or thrombophlebitis (see p. 432).

- Avoid fatigue, stress, and altered rest and dietary habits; particularly avoid missing meals in the last half of pregnancy, to prevent ketosis or premature labor (see p. 81).
- If traveling in the last months, a woman should realize that she may need alternative delivery plans; women traveling to remote areas should realize that they may find themselves removed from conventional maternity care.

mother who is interested can ask her doctor or midwife to point out the baby's head, rump, front, and back so that she can distinguish them herself.

Somewhere between 36 and 40 weeks, the doctor or midwife may also do a vaginal exam to look for signs that labor is nearing. The practitioner will check to see if the cervix is beginning to *efface*, or thin, and *dilate*, or widen. At the same time he or she will feel internally to see if the baby's head (or whatever part is nearest the cervix) has engaged and dropped down. In the last weeks some doctors routinely do a more extensive physical exam to reevaluate the size and shape of the mother's pelvis in light of how much the baby has grown and how much the pelvic ligaments have stretched. Also the doctor or midwife will probably do another hemoglobin test to make sure the mother has not become anemic, and another urine test to rule out the possibility of a urinary tract infection.

Diagnostic Tests Sometimes Used During Pregnancy

Over the last twenty years medical technology has made incredible progress in its ability to test for potential serious problems while the infant is still in utero. Out of this has grown a whole new field called *perinatology*. It combines the roles of obstetrician and pediatrician in dealing with the growing baby before birth.

A number of perinatal tests and procedures have become common enough that they need to be included in a lay pregnancy book such as this. It's important to note that not all tests will be used on every mother. In general, there are specific criteria for each of the tests, although doctors vary widely in how broadly they apply these criteria. Thus one doctor may use a particular test rather frequently, while another doctor will use it only under very limited circumstances. Often a doctor will talk with parents and make the decision to use a test in consultation with them.

Despite the frequency with which some of the tests are used, the conditions the tests screen for are generally uncommon or rare.

The point is not that the incidence of these problems has risen during recent years but that doctors can now screen for conditions that formerly couldn't be diagnosed before birth. As a result, they tend to use the tests fairly widely. For mothers, the technical nature of these procedures, combined with their unknown outcome, may make them seem frightening. The more parents know about the tests and the more they realize how low the incidence of problems actually is, the more reassured they are likely to be.

ULTRASOUND

Ultrasound or *pulse-echo sonography* is a procedure in which high-frequency sound waves—vibrations that can pass through air, liquids, or solids—are used to build up a visual image of the baby in the uterus. Sound waves above 20,000 cycles per second, which are above the range of the human ear, are referred to as *ultrasound waves*. Like all sound waves ultrasound bounces back when it encounters material of a different density. This is the way a ship's sonar works, as well as the way bats navigate.

In medical ultrasound a sound wave of 2 million cycles per second is produced by sending a small burst of electricity through a quartz crystal. The wave bounces back to the crystal as soon as it hits a change in density in the mother's body and causes the crystal to send out a tiny burst of electricity in return. It is this burst of electricity that is picked up and translated into a dot of light on a screen. By scanning the mother's abdomen and building up a series of dots, a picture of the baby emerges.

Ultrasound sonograms have three important advantages over previous diagnostic techniques. First, they are noninvasive; that is, they gather information without directly entering the uterus. Second, their imaging does not involve X-ray radiation, which is known to be dangerous to the fetus. Third, ultrasound is a fast, easy, procedure that causes the mother no discomfort. Sonograms do take considerable skill and experience to read, however, and they should only be done by a *sonologist*, a doctor who has had special training in the technique. Even so, it is not unusual for the results of a sonogram reading to be unclear. In such cases the test is repeated at a later date, often by a more experienced sonologist.

There are two types of ultrasound examinations used during pregnancy. A *stage 1 ultrasound* is a short, simple exam that basically involves measuring the widest diameter of the baby's head, the *biparietal diameter* (see p. 294). The biparietal diameter increases steadily during the first 26 weeks, and then its growth rate slows markedly. Until this time the biparietal diameter provides a good indication of the baby's gestational age.

In addition to visualizing the biparietal diameter, stage 1 ultra-

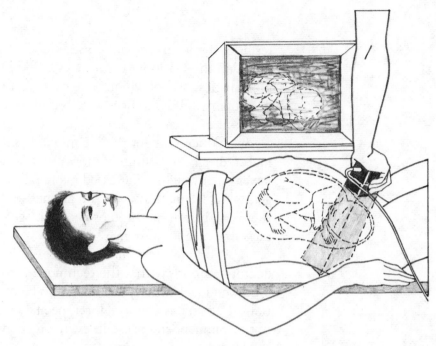

Ultrasound is a technique in which high-frequency sound waves are used to build up a visual image of the baby. It is a commonly used diagnostic procedure because it is noninvasive and doesn't involve radiation.

sound can reveal the location of the placenta, the position the baby is in, the location and amount of amniotic fluid in the uterus, and the baby's heartbeat. Because of the information it can provide on the location of the baby and the amniotic fluid, the most frequent use of ultrasound is to help the doctor do an *amniocentesis* test. Stage 1 ultrasound is also used to verify fetal growth if the baby seems to be growing very rapidly or very slowly, to verify gestational age in planned cesareans, to confirm the diagnosis of twins, and to locate the placenta in instances of third-trimester bleeding.

Stage 2 ultrasound is a longer exam that is performed if there is a *possibility* of a problem in the pregnancy. It is used both to answer any questions raised by a stage 1 exam and to rule out the presence of certain congenital malformations in babies who may be at risk.

During a stage 1 or 2 ultrasound exam, the mother's abdomen is covered with a special mineral oil that enables the ultrasound waves to be conducted directly into her abdomen. Otherwise they would be lost in the air between her skin and the *transducer* or wavemaker. The transducer box is moved slowly back and forth across her abdomen while the doctor views the resulting image on an *oscilloscope screen*. Polaroid shots are often taken of the best images and used for later study. Generally, the doctor shows the mother and father the screen and explains what they are seeing. Many parents enjoy the test and are very excited at seeing the baby move, just as they are excited to hear the fetal heartbeat or feel the baby kicking.

The Safety of Ultrasound

There has been much debate about the relative safety of ultrasound. During the twenty-five years that ultrasound has been used on humans, no problems have been observed in patients or operators as a result of the levels presently used. In the largest human study to date, in which the National Institute of Child Development followed 1952 pregnancies, 303 of which were exposed to ultrasound, no physical or developmental differences were found between the two groups of babies at one year of age.

Concern about the technique has arisen from the fact that animal studies have definitely shown that *high levels* of ultrasound cause lower birth weights, increased neonatal mortality, and increased congenital malformations. Several animal studies have also found that there can be minor chromosomal damage called *sister chromatid exchanges* at normal human dosages.

No long-term human studies of ultrasound are yet available, so doctors cannot say that the technique is totally safe. But at present ultrasound is definitely considered to be of greater benefit than potential risk *when it is indicated* for a specific medical reason. However, it is not recommended for use in every pregnancy or for merely visualizing the baby.

AMNIOCENTESIS

Amniocentesis is the most important test that can be done before birth to diagnose serious, nontreatable hereditary diseases and congenital malformations in the fetus. In this procedure 25 to 35 cubic centimeters of amniotic fluid are withdrawn from the uterus during pregnancy. From the sample a laboratory can grow fetal cells in a tissue culture.

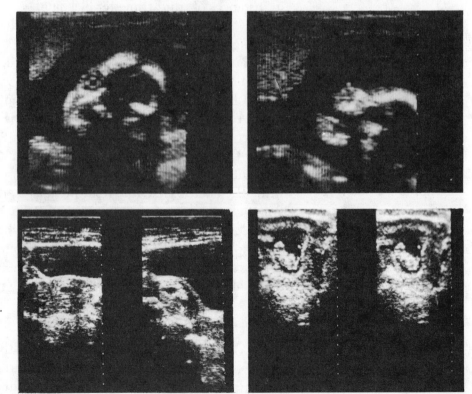

Ultrasound is a diagnostic technique that uses sound waves to build up a picture of the baby in utero. Photo courtesy of Dr. Jon Schwartz. Top left, front view of face; top right, side view of face. Lower left, 5–6 week fetus; lower right, 11 week fetus.

The chromosomes in the cells can be checked, and various biochemical *assays* or tests can be done if indicated.

Doctors have known how to remove amniotic fluid from the uterus for over a hundred years, but it was not until 1970 that researchers discovered that the amniotic fluid could be used for accurate tests that reveal genetic diseases and malformations. These tests, coupled with the liberalization of abortion laws that occurred in the late 1960s, made amniocentesis a primary tool for genetic counseling. The new procedure was widely covered in the media, and parents with a history of genetic disorders began to ask their doctors to perform the test.

Indications for Amniocentesis

At present 80 to 90 percent of all amniocentesis tests are done for *advanced maternal age.* As the mother's age goes up, there is an increase in the number of babies with *Down's syndrome* (formerly called mongolism), as well as of babies with other, rarer chromosomal abnormalities that also result in congenital malformations. Currently only 5 to 6 percent of the 150,000 mothers over age thirty-five who give birth in the United States each year actually make use of the test, although the number is growing. By 1978 over 40,000 tests had been done, including 15,000 in that year alone.

Down's syndrome, or *trisomy 21,* is a genetic disorder in which the affected individual has 47 chromosomes rather than the normal 46. A person with Down's syndrome has an extra number-21 chromosome. In addition, there are a whole group of physical characteristics that distinguish the syndrome, including short stature and a special facial structure with an *epicanthal fold* at the outer corner of the eyelid. But the most constant feature of Down's syndrome is mental retardation, with IQs of affected individuals varying from 20 to 80, though most range from 45 to 55, which is considered moderate retardation.

Doctors do not know why Down's syndrome is more prevalent among children of older women, although some researchers speculate that the mother's eggs, which have remained in the middle of a cell division since before her birth (see p. 55), tend to complete the division less perfectly as they age. Other researchers think that trisomy 21 may be caused by maternal thyroid abnormalities or exposure to radiation or viruses.

The overall incidence of Down's syndrome in the United States is 1 in 800 live births. The risk increases as the mother's age goes up: at age twenty-five the mother's risk is 1 in 1205, at thirty it is 1 in 885, at thirty-five it is 1 in 365, at forty it is 1 in 109, at forty-five it is 1 in 32, and at forty-nine it is 1 in 12. When amniocentesis first came into general use, research geneticists recommended it for every mother over the age of forty. Now the age has arbitrarily been lowered to thirty-five. No significant change occurs at the age of thirty-five, but doctors feel that the procedure is safe enough to justify its use even in this younger age group.

In addition to its use with advancing maternal age, amniocentesis is performed in situations in which the family is thought to be at risk for a specific, detectable hereditary disorder or congenital defect. This category covers a broad range of diseases. First, doctors will test mothers who have already given birth to babies with chromosomal abnormalities. Second, they will do an amniocentesis if either parent is known to have a mild chromosomal alteration. Third, they will test mothers who have had three or more spontaneous abortions, miscarriages, or stillbirths. Over half of all fetuses or embryos that are lost in the first trimester have chromosomal abnormalities, as do 5 percent of all stillborn infants.

Amniocentesis can also be used to detect certain diseases that result from abnormalities in a single gene or group of genes, as opposed to an entire chromosome. These diseases are detected with *biochemical assays* that measure chemicals present in the amniotic fluid. The diag-

Risk of giving birth to a Down's syndrome infant by maternal age

MATERNAL AGE	FREQUENCY OF DOWN'S SYNDROME INFANTS AMONG BIRTHS
30	1/885
31	1/826
32	1/725
33	1/592
34	1/465
35	1/365
36	1/287
37	1/225
38	1/176
39	1/139
40	1/109
41	1/85
42	1/67
43	1/53
44	1/41
45	1/32
46	1/25
47	1/20
48	1/16
49	1/12

nosis of a particular disease or defect is based on the presence of too much or too little of a specific chemical made by the baby.

The list of detectable *metabolic diseases* is growing and now includes literally hundreds of conditions. In diseases that are caused by *inborn errors of metabolism,* an important metabolic enzyme is missing. One such disease is *Tay-Sachs.* In this case the missing enzyme is essential to the breakdown of a kind of fat called *sphingolipid.* When this fat accumulates in the body, it interferes with neurological development. Tay-Sachs is a tragic disease that appears in otherwise healthy infants at about two to six months of age. It begins with symptoms of apathy and listlessness, followed by loss of motor and visual function, and progresses to seizures and death by the age of four. Genes for this very rare disease are carried by 1 in 300 people in the non-Jewish population, and by 1 in 27 among Ashkenazi Jews from Eastern Europe. When both parents carry the gene, each of their offspring has a one in four chance of developing the disease. Because of these statistics, many Jewish couples now take advantage of a simple blood test that will reveal the presence of the gene. Unfortunately, if a woman is already pregnant, she can have a false positive blood test result. However, this can be checked by another test called a *leukocyte assay.* When both parents are proved to be carriers, amniocentesis can determine whether or not the developing baby has the disease.

Amniocentesis and biochemical assay can also be used to diagnose certain congenital defects of unknown cause. Such defects include incomplete closure of the developing neural tube, which results in diseases such as *anacephaly* and *spina bifida.* Babies with anacephaly are stillborn or die shortly after birth, whereas babies with spina bifida can survive but have numerous congenital malformations and resulting medical problems. Genetic counselors recommend that parents who have had a baby with either condition have amniocentesis with all future pregnancies because of a 2 percent chance of having another baby with neural tube defects. Although this risk isn't high, it is much greater than that among the general population.

Babies with neural tube defects (as well as other rare congenital malformations) show higher than normal levels of a chemical called *alpha fetoprotein (AFP).* This substance crosses the placenta and can be picked up in the mother's blood at about 16 to 18 weeks of gestation, but the maternal test can show many false positives. Such testing is widely done in England, where the incidence of neural tube defects is much greater than in the United States. Amniocentesis, which tests the baby's cells, is much more accurate than maternal tests.

The Amniocentesis Procedure

Pregnant women are often hesitant to have amniocentesis. They naturally tend to feel protective of the baby, and the idea of withdrawing fluid through the abdominal wall with a needle may be upsetting. Some women fear the procedure will hurt the baby or be painful. Others fear the test because it focuses on the possibility that their baby may not be healthy. Learning about the procedure helps to reassure most women.

Amniocentesis is done at 16 weeks of gestation. By this time there is a significant amount of amniotic fluid and enough living cells from the baby's skin to make it easy to check the chromosomes. It takes only a week or so to do biochemical assays, but it takes 3 to 4 weeks to grow the fetal cells for the chromosomal tests.

Amniocentesis is almost always preceded by a stage 1 ultrasound (see p. 236), which shows the baby's position and the location of pockets of amniotic fluid. There is some controversy about the usefulness of ultrasound in this case, both because the doctor can judge the baby's position by physical exam and because the fetus is in constant motion at this age. No study has demonstrated that ultrasound lowers the risk factors for amniocentesis, but most doctors prefer to use it to visualize the baby.

Depending on where the most amniotic fluid is, one of several

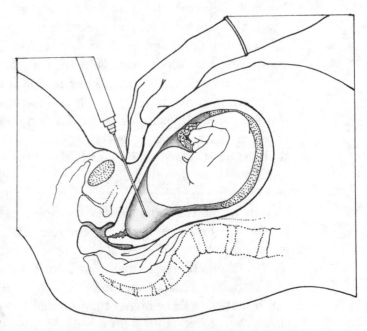

Amniocentesis is a procedure in which amniotic fluid is withdrawn from the uterus using a long thin needle. It is the major technique used to screen for a variety of genetic disorders. It is most commonly used in mothers over age 35 to detect those rare babies who have Down's syndrome.

areas on the mother's abdomen will be chosen from which to withdraw the sample of fluid. First, the area will be wiped with an antiseptic, and sterile drapes will be put around the rest of the abdomen. Using a very small needle, the doctor will insert a small amount of local anesthetic, such as *lidocaine,* to numb the area. This amounts to a small prick and a burning sensation. Then the doctor will gently insert a long, thin needle through the abdominal wall, moving it up and down slightly until a total of 20 to 30 milliliters of amniotic fluid is obtained. If the syringes are small (10 mm.), the needle will be left in and the syringe will be replaced so that one or two more tubefuls can be withdrawn. At 16 weeks there is roughly 250 milliliters of amniotic fluid in the uterus, and more is being made rapidly all the time (see p. 69). Thus only a small percentage of the total fluid is withdrawn, and it is quickly replaced.

Between 5 to 20 percent of the time the amniotic fluid withdrawn will contain blood, which does not interfere with the culture and is not a cause for concern. This whole part of the procedure takes about three minutes and has been described by mothers as being no more uncomfortable than getting a regular shot. Once the fluid is obtained, the needle is withdrawn and a small bandage is put over the site. Occasionally no amniotic fluid can be obtained as the needle is first positioned, and the doctor will reinsert it in a new location. One to 10 percent of the time the culture will not grow, and the procedure has to be repeated at a later date. In a situation in which the mother is Rh-negative and the father is Rh-positive, the mother is routinely given a follow-up shot of *Rh-immune globulin (Rhogan).* This is done because there is a possibility that some of the baby's cells might have entered the mother's bloodstream, causing her body to make antibodies against the baby's blood.

Before the mother leaves, the doctor observes her for a brief time and listens to the baby's heartbeat. After she leaves the mother can go about her normal activities, but as a routine precaution, she is told to call if she experiences persistent cramping, vaginal bleeding, leakage of amniotic fluid, or fever. These complications are uncommon and usually do not signal a problem, but the doctor should be made aware of them.

The Safety of Amniocentesis

Three major studies have shown that amniocentesis is a remarkably safe procedure for both mother and baby. From 1971 to 1973 the National Institute of Child Health and Human Development ran a large study of amniocentesis to assess the risk of injuring the fetus or causing maternal infection or hemorrhage. Of 1040 women who underwent diagnostic amniocentesis at nine centers, there was no statistical difference in their pregnancies as compared to a matched group who did not have amniocentesis. There was no increase in fetal loss rate, perinatal problems, birth weight, neonatal complications, or birth defects in the amniocentesis group. There were also no differences among the babies in growth, development, or behavior at one year.

The spontaneous abortion rate for the second trimester was 3.5 percent among women who had had amniocentesis, only slightly higher than the overall rate of 3.2 percent. A study done by the Medical Research Council of Canada found no difference in the rate of spontaneous abortion among a group of 1223 mothers who had amniocentesis, whereas a study in England found a 1.0 to 1.5 percent increase in abortion among mothers who had had the test. However, the English study has been criticized because the mothers in the control group were younger and had had fewer children. When this discrepancy was adjusted, there was no difference between the group that had had amniocentesis and the one that had not. From these studies researchers have concluded that if there is any increase in the risk of spontaneous abortion, it is probably in the range of .5 percent.

The relative safety of amniocentesis accounts for why it has become increasingly common and is now recommended for women between the ages of thirty-five and forty as well as for those over forty. The estimated increased risk of spontaneous abortion is only slightly higher than the .3 percent risk of Down's syndrome among mothers at age thirty-five, but is much lower than the 1 percent risk of Down's syndrome among forty-year-old mothers.

The Question of Abortion

In the rare instances when amniocentesis reveals the presence of Down's syndrome or some other serious genetic defect, parents face the difficult decision of whether to abort the baby at about 17 to 20 weeks. Their decision will be based on the seriousness of the genetic condition, the gestational age of the baby at the time of diagnosis, and their religious or moral convictions about abortion. Many parents have strong personal or religious feelings against abortion, particularly in the second trimester when the baby is fully formed.

By 20 weeks the baby weighs about ¾ pound (100 grams) and is 6½ inches (16 centimeters) long. The fetus is still not viable outside the uterus and thus can legally be aborted. In many states the latest an abortion can be performed is 24 weeks. Two kinds of abortion are possible at this stage of pregnancy. Saline can be injected into the amniotic fluid, which induces contractions and the mother delivers the fetus vaginally after several hours of labor. However, some centers and doctors elect to do a procedure in which the baby is scraped out of the uterus.

The emotional trauma of a second-trimester abortion has to be balanced against the trauma of raising a child with mental retardation or severe congenital defects. It is best if the decision is undertaken only after the parents have had intensive genetic and psychological counseling. The dilemma of the parents' decision extends to the medical staff as well, and some centers are refusing to do 20-week abortions, based on the rationale that as the fetus approaches 24 weeks, there is the possibility of a live birth after a saline abortion. *Chorionic-villus sampling,* a new test that can be done earlier than amniocentesis, avoids the turmoil of a second-trimester abortion for parents and the possible medical-legal problems for the doctor and hospital. It involves taking a sample of the placental membranes through the cervix and allows chromosomal tests to be made much sooner. It is still in the experimental stages because its safety has not been proved on a broad scale, but it is being used at university centers.

Fetal Well-being Tests During Pregnancy

Perinatologists have developed several tests that obstetricians use in certain high risk or complicated pregnancies to assess the baby's general health while in utero. It is interesting to note that the results of the tests are usually reassuring and show that the baby is doing well. The three most common fetal well-being tests are the *fetal activity test* (FAT), the *nonstress test* (NST), and the *oxytocin challenge* or *stress test* (OCT). All involve fetal monitoring. Two newer tests, which are less frequently used, involve ultrasound. They are the *fetal breathing movement* test (FBM) and an *amniotic fluid volume* test (AFV).

Many doctors feel that no single test can definitely identify a baby at risk and that an accurate assessment emerges only when the

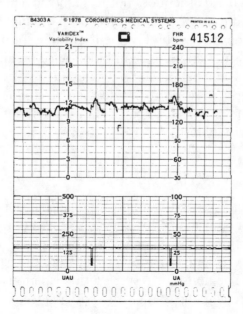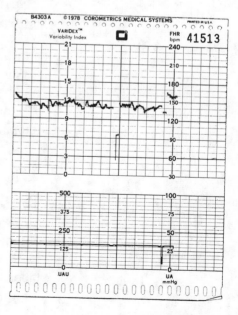

The stress test and the nonstress test use fetal heart tracings to assess the state of the baby's health in the uterus. Tracings courtesy of Dr. Jon Schwartz.

results of several tests are combined. Basically all these tests measure the baby's response to stress or lack of oxygen. The baby's breathing, heart rate, and movement are all controlled by its central nervous system, which is very sensitive to oxygen deprivation.

THE FETAL ACTIVITY TEST

The fetal activity test is the simplest of the prenatal tests. Basically it involves monitoring the baby's movements for a 30- to 60-minute period. There are several ways to conduct the test. The most informal is to have the mother lie down and keep a record of the baby's movements over a given period of time. More sophisticated versions of the test keep track of the baby's movements with an ultrasound machine or an electronic monitor that is strapped around the mother's abdomen to record pressure changes.

Most women first become aware of fetal movements between 16 and 20 weeks of pregnancy. Initially the movements are weak and fluttery and sometimes difficult to distinguish from gas pains. But as the baby grows, the movements become stronger and more discernible. The baby's movements peak in strength and frequency at about week 32. The *average* number of movements is 200 per day at 20 weeks, increasing to 375 at 32 weeks, though there is tremendous variability in the numbers that different mothers report. In fact, the same baby can range from 200 to 700 movements within a period of several days. As all mothers are aware, fetal movement varies with the time of day, generally reaching the highest levels in the evening. It is also interesting to note that babies' movements have been shown to vary with light, sound, and touch. Researchers have observed that ultrasound causes fetal movements to increase.

If a mother does not feel any movements during a test, it is assumed that the baby is asleep. An attempt will then be made to wake the baby with movement or noise, or by sending the mother for a meal since an increase in blood sugar usually awakens the baby. A *very* low number of fetal movements can be a sign of fetal distress. The number of movements would then be correlated with other test results. The nonstress test, in particular, is often done in conjunction with the fetal activity test.

THE NONSTRESS TEST

The nonstress test is simply *external fetal monitoring* using a Dopler ultrasound machine for a specific length of time (see p. 356 for a description of the procedure). The machine is the same external monitor that is sometimes used to measure the baby's heart rate during labor. The nonstress test is routinely performed in the doctor's office for a broad group of high-risk patients (see chart) at about 34 weeks.

The mother is positioned on her back but tilted slightly to the left to relieve pressure on her vena cava and to ensure optimum blood flow to the baby. Two belts are strapped around her abdomen: one contains a transducer that measures the baby's heart rate, the other measures uterine movements. In labor the second transducer is used to measure contractions. During the 30 to 60 minutes that the mother is monitored, she may be asked to keep a record of when she feels a movement, or a nurse may mark it on the pressure chart. The point of the test is to verify that whenever the baby moves, its heartbeat increases at a normal rate, just as an adult's does with exercise. If the mother has a particular medical condition such as diabetes or heart disease, the test is repeated once a week from 34 weeks until delivery.

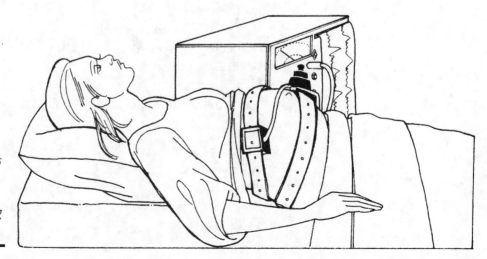

The stress and nonstress tests are done with the same kind of electronic fetal monitor that is sometimes used during labor.

THE STRESS TEST

The oxytocin challenge test (OCT) is done on women who have had a nonstress test that yielded negative or questionable results. It is very similar to the nonstress test, with one important difference: in the OCT the mother is given small amounts of the drug oxytocin through an IV to stimulate uterine contractions. Oxytocin is continued until she experiences three regular contractions of 40 to 60 seconds duration within a period of 10 minutes. The purpose of the test is to see how the baby will deal with the stress of normal labor, because contractions tend to cut down on the baby's oxygen supply by compressing the placenta. The doctor watches the baby's heart rate to see if any pattern of deceleration takes place *after,* as opposed to during, the contractions (see p. 358).

This test is only performed after 34 weeks, when a baby could easily survive should the test prematurely induce labor. Because of the slight risk involved in giving oxytocin to a high-risk baby who might not be able to withstand contractions, the stress test is always done in a hospital and it is never used on mothers with complications that make it important not to risk the possibility of unexpectedly inducing labor.

Currently the trend is to replace the stress test with the nonstress test for initial screening, since many doctors consider the nonstress test to be equally or more reliable without having the risks of the stress test. Also another, less invasive form of the stress test has been developed. It is called the *nipple stimulation test.* In this test contractions are triggered by having the mother rub her nipples, which

Criteria for administering stress test

- Diabetes (in some cases)
- High blood pressure
- Toxemia
- Mother over 40
- More than 2 weeks past due date
- Suspected low-birth-weight baby
- Severe heart disease
- Hyperthyroidism
- Meconium staining of amniotic fluid

MEDICAL REASONS NOT TO ADMINISTER STRESS TEST

- Third trimester bleeding
- Threatened premature labor
- Previous cesarean with classical incision
- Twins or triplets

causes her body to secrete its own oxytocin. This technique has many of the advantages of the stress test, but with less risks.

Both the stress and the nonstress tests have been shown to reflect the well-being of the baby accurately. One study found that a baby who does poorly on both tests has an 83 percent chance of experiencing fetal distress during delivery. For this reason such babies are very carefully monitored in a vaginal delivery or are delivered by cesarean section.

THE FETAL BREATHING MOVEMENTS TEST

It has only been possible to monitor fetal breathing since the advent of ultrasound technology. Using constantly scanning ultrasound to convey an image onto a screen, doctors today can actually observe the baby's breathing movements in utero. The procedure for doing the test is similar to a diagnostic ultrasound test that verifies the size and age of the baby (see p. 236). The breathing movements test is being experimented with in research centers and is done around 34 weeks, in conjunction with other tests such as the nonstress test.

Although doctors aren't certain, they believe that such movements help prepare the baby for breathing air after it is born. Like general body movements, breathing movements vary widely at different times of the day and from one baby to another. On the average, a 34-week baby makes breathing motions 30 percent of the time, but can vary normally from making no movements to making breathing motions 86 percent of the time within a given hour.

It is interesting to note that breathing patterns are quite different from body movement patterns in their biological rhythm cycles. Breathing motions have been found to peak between 4 and 7 A.M., with another predictable rise when the mother's blood sugar increases after a meal. Caffeine and maternal exercise also increase the baby's breathing motions, while smoking, alcohol, and sedatives cause a decrease.

THE ESTRIOL TEST

Before ultrasound was broadly employed, the most widely used test for evaluating fetal condition before delivery was the *estriol test*. This test is still used in conjunction with others, but decreasingly so. The estriol test measures the amount of a particular kind of estrogen, called estriol, which is made by the baby's adrenal glands and crosses the placenta to be found in the mother's blood and urine.

A mother will show only low levels of estriol during the first and second trimesters, with a gradual increase after 32 weeks, and a sharp increase after 36 weeks as the baby's adrenals make more and more of the hormone (see p. 34). Estriol amounts can be judged either through a simple blood test or through a 24-hour collection of urine. The amount of estriol measured gives an indication of the baby's health and development as well as of the efficiency of the placenta. The test is accurate in diagnosing fetal distress 70 to 80 percent of the time.

Medical Concerns During Pregnancy

Many birth educators feel that descriptions of complications that *occasionally* occur during pregnancy may unnecessarily frighten expectant mothers and cause them to worry needlessly. However, most pregnant women have sketchy information about these conditions anyway and they are often reassured when they can get accurate information and learn how unusual most of these complications are. In fact, most complications except early miscarriage are quite rare.

The great majority of pregnancies occur without complications. Yet most pregnant women know of a few mothers who have had problems. Also, doctors and midwives generally tell mothers about a group of symptoms that could indicate problems and that should be reported promptly if they occur. These symptoms relate to some of the complications we will discuss.

Since most of the concerns included in this section require diagnosis and treatment by a doctor, we are including only brief descriptions, which will enable a mother to understand the reason for reporting her symptoms. If a particular description causes a mother any concern, she should discuss it with her doctor or midwife, who will most likely reassure her.

It's important to point out that the figures given for the incidence of a particular condition take into account *all* pregnancies, including those mothers known to be at high risk for a specific condition. The incidence for a healthy mother who is not in any high-risk category would be much, much lower. And, of course, even most of the mothers in a particular high-risk category will not develop a problem.

PREGNANCY OVER 35

In recent years the number of older mothers has been on the rise. In 1981 over 50 percent of all births to white women in Washington, D.C., were to women over thirty. In 1978 in the U.S. more than 150,000 women over age thirty-five delivered babies, which amounted to 4.5 percent of all babies born that year. A number of sociological and medical factors seem to be responsible for this increase: many women are choosing to delay motherhood until their careers are well established; others are having second families with a new father; and still others are having children after being treated for infertility problems.

Maternal age over thirty-five is usually considered to be a risk factor in that most obstetricians will take note of it and keep an eye out for problems that are more likely to arise in older mothers. Yet pregnancy is currently so safe that actual risks, even for mothers over thirty-five, are extremely low. When doctors speak of a risk factor, they do not necessarily mean a *significant* risk; they simply mean that the risk is somewhat greater, even if only minimally, than for an "average" pregnancy. Perhaps the most significant risk to increase with maternal age is the chance of having a *Down's syndrome* baby, although the odds are less than many mothers think. At age forty a woman still has greater than a 99 percent chance of giving birth to a baby who does not have Down's syndrome.

Past research indicated that mothers over the age of thirty-five had more problems with pregnancy and labor than did younger mothers. A 1980 study by Harvard obstetricians Cohen and Friedman showed that first-time mothers, in particular, had a higher-than-average incidence of slow labor in the second stage. Other studies have shown an increased prematurity and infant mortality rate among older mothers. But several recent studies have brought these results into question and, in fact, have indicated that pregnancy in mothers over thirty-five is as safe as pregnancy for younger mothers. A study by Ann Stein at the nurse-midwifery service of Roosevelt Hospital in New York found that not counting mothers who had major medical problems, 87.5 percent of the mothers *over* thirty-five had spontaneous vaginal deliveries, as compared with 90.2 percent of the mothers *under* thirty-five. Neither was any increase in perinatal mortality or morbidity found among the babies of women over thirty-five. In an Israeli study of 402 mothers, 55 of whom were over thirty-five, the older mothers showed no difference in length of labor, congenital malformations, or infant mortality, although they did have a higher incidence of cesarean section.

A study by Grimes of the United States Center for Disease Control on the records of 26,000 women under age thirty-four and 788 women age thirty-five and older who gave birth at Grady Memorial Hospital in Atlanta found that infant mortality was the same for both groups *if* mothers with hypertension were eliminated from the study. Studies like this have led doctors to believe that *preexisting medical conditions* are more important than age in determining whether the mother or baby is at risk. However, this study also showed that older mothers had a higher cesarean rate, although Grimes could not determine the reason for this from the records.

Finally, a study by Kearn in Washington, D.C., found that among a group of 83 mothers between the ages of thirty-eight and forty-nine, of whom one-third were first-time mothers, 80 percent delivered vaginally, 58 percent without any kind of medication. A number of the mothers believed they had done well in labor because they were more familiar with their bodies than they had been when they were younger. When they were interviewed by Kearn, these mothers said that they had had a more positive experience than they had dared to imagine. They said that they were in a better economic and psychological situation than when they were younger, although they admitted to having less physical energy.

High-Risk Pregnancies

Obstetrics has undergone radical changes in recent years, especially in the management of high-risk pregnancies. The decade from 1970 to 1980 has even been called the era of scientific obstetrics. Comparison of a recent obstetrical textbook with one that is more than ten years old reveals a striking difference in the topics covered. Most of the new material relates to perinatology, a new subspecialty that deals with maximizing the welfare of the fetus during pregnancy and delivery. In the nineteenth century the central problem of obstetrical care was maternal mortality. Now obstetrical advances have reduced the risks of pregnancy and delivery for the mother to such an extent that the focus of obstetrics has shifted to the baby.

As Dr. T. Chard, an English obstetrician, points out, perinatology is quite different from other medical specialties because the patient, who is the fetus, is basically inaccessible to normal diagnostic exams or techniques. Therefore both tests and treatment must be indirect. The focus of perinatology is on identifying patients who are at risk and on taking preventive steps to avoid problems before they arise.

The term *high-risk pregnancy* simply means that the risks for the mother and baby are higher than average, not necessarily that the actual risk of a given complication is high. Because the average risks are very small, a mother at increased risk is still likely to have very low odds of developing a serious medical condition and very high odds of delivering a normal baby.

Perinatologists rely on wide screening and the identification of broad risk factors. For example, a mother who has had a stillbirth has good odds of having a subsequent healthy baby, but she is generally considered to be in a high-risk category because her odds of having another stillbirth are three times that of the average woman. The point we want to make is that mothers should not be depressed or frightened at being told they are in a high-risk category. It generally does not mean they are actually at great risk, simply that it is prudent to monitor their pregnancy carefully.

It is also important for parents to realize that the individual classifications of high-risk pregnancies vary greatly among different medical centers and different doctors. A number of risk factors are so broad that if they were strictly applied, as many as 40 percent of all mothers would be considered at high risk. Although this may seem strange at first, when analyzed it makes more sense. The great majority of babies with problems are born to mothers in this category rather than to mothers in the low-risk category. A more typical estimate of the number of mothers in the high-risk group is under 20 percent. This estimate is still based on very broad criteria, but a great deal of all perinatal problems come from this group.

There are some specific as well as general conditions that have been found to be statistically significant in assessing a pregnant woman's risk. The broadest conditions are poverty, unwanted pregnancy, and a maternal age under twenty or over thirty-five or forty. Specific conditions that are associated with increased risk are previous obstetrical problems such as stillbirth, known maternal illnesses such as diabetes or high blood pressure, specific complications during pregnancy such as bleeding, and complications during labor such as fetal distress.

Factors indicating high-risk pregnancy

MATERNAL ILLNESS

- Diabetes mellitus
- Heart disease
- High blood pressure
- Thrombophlebitis
- Thyroid condition
- Anemia
- Asthma
- Kidney disease
- Hepatitis
- Lupus
- Tuberculosis
- Epilepsy

PREVIOUS OBSTETRICAL PROBLEM

- Three or more consecutive spontaneous abortions
- Incompetent cervix
- Previous cesarean section
- Previous baby with congenital malformation
- Previous stillbirth
- Previous premature labor
- Uterine abnormality
- Maternal age less than 17 or greater than 35 (see above)

There are also a group of factors that relate to the baby, including low birth weight and prematurity.

A woman may be identified as being at high risk during her initial exam, at some point during her pregnancy, or during labor and delivery. As soon as the doctor or midwife identifies a specific condition or potential problem, he or she will explain these findings to the mother. Most doctors and midwives will not concern the mother with *very* low risk factors, such as poverty or maternal age over thirty-five, but will take note of them and watch the mother more carefully. Doctors and midwives *will* discuss with the mother and father any conditions that will need special checkups or treatment during pregnancy and birth.

INFECTIONS

Colds and Flu

Although all pregnant women try to stay as healthy as they can throughout their pregnancy, occasionally they will catch a cold or a flu. In fact, women may be slightly more susceptible to infections during pregnancy, so common sense would dictate that they should avoid getting rundown or exposing themselves unnecessarily to illness. If she has young children, this may not be entirely possible, but a mother can try not to become fatigued and can practice extra cleanliness in hand washing and food preparation. Should an expectant mother catch a cold, it is most important that she continue to eat well and keep herself hydrated. As long as she does not become seriously ill, she can be reassured that her cold will not be dangerous for the baby.

Although a pregnant woman with a cold feels just as sick as a nonpregnant woman with a cold, most doctors and midwives would advise her to forego *any* over-the-counter preparations. However it is reassuring to learn that statistically these preparations pose very little danger to the baby (see p. 130). For this reason practitioners vary widely in their advice on over-the-counter drugs. Some won't hesitate to tell an uncomfortable expectant mother to take aspirin or nonaspirin compounds like Tylenol. However, there are alternatives that may make the mother feel better without any risk, and they should be tried first (see chart).

In certain situations a pregnant woman should consult her doctor. If she runs a high fever, her doctor may advise her to take something to bring the fever down. If she develops an ear infection or a strep throat, her doctor may prescribe an antibiotic that has been used safely by other women during pregnancy (see p. 130).

While most infections rarely have any effect on pregnancy, certain ones can be serious. The three most common are *rubella, herpes simplex,* and *toxoplasmosis.* In addition to affecting the mother, these

Alternatives to drugs

DRUG	ALTERNATIVE TREATMENT
Aspirin	Take lukewarm sponge bath; take clothes off.
Cough syrup	Take lots of liquids, or honey and water.
Decongestants	Take liquids; rest; use vaporizer.
Laxatives	Increase fruits, liquids, and bulk in the diet.
Antacids	Drink milk, soda; eat bland crackers; rest.
Antidiarrhea drugs	Stop solid foods initially; later eat rice and dry toast.
Skin drugs	Gently wash area, pat dry; give sunlight and air exposure if irritated area is wet, oil if area is dry.
Eyedrops (nonprescription)	Use dropper or cup to wash eyes with water. Add ½ teaspoon of salt per 1 quart of water to make saline eyewash.

infections have the potential to cause congenital malformations or serious illness in the newborn.

Rubella

Rubella, or German measles, is a virus that has a 20 percent chance of causing a congenital syndrome in the fetus if a pregnant woman becomes ill during the first trimester. The syndrome includes cataracts, deafness, heart defects, and central nervous system effects. However, rubella is not the problem it once was because over 85 percent of all pregnant women in the United States now have either had rubella or have acquired immunity to it through vaccination.

During one of the early prenatal visits many doctors routinely do a rubella *antibody titer*, a test that picks up the presence of antibodies, thereby confirming that the mother is already immune to the disease. Once a woman is pregnant she cannot be immunized even if she is exposed to rubella, because the vaccine itself poses a danger to the fetus. In fact, a woman should not have the vaccine within three months prior to becoming pregnant.

If a pregnant woman is not immune and believes she has been

exposed to rubella, she should do two things. First, she should have her titer level checked immediately and again four weeks later. If the second titer is higher, it indicates that she has had a recent infection. Checking titers is the only way to rule out a recent infection, since one-third of people who get rubella do not show the usual symptoms of rash, fever, and swollen lymph nodes. Doctors also advise pregnant women who think they have been exposed to ask their contact to have a titer check if there is a question as to whether the person actually had German measles.

Those few mothers who have proved rubella infections during early pregnancy face a difficult decision if they do not spontaneously abort. Of babies exposed during the first month in utero, 50 percent have malformations. During the second month the rate is 22 percent; during the third month, 10 percent; and during the fourth and fifth months, 6 percent. Because of the high incidence and seriousness of the malformations, a decision to have an abortion is often made by the mother and father in consultation with their practitioner (see p. 244).

Genital Herpes Simplex

Herpes simplex is now one of the most common venereal diseases in the United States. Its present incidence has been estimated at 300,000 to 5 million new cases per year among the general population, and at .1 percent to 1 percent among pregnant women. There are actually two kinds of herpes: Type I causes cold sores around the mouth and nongenital skin lesions; Type II causes genital lesions or sores. Only genital lesions are of importance to a pregnant woman because if she has a herpes infection at the time of delivery, the baby can become infected during passage through the birth canal. Unlike the mother, the newborn can develop a total systemic infection that can often be life-threatening.

Genital herpes (HSV2) is spread through sexual contact with someone who has an *active* infection, that is, a herpes lesion or sore. Within 3 to 6 days after exposure, people who have become infected will notice pain and tenderness in the genital area. Raised, reddened areas appear, which turn into blisters filled with clear fluid. The blisters pop within 48 hours, leaving shallow sores or ulcers that scab over and eventually heal without scarring. Men develop lesions on the shaft of the penis, while women can develop blisters on the labia, vagina, cervix, or perineum. Women sometimes notice pain on urination or rectal pain. Many people have recurrent outbreaks of lesions, with symptoms usually being milder with subsequent outbreaks. Unfortunately, some people who have herpes have no noticeable symptoms and therefore do not realize that they can spread the virus.

Genital herpes is diagnosed by a visual examination of the lesions and a viral *culture* or an antibody test. A culture involves taking a smear to see if the virus will grow in the presence of nutrients; it takes 1 to 3 days and is quite reliable. Since herpes poses such a potential danger to the baby, doctors screen those pregnant women who show herpes symptoms, who have a history of herpes, or whose mate has a history of herpes. Doctors specifically advise women not to have intercourse during the last trimester when their mate has active herpes sores.

If there is a history of herpes the doctor will do viral cultures on the mother at 32, 34, and 36 weeks and weekly thereafter. Provided the mother has no visible lesions and has negative results on the last two tests before delivery (one test being less than 7 days old), she is considered eligible for a vaginal delivery. If a woman has active lesions or a positive culture, the doctor will deliver the baby by cesarean section in order to prevent the possibility of the baby becoming infected. An exception is made, however, if a woman's membranes have been ruptured for *more* than four hours prior to her arrival at the hospital. In this case it is assumed that the baby has already been exposed to the virus. Should the mother check into the hospital less than four hours after the membranes have ruptured, most doctors will deliver the baby by cesarean section.

Despite the prevalence of genital herpes among women and the number of cases that are asymptomatic, infection of newborns is extremely rare. This *may* mean that the risk of infection for the vaginally delivered baby is actually very small, but because of the severity of newborn infections when they do occur and the lack of research data, the American Academy of Pediatrics advises that cesarean sections "should be considered" for women with active herpes.

The Academy of Pediatrics also recommends special care for infants born to mothers with active herpes. Babies born by cesarean from an infected mother are watched closely for several days and are often kept in a special nursery if they can't room in with the mother. The mothers are given special gowns and instructions on cleanliness and hand washing. Babies born vaginally to an infected mother will be put in a special isolation nursery for up to two weeks and are closely monitored for signs of infection.

Toxoplasmosis

Toxoplasmosis is a common infection caused by a large microorganism called a protozoa. In the United States 25 percent of women have antibodies that show evidence of prior infection. Only .2 percent of women become infected for the first time during pregnancy, and only they can pass the infection on to their baby. The protozoa crosses the placenta when the mother becomes infected.

As the pregnancy advances, the chances of passing on the infection increase, but the results tend to be less serious. Most newborns with congenital toxoplasmosis are asymptomatic or have problems that disappear in the first year of life. However, 8 percent of infected newborns have severe eye and central nervous system damage (that is, about 8 per 10,000 babies).

Unfortunately, 80 percent of pregnant women who develop toxoplasmosis show no symptoms and only 20 percent have mild viral symptoms with swollen lymph nodes. Interestingly, the parasite is harbored by mice who pass it on to other animals through their feces. People get toxoplasmosis either by eating or handling uncooked lamb or beef from animals that have grazed in mouse-infected fields, or by handling the litter of cats that have caught infected mice. Pregnant women who aren't immune to toxoplasmosis can prevent exposure by not eating raw meat and by having someone else in the family change the cat litter at frequent intervals.

FIRST TRIMESTER BLEEDING OR SPONTANEOUS ABORTION

It is very common for women to spot or bleed during the first trimester of pregnancy. Doctors estimate that this occurs 20 to 25 percent of the time. Such bleeding may range from spotting to heavier flow and may last for days or even weeks. Most commonly, a woman has bleeding or spotting about the time of her first missed period—17 days after conception, or 4½ weeks after the last menstrual period. Such bleeding is referred to as *Hartman's placental sign* and is thought to be due to the breakdown of small blood vessels in the wall of the uterus as the embryo becomes embedded.

Another frequent cause of bleeding in the first trimester is lesions or abrasions of the cervix. The cervix is highly vascular during early pregnancy and often bleeds in response to being bumped during intercourse. Although any bleeding should be reported to the doctor, this kind goes away by itself and poses no danger to the pregnancy.

A mother may also bleed during the first trimester due to threatened *spontaneous abortion* or *miscarriage.* Symptoms include cramping abdominal pain that may be rhythmic and may be associated with low-back pain. Less than half of those women who bleed during the first trimester actually have a miscarriage. Yet it is true that spontaneous abortion is quite common; it occurs in at least 10 to 15 percent of all recognized pregnancies. If one includes spontaneous abortions that take place before a woman even knows she is pregnant, the figure may be as high as 75 percent. Of reported spontaneous abortions, 75 percent occur before 16 weeks, and of these, the great majority occur before 8 weeks. Miscarriage is a very upsetting event for most women, but it seems to be a natural part of the reproductive process. Doctors have come to realize that reproduction is incredibly delicate and has a high rate of error built into it.

Spontaneous abortion is almost always caused by death of the embryo, which subsequently becomes detached from the placenta and is expelled as a miscarriage. At least 60 to 80 percent of such embryonic deaths are due to significant defects in the fertilized egg, the most common of which by far are abnormalities in the number of chromosomes. Chromosomal abnormalities mean that the problem actually arose *before* conception or in the earliest mitotic divisions of the fertilized egg (see p. 55). Such a *blighted embryo* may be aborted with the first menstrual period or may persist for a longer time, but there is no way that such an embryo could viably develop. Abnormalities in the placenta and nonchromosomal defects in the embryo can also cause early first trimester abortions.

Spontaneous abortions late in the first trimester or early in the second are more likely to be caused by severe maternal illness, trauma, toxic factors, or uterine conditions such as incompetent cervix. But doctors currently estimate that less than 15 percent of all miscarriages are due to maternal factors of any kind and almost none are due to anything the mother could have prevented. Occasionally a mother will fear that one specific incident has caused her miscarriage, but usually the embryo has not been viable for some time and the actual process of aborting the fetus has taken place over several weeks.

The doctor or midwife should be advised of all cases of first trimester bleeding. A vaginal exam will be done to determine if the bleeding is from the uterus or the cervix, and a *hemoglobin test* will also be done to determine if the mother has become anemic as a result of the bleeding. The mother is usually told to restrict her activities and not to have intercourse for several weeks.

The doctor may also do an *ultrasound test* (see p. 236) if the mother has been pregnant for 7 weeks. This procedure enables the doctor to visualize the embryo and the placenta, determine what is happening, and inform the mother immediately. More than half of the time the embryo will be viable, in which case the mother has over a 90 percent chance of successfully carrying the baby to term.

If the embryo is not alive, the mother will either spontaneously abort or be hospitalized for a *D & C* (*dilatation and curetage*), a procedure in which the lining of the uterus is scraped out to make sure that no placental fragments remain to cause infection. A mother who miscarries should be reassured that she will be able to become pregnant again soon.

ECTOPIC PREGNANCY

An ectopic pregnancy is one in which the fertilized egg implants *outside* the uterus, most commonly in a fallopian tube (90–95 percent) or occasionally in the cervix, abdomen, or ovary itself. Ectopic pregnancy is rare, occurring in one out of every hundred pregnancies. In recent years, however, the number of ectopic pregnancies has risen as a result of tubal infections caused by gonorrhea, IUDs, or undetermined complications. Such infections can cause local swelling and scarring of the tubes, which seems to impede the passage of the egg.

The classic symptoms of a tubal pregnancy are abdominal pain and vaginal bleeding within the first 8 or 12 weeks of pregnancy. Although the symptoms can vary widely, a woman generally has sudden, severe lower abdominal pain that is sharp, stabbing, or tearing. She may also have dizziness and faintness. These symptoms can occur either before a woman has missed a period or after. If a woman has very light bleeding she may suspect that she is pregnant but miscarrying.

Unlike a threatened spontaneous abortion, an ectopic pregnancy becomes a true medical emergency because the tube eventually ruptures and causes internal bleeding. Thus if a mother has any of the symptoms of ectopic pregnancy she should call a doctor *immediately.*

The doctor will do a vaginal exam. A blood sample will be taken for a pregnancy test if one has not already been done, and a hemoglobin test will also be done to determine if the woman has lost blood. The doctor will also do an ultrasound test to confirm the presence of an embryo and visualize where it has implanted.

If the tests verify that the woman has an ectopic pregnancy, the doctor will operate and remove the embryo. The earlier an ectopic pregnancy can be diagnosed, the more likely the operation can be done before rupture of the *gestational sac* containing the embryo and membranes. This is significant in terms of future pregnancies because it is much more likely that the tube can be saved if the gestational sac has not ruptured.

THIRD TRIMESTER BLEEDING

In 3 to 10 percent of all pregnancies women have some vaginal bleeding in the last three months. In most cases the bleeding is minimal and there is no threat to the baby or the mother, but in rare instances there can be enough bleeding to be dangerous. For this reason the

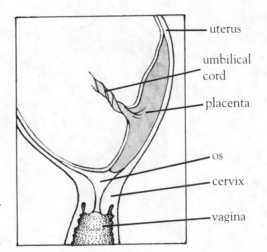

uterus

umbilical cord

placenta

os

cervix

vagina

Placenta previa is a rare condition in which the placenta is abnormally situated near the bottom of the uterus. Placenta previa can be a cause of third-trimester bleeding.

practitioner should always be called about bleeding in the latter part of pregnancy. In over 90 percent of mothers hospitalized for third-trimester bleeding, the bleeding stops by itself within a day or so.

The two causes of significant bleeding that the practitioner is concerned about involve problems with the placenta. Premature separation of the placenta or *abruptio placenta* is a situation in which the placenta is normally situated at the top of the uterus but separates abnormally before the baby is born. This condition is rare, occurring in only 1 pregnancy out of 120, a figure that includes both very mild cases and cases that occur during labor. Premature separation of the placenta tends to be more common in women who have high blood pressure during pregnancy, who have previously experienced it, or who are having second or third children. Thus the frequency of this condition is even lower than 1 in 120 among women who don't have high blood pressure or who are having their first child. The signs of premature separation of the placenta are vaginal bleeding and the sudden onset of abdominal pain. In rare cases there is little or no bleeding, and the main symptom is pain.

In placenta previa the placenta is abnormally situated near the bottom of the uterus. The condition ranges from a placenta that lies near the cervix to one that totally blocks it. All forms of this condition are very rare, occurring in only 1 out of every 260 pregnancies. Unlike abruptio placenta, the symptoms of placenta previa are sudden, profuse, painless bleeding, caused by blood vessels in the placenta shearing away from the uterine wall. The bleeding generally stops by itself, but it can reoccur. Placenta previa is most common among women who have had a number of babies.

In any case of third-trimester bleeding the doctor will want to follow the mother closely. If the bleeding is significant, the mother will be hospitalized for observation. Whether the doctor suspects placenta previa or abruptio placenta, he or she will do an ultrasound test to help diagnose the problem.

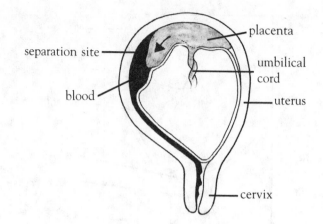

placenta

separation site

umbilical cord

blood

uterus

cervix

In abruptio placenta the placenta separates from the uterine wall before the baby is born. This condition is a serious but very rare cause of third-trimester bleeding.

In both premature separation of the placenta and placenta previa, treatment depends on how severe the bleeding is and how close the baby is to its due date. If bleeding is light and the baby is early, the doctor will prescribe bed rest and watch the mother carefully. If bleeding is more significant or the mother is due, the baby will be delivered, generally by cesarean section.

PREMATURE LABOR

Premature labor or *preterm labor* is one of the most significant complications of pregnancy in that it has far-reaching effects on both the baby and the parents. Its incidence is only 6 to 8 percent, but it is responsible for a great amount of newborn health problems. Premature labor is the onset of labor *prior to 37 weeks.* It is defined as contractions that dilate the cervix to 2 centimeters or more or that last 30 seconds or more and continue for a period of 4 to 20 minutes. Treatment to stop premature labor must be started quickly to be effective, so if a woman even suspects that she might be in premature labor, she should call her practitioner immediately.

The majority of women experience contractions throughout pregnancy, but these contractions do not usually become frequent, regular, or strong until the last several weeks. In some expectant mothers it may be difficult to tell premature labor from *false labor* or Braxton-Hicks contractions (see p. 272), but it is important that the mother call her doctor or midwife and be examined. The practitioner can distinguish premature labor by whether or not the cervix is dilating in response to the contractions, and by whether regular contractions persist for an hour or more.

The specific cause of premature labor is generally unknown, but it is more common among women who are at high risk, which is one

> ## Signs and symptoms of preterm labor for mothers at risk
>
> - Menstrual-like cramps
> - Dull low backache that is new or changed in character
> - Pelvic pressure
> - Increase or change in vaginal discharge
> - Intestinal cramping with or without diarrhea
> - Regular contractions, either painless or painful, that persist for an hour

of the reasons they are followed so closely. High-risk mothers include those who have high blood pressure, untreated or poorly treated endocrine disorders, kidney infections, excess amniotic fluid, abruptio placenta, or placenta previa. Mothers are also at higher risk if they have had previous preterm pregnancies, three or more induced abortions, or smoke cigarettes. Premature labor follows premature rupture of the fetal membranes 15 to 30 percent of the time (see p. 264).

Premature labor is taken seriously because it is a significant threat to the health of the baby. Even with the tremendous progress that has been made in neonatal care, prematurity is one of the major causes of newborn morbidity and mortality. The premature baby commonly has difficulty breathing due to the immaturity of its lungs and may have a number of other problems (see p. 70).

If the mother is not dilated when she is examined, the doctor will generally follow her progress with an external monitor for an hour. Provided the contractions do not persist and there is still no dilatation, it is assumed that the mother is in false labor and she is sent home. But if the mother is dilating or if the contractions continue, she will be hospitalized and treated.

The way premature labor is dealt with depends upon the gestational age of the baby and the health of the mother. Doctors try to let the baby continue to mature within the uterus as long as the uterine environment is safe. When the baby is very early (20 to 35 weeks), the mother is less than 3 to 4 centimeters dilated, and it is considered advantageous for the pregnancy to be maintained, the doctors will either prescribe bed rest and/or sedation, or they will administer intravenous *tocolytic agents*, drugs that actually slow or inhibit uterine activity. If labor can be successfully shut down, the mother will be released from the hospital and sent home.

Dr. Robert Creasy, an expert on preterm labor, believes that early detection is the key to reducing the incidence of preterm birth. He advocates teaching all women at risk of premature delivery to recognize the subtle signs of preterm labor. These include menstruallike cramps, a dull backache that is new or different from previous sensations, a sense of pelvic pressure, an increase in vaginal discharge, and intestinal cramping. He also teaches mothers at risk to detect "silent" uterine contractions by feeling their abdomen. They are told to call if such contractions continue for up to an hour. Creasy's staff are educated to respond promptly to patients' calls about signs of preterm labor. If there is any question of labor, the mother is examined and watched for a brief time. Mothers who are actually in early labor are treated conventionally with drugs to shut down their contractions. Creasy found a 50 percent decrease in preterm birth among mothers at risk who participated in his program.

In certain situations doctors may feel that delivery rather than maintenance of pregnancy is in the best interest of the baby or mother. Such circumstances include maternal high blood pressure, abruptio placenta, placenta previa, maternal infection, or severe growth retardation of the baby, which may indicate problems with the placenta. When doctors feel the baby is better off outside the uterus or when they cannot shut down labor, they deliver the baby.

Preterm babies are generally much more delicate to deliver than full-term ones. They are more susceptible to lack of oxygen during contractions and to the depressant effects of anesthetic drugs the mother may be given. Their skulls are weaker and more vulnerable to the pressure of contractions and preterm babies are frequently in difficult delivery positions. For these reasons every attempt is made to monitor the premature baby's birth and make it as rapid and easy as possible. Depending on the age, weight, and presentation of the baby, the doctor will decide whether a vaginal birth is safe. When a vaginal birth is chosen, it is done with a minimum of drugs, an internal monitor, and a large episiotomy. A cesarean delivery is frequently chosen, particularly if the baby is in a breech or transverse position.

PREMATURE RUPTURE OF THE MEMBRANES

Premature rupture of the membranes is defined as rupture of the fetal membranes or breaking of the bag of waters *before* the onset of labor. This situation arises in 7 to 10 percent of all pregnancies. Premature rupture of the membranes is largely of unknown origin, although it can follow trauma, excess amniotic fluid, uncommon presentations, or uterine infection. Whenever an expectant mother experiences premature breaking of the bag of waters, she should call her doctor or midwife.

There are two problems associated with premature rupture of the fetal membranes. First, premature breaking of the bag of waters often starts labor, which is a problem if the baby is very early (see previous discussion). Second, it opens the uterus to bacteria present in the vagina, which can cause the baby or mother to develop an infection.

The handling of premature rupture of the membranes is currently a controversial topic in obstetrics, because individual studies show differing rates of infection depending on the time that elapses between rupture and delivery. Some studies show increased incidence of infection after only 12 hours, some not until much later; other studies show higher incidences of infection among full-term babies than among premature babies. Thus the practitioner is not only faced with the problem of whether or not the baby is mature enough for delivery; he or she must decide whether to speed up or induce labor in an effort to avoid infection.

Depending on their philosophy and training, doctors and midwives may want the baby to be born within 12, 16, 24, or 72 hours after the bag of waters breaks. Others will not set any time limits at all. If it does not appear that the baby will be born within the time frame they adhere to, most doctors will induce contractions with intravenous *pitocin*.

Past 35 or 36 weeks, more than 80 percent of mothers with ruptured membranes will go into labor within 24 hours. Because the baby at this stage is essentially full-term and has sufficient lung development, the doctor will not attempt to shut down the mother's contractions. But if the baby is less than 35 or 36 weeks, the doctor may simply hospitalize the mother, put her in bed, and follow her temperature and white blood cell count to make sure she is not developing an infection. Some doctors will also do *ultrasound* and *fetal lung-maturity tests* (see pp. 236 and 379) to verify the baby's gestational age. If the mother does not go into labor and does not develop an infection, she may be sent home. In this case she will be told to rest and refrain from intercourse. Some doctors will then wait until contractions begin of their own accord; others will induce labor with IV pitocin when further tests indicate that the baby's lungs are mature.

HIGH BLOOD PRESSURE DURING PREGNANCY

High blood pressure during pregnancy is part of a complicated condition that arises rather suddenly 5 to 10 percent of the time in the latter half of pregnancy. The condition may also include protein in the urine and/or swelling of the face, hands, and feet. It used to be called *preeclampsia* or *toxemia*, but these terms are less commonly used now. More recently it has been referred to as *gestational edema-proteinuria-hypertension complex (GEPH)*.

If untreated, GEPH can pose real dangers for the mother as well as the baby and in rare cases can lead to maternal convulsions referred to as *eclampsia*. Prevention of high-blood-pressure complications is one of the most important reasons for frequent prenatal checkups, especially during the second and third trimesters. Without

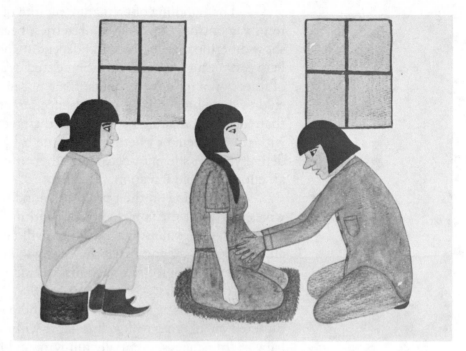

Prevention of complications of high blood pressure is one of the most important reasons for frequent prenatal checkups. Pregnant Woman Visiting the Doctor, *Arlo Nuvayouma. Watercolor painting, 11" x 14½". Museum of the American Indian, Heye Foundation.*

checkups and laboratory tests, a pregnant woman may be unaware of high blood pressure or proteinuria. Some swelling of the face, hands, and feet is not uncommon in late pregnancy and, by itself, does not necessarily indicate a problem.

A nonpregnant woman's blood pressure averages 120/80 at the age of twenty, 123/82 at thirty, and 126/84 at forty. A pregnant woman's blood pressure is considered high if it is above 140/90 *or* if it rises more than 30 points in the upper figure *(systolic pressure)* or more than 15 points in the lower figure *(diastolic pressure)*. Because blood pressure normally rises when a person is anxious or under stress, a diagnosis of high blood pressure is not made unless the rise is constant or is confirmed by two readings within 6 hours. If a woman has mild high blood pressure before she becomes pregnant or develops it during the first half of pregnancy, the doctor will not diagnose GEPH unless there is a significant rise in the systolic or diastolic blood pressure. In fact, women who have *mild* high blood pressure generally do not have problems during pregnancy.

Edema or swelling of the legs is normal for many pregnant women. It is not of particular concern unless it is associated with edema of the face and hands and with high blood pressure. Women who experience this kind of swelling may also show a sudden weight gain of more than 2 pounds per week. One late symptom to appear may be the presence of protein in the urine. If the illness is untreated, the mother can develop severe symptoms, including blurred vision and headache.

If a woman is diagnosed as having high blood pressure–edema–proteinuria, she is hospitalized, given bed rest, sometimes sedated, and followed closely. Often this treatment will bring the mother's blood pressure down. Drugs can be given to prevent severe complications, but the only way to stop the illness itself is to deliver the baby.

If the mother is 36 or more weeks pregnant, the doctor will induce labor with IV pitocin. If she is less than 36 weeks pregnant and her blood pressure goes down, she will be watched until the baby is more mature and then labor will be induced. When the mother is earlier than 36 weeks but the doctors cannot control her blood pressure, the baby will be delivered in a hospital with a neonatal unit. In this case the baby is often delivered by cesarean section.

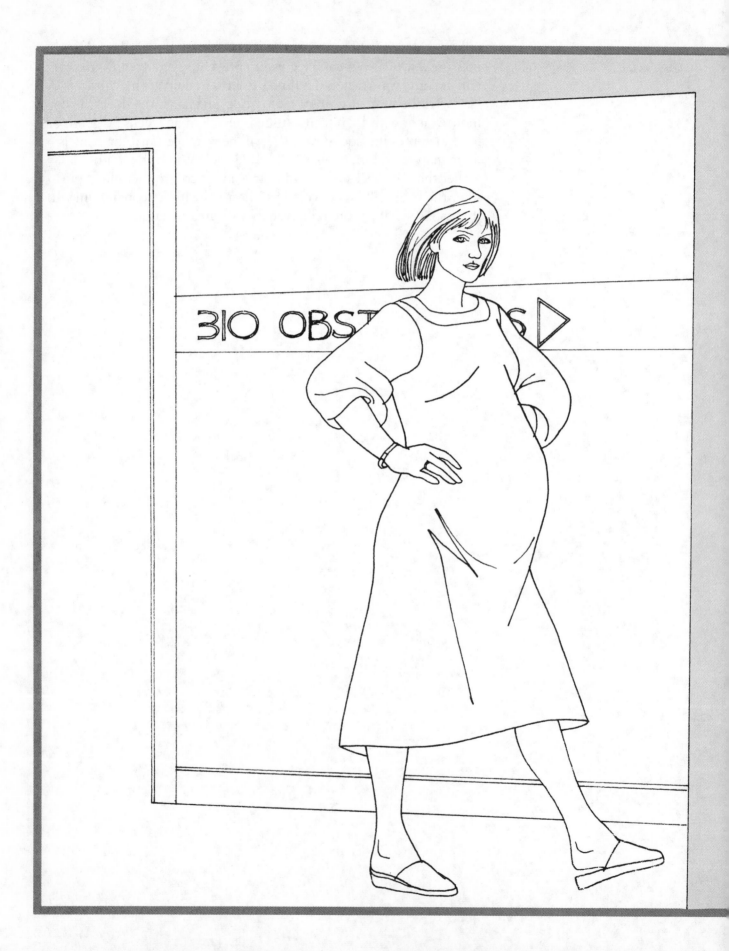

SECTION
III

Labor
and
Delivery

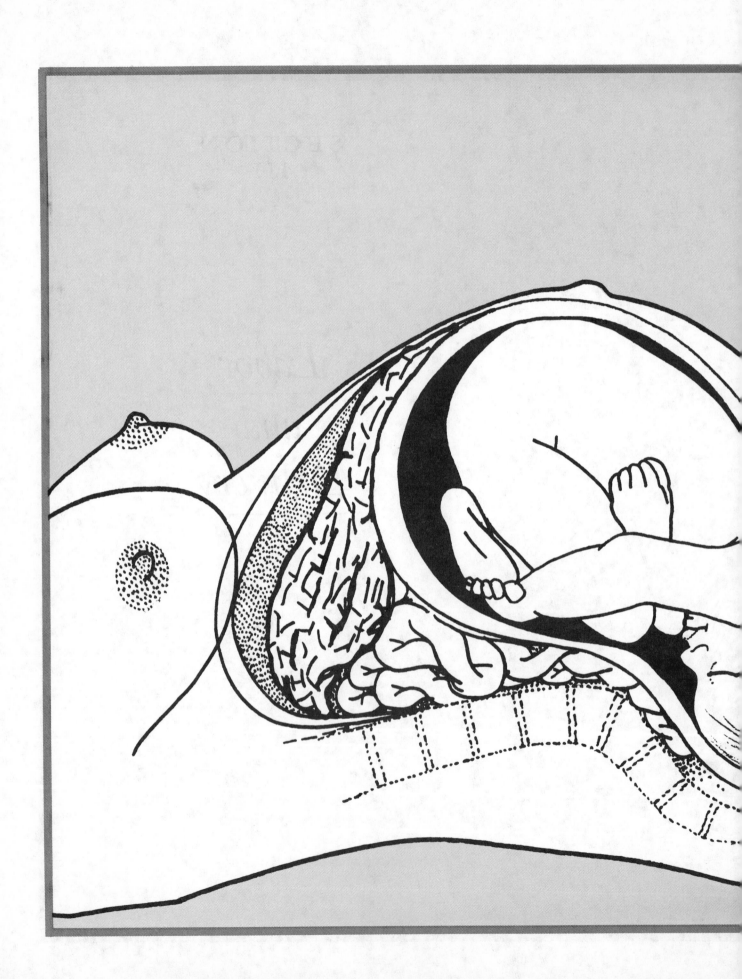

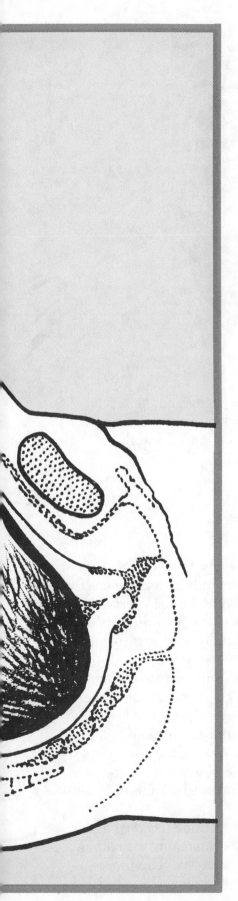

The Physiology of Labor

Labor as a Natural Bridge

All the hormonal and physical changes of the nine-month gestational period culminate in labor, an incredible and complex series of anatomical, physiological, and endocrine events that work together to separate mother and baby from one another physically. Both mother and baby must undergo important changes in order to make the transition from the baby being nurtured within the uterus to it being nurtured in the external world. Thus labor functions as a natural bridge leading to delivery. Considering the fact that women have been giving birth for thousands of years, it is extraordinary that doctors have only recently begun to analyze what starts labor and determines how it progresses.

For nine months the mother's anatomy, physiology, and endocrinology have all been geared to promoting the baby's remarkable growth and development within. During labor everything becomes geared to getting the baby safely out of the uterus. The upper part of the uterus, which is made of smooth muscle, has for a period of months been expanding to accommodate the growing baby. During the last few weeks of pregnancy it stops enlarging and begins to contract. At the same time the lower part of the uterus begins to stretch, preparing the cervix to open so the baby can finally emerge. Basically, the hard work of labor consists of muscular contractions that push the

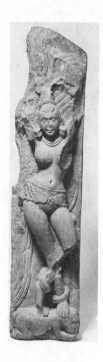
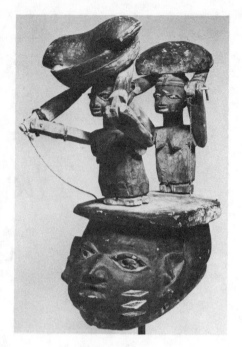

baby downward, thinning the bottom of the uterus and the cervix. The contractions help to pull the cervix back over the baby, who is eventually thrust down the birth canal and out into the world.

Early Signs of Labor

BRAXTON HICKS CONTRACTIONS

Labor is actually a progressive action that begins slowly during the ninth month and then gathers speed. After months of relative inactivity, the uterus contracts more and more often in the weeks before birth. Occasional uterine contractions have taken place throughout pregnancy, but they have been so sporadic and weak that they have had no effect on the cervix.

Contractions during the ninth month still tend to be brief, irregular, and imperceptible to the mother, but they are more frequent and coordinated than earlier ones. These contractions were first described by an English doctor named John Braxton Hicks in 1872, and hence they became known by his name. During the last several weeks of pregnancy they increase tremendously in frequency and may even become somewhat rhythmic. The period in which this happens is called *prelabor*.

Prelabor contractions work toward shortening (*effacing*) and widening (*dilating*) the tube-shaped cervix and stretching the bottom of the uterus. The contractions also soften the cervix. This process is called *ripening*; it indicates that the cervix is becoming ready for labor.

The "lip-soft" cervix of pregnancy now becomes "pudding-soft." Thus women enter labor with varying amounts of the work of delivery already done in prelabor. By the final weeks of pregnancy many women have dilated their cervix about 2 centimeters and have thinned and shortened it between 20 and 60 percent. In general, the more work done in prelabor, the shorter the mother's actual labor tends to be, although, as we shall see, labor never proceeds at a fixed rate, and much of the visible progress takes place in the last several hours before delivery.

If Braxton Hicks contractions increase and become rhythmic late in the pregnancy, they are referred to as *false labor*. What distinguishes false labor from real labor is simply that after a point, false labor does not progress and it eventually stops. The determination of whether labor is false can only be made in retrospect; there is still no test that can distinguish it from real labor. Many obstetricians and midwives say there is actually no difference between the two. Not only are the types of contractions indistinguishable, they serve the same purpose; that is, they prepare the cervix and the uterus for delivery.

LIGHTENING

Lightening or *dropping* is another event that helps to prepare for birth and signals its approach. Lightening refers to the baby gradually dropping down into the pelvis, due to the thinning and stretching of the bottom of the uterus. Among women who've previously had babies, it does not occur until shortly before labor begins, but it occurs two or three weeks before delivery in first-time mothers.

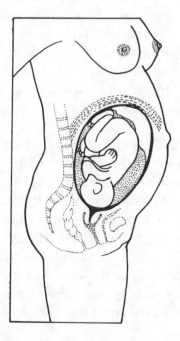 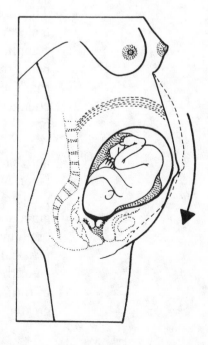

Lightening takes place when the baby drops down into the pelvis. It is one of the signs that occur before labor, usually preceding a first delivery by two or three weeks and subsequent deliveries by hours or days.

Lightening causes a number of physical changes that mothers notice. The mother's abdomen protrudes further out and lower down, which relieves pressure on her diaphragm, making her breathing easier and lessening heartburn and stomach fullness. At the same time lightening causes increased pressure on the mother's pelvis, which in turn results in increased frequency of urination, constipation, and low backache. It can also make walking more difficult and contribute to swelling of the mother's feet and legs. But most women are happy with the trade-off in symptoms because it graphically demonstrates that the end of pregnancy is at last in sight.

SHOW

Another event, called *show*, signals the onset of labor by hours to days. From soon after conception until shortly before delivery, the mother's cervix is sealed with a mucous plug. As the cervix dilates and stretches, the opening becomes too wide to maintain the plug, and it slips out. The mother will notice a brownish or blood-tinged mucous discharge when this happens. Occasionally the show may be confused with blood-tinged mucus caused by a pelvic exam or intercourse. Women normally have a profuse vaginal discharge at this time, and jarring the cervix can cause part of the plug to separate prematurely or cause slight bleeding by abrading the cervix, which has now become very soft.

The Beginning of Real Labor

There are several medical theories about what causes labor to begin. The most recent ones, rather fittingly, accredit the baby with the major role in initiating labor. To be more exact, labor is the result of a complicated interaction within the *fetoplacental unit* that includes the baby, the placenta, and the mother. Not surprisingly, doctors believe that the causal agents behind these interactions are hormones, the chemical messengers that cause physiological changes throughout the body.

Based on animal and human studies, researchers think that the baby's *hypothalamus*, the hormone control center in the brain, initiates labor. Why it does so remains a mystery. The hypothalamus may be programmed for a nine-month maternity cycle, much as it is programmed to produce a twenty-eight-day menstrual cycle, or the baby's brain may pick up signals, such as chemical indicators of maturation, physical indicators of size, or a combination of such factors. In any case, the baby's hypothalamus sends a hormone to the pituitary, which in turn causes its very large and active adrenal glands to make even greater amounts of a chemical that the placenta turns into estrogen.

Animal studies show that there is a marked increase in the production of estrogen starting about twenty-four hours before the onset of labor. High levels of estrogen cause the placenta to produce special on-site hormones called *prostaglandins*, which stimulate the nearby uterine muscle cells to contract.

It is thought that the placenta simultaneously slows its production of progesterone, the hormone that throughout pregnancy has kept the uterus relatively inactive by preventing contractions from spreading to adjacent cells. When there are high levels of estrogen and prostaglandins along with low levels of progesterone, the calcium stored in uterine muscle cells is freed. The free calcium enables little hooks within the muscle cells to grab onto one another, shortening the cells and contracting uterine muscle fibers. Through this complicated sequence of chemical reactions, the baby ultimately causes the uterus to contract and go into labor.

The Autonomic Nervous System and Labor

Like the heart, diaphragm, and digestive tract, the uterus is made up of smooth muscle tissue. Basically, smooth muscle works automatically: the muscle cells contract by themselves; no motor nerve under voluntary control stimulates them to contract. Thus a woman in labor does not *consciously direct* contractions as she would direct her muscles to lift a weight time after time. Rather, she *experiences* uterine contractions much as she feels her heart beating or her lungs expanding

Even though uterine contractions are basically involuntary, there is no doubt that a woman's thoughts and feelings can affect her labor. Relaxation tends to promote effective rhythmic contractions, whereas tension tends to make contractions irregular and unproductive.

Draped Reclining Figure, Henry Moore, 1951. Aquatint and engraving, 6¹/₁₆" x 8". Collection, The Museum of Modern Art, New York. Gift of Gerald Cramer.

Statuette of a Woman, Cycladic, 300 B.C. The Metropolitan Museum of Art. Fletcher Fund, 1934.

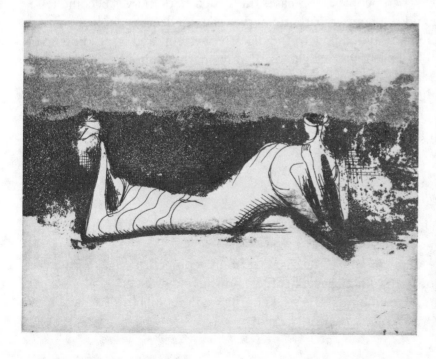

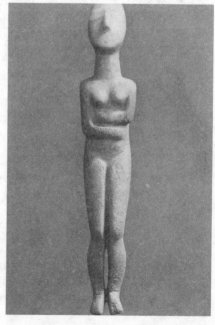

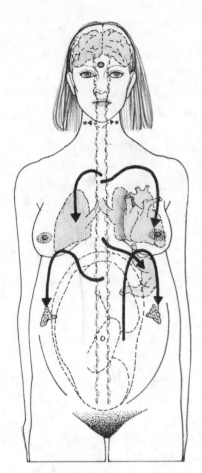

Thoughts and feelings affect labor through the autonomic nervous system. Relaxation tends to promote rhythmic, effective contractions, whereas high levels of anxiety tend to make contractions less regular and less effective.

when she inhales. However, a woman's thoughts and feelings do stimulate nerves that affect the way in which smooth muscle contracts.

When people are relaxed and happy, their heart beats slowly and evenly; when they are tense or frightened, their heart beats more rapidly, making more blood available in case they should need to deal with something perceived to be threatening. Actually, we all know these sensations from personal experience. This involuntary response to a perceived threat was discovered years ago by the renowned physiologist Walter Cannon, who called it the *fight-or-flight response* (see p. 138). Such smooth muscle responses are initially mediated by a special part of the nervous system. Cannon's work gave the first scientific demonstration of how the *autonomic nervous system,* the automatic or unconscious part, is affected by the rest of the brain.

The autonomic nervous system innervates all the body's organs, including the heart, lungs, stomach, intestines, liver, bladder, uterus, and adrenal glands. It doesn't cause these organs to act; it simply speeds up or slows down the work they do. Essentially, it serves as a regulator that maintains the body's physiological balance and sets appropriate rates for different functions.

The autonomic nervous system has two parts. The *sympathetic* nerves basically alert the body and prepare it for fight or flight; the *parasympathetic* nerves cause the body to carry on maintenance functions such as digestion. When people become frightened, thoughts in their brain stimulate the sympathetic branch of the autonomic nervous system, which causes increased heart rate, increased blood flow to muscles in the arms and legs, dilation of the lung passages, and increased *metabolism* or energy production.

When people are at ease, the sympathetic nerves become less active and the parasympathetic nerves cause a decrease in heart rate, an increase in blood flow to the digestive system, and a speeding up of the work of the digestive glands. Parasympathetic arousal and sympathetic dampening lead to the *relaxation response,* a restful state similar to meditation, in which the body heals and maintains itself.

Fearful or happy thoughts not only cause an immediate response from the autonomic nervous system, they also cause a sec-

How emotions affect labor

- The uterus is an autonomic nervous system organ and thus responds to stress.
- In large amounts, the stress hormone epinephrine makes uterine contractions less effective and thus slows labor.
- In large amounts, the stress hormone norepinephrine results in long or overtense contractions.

ondary response that is hormonal and takes place more slowly. Autonomic nerves stimulate the adrenal glands to produce hormones that slow down or speed up metabolism, thereby reinforcing the effects of the relaxation or fight-or-flight responses. This secondary response is significant in situations in which fears or anxieties last for hours or days, because it has important effects on both mother and baby during pregnancy (see p. 142 and p. 147) and during labor, as we shall see.

Although the contractions of labor are basically involuntary, for years women have observed that their contractions tended to slow down when they traveled to the hospital, when someone entered the room to examine them, or when they became anxious for any reason. By contrast, women have sometimes noticed that they dilated very quickly after being reassured that they were making good progress at some point in labor. Mothers and midwives have acknowledged such reactions, but doctors have frequently tended to minimize their importance because they didn't have a clear scientific model or studies to back them up. Only fairly recently have animal and human studies begun to demonstrate the effects of emotional states on labor.

It is unfortunate that so little attention has been paid to autonomic effects on the uterus. Many obstetrical textbooks have entire chapters on the physiology of labor but not one sentence on the role of the autonomic nervous system in regulating contractions. In a sense, that information is at the heart of this book. While it is true that the physiological mechanisms are complex and not easily grasped, the persevering mother will be rewarded by the effect her knowledge will have on her attitude toward labor and delivery.

Ironically, there is a vast amount of literature on autonomic effects on the heart, blood vessels, and other organs. In fact, *behavioral medicine* is a new field that specifically deals with how people can *consciously* control autonomic effects to relieve high blood pressure, ulcers, migraine headaches, asthma, and diabetes. At the heart of these attempts to consciously affect the autonomic nervous system are stress reduction techniques, relaxation, and biofeedback.

Relaxation techniques have been used for years in obstetrics to make women's labor more comfortable (see pp. 154–55), but little notice has been paid to how these techniques could be used to treat labor problems or control the rate or strength of contractions. Paradoxically, the growth in popularity of natural childbirth in the West stems directly from Pavlov's research in Russia in the late 1800s on the conscious control of the salivary glands, which are autonomically regulated. Over the years, through multiple translations and misunderstandings, the relationship between Pavlov's theories and the physiological mechanisms of labor became lost and the concept of controlling labor was replaced by the concept of moderating pain and discomfort. The initial impetus for using natural childbirth in the United States came basically from consumer pressure, not from scientific studies of mechanisms or effects. As a result, there is still very little scientific information on how natural childbirth can work for pain control and no information on how it can work to increase control of labor.

A woman's uterus, vagina, ovaries, and Fallopian tubes are extensively innervated by nerves from the autonomic nervous system. Both sympathetic and parasympathetic nerves leave the spinal cord at several points, ending in weblike structures that cover the reproductive organs. There are two types of nerve fibers: involuntary *motor fibers* that affect muscle cell contraction, and *sensory fibers* that relay sensations of pleasure or pain to the brain.

The autonomic nerves are quite unlike the voluntary motor and sensory nerves that innervate the muscles of the arms and legs. Autonomic motor nerves to the uterus terminate on the surface in ball-shaped endings that release a hormone called *norepinephrine.* It is similar to *epinephrine,* the hormone released by the outer layer of the adrenal glands. Both these hormones basically stimulate the fight-or-flight response, but they influence contractions in subtly different ways.

Uterine muscle cells have two types of receptors that pick up these hormones: *alpha* and *beta* receptors. Norepinephrine is only picked up by alpha receptors; epinephrine can be picked up by either alpha or beta receptors. Estrogen, which is present in large amounts during labor, increases the amount of norepinephrine and the number of alpha receptors that pick it up, basically causing uterine cells to contract. Progesterone, the levels of which decrease during labor, causes an increase in beta receptors, which tends to make the uterus relax. Thus when labor is active, the uterus tends to pick up more norepinephrine at alpha receptors, resulting in more frequent and stronger contractions. When labor slows or doesn't progress, more epinephrine is being picked up at beta receptors.

In recent years research has been done on the effects of all these hormones. Studies on norepinephrine have shown that in high doses it improves uterine tone and increases the frequency of contractions, producing strong but uncoordinated nonrhythmic contractions. Epinephrine has been shown to diminish contractions, increase the time between them, and decrease the tone of the uterus. Studies have found high levels of epinephrine in women who had long, painful labor and in women whose labor slowed or stopped. Epinephrinelike compounds have been given to women in premature labor to shut down their contractions and allow them to carry the baby to term.

Stress and anxiety are known to produce elevated levels of both epinephrine and norepinephrine. high levels these hormones tend to slow labor or make it ineffectual when accompanied by low levels of estrogen and high levels of progesterone. Studies on animals have shown that in addition to affecting muscle contraction, both epinephrine and norepinephrine tend to clamp down blood vessels, reducing blood flow to the uterus by 65 percent or more. Researchers have theorized that such reactions might have evolved as the ultimate fight-or-flight response, in which a female in labor, confronted by a dangerous situation, would be able to shut down labor hormonally and flee. Naturalists have observed in the wild both new mothers and new-born animals are particularly vulnerable to attack.

Under ideal conditions there are high levels of neither epinephrine nor norepinephrine during labor, and labor takes place *by itself*. When a woman is anxious or frightened, the sympathetic nervous system is turned way up, whereas when she is relaxed or perceives pleasure, it is turned down. The effect of thoughts and feelings on contractions underscores the tremendous potential for control over labor that women have. By minimizing fear and tension, a mother can help her contractions to proceed steadily and effectively, neither stopping nor becoming too strong or uncoordinated.

A physiological model postulating how the autonomic nervous system affects uterine contractions was suggested in 1933 by one of the pioneers of natural childbirth, Grantly Dick-Read, years before studies confirmed the existence of alpha and beta receptors or the effects of estrogen and progesterone on nerve transmitters. His ideas stemmed from his clinical and personal experience as well as from research. In particular, he was profoundly affected by one mother who refused his offer of chloroform anesthesia, then gave birth totally without pain, explaining afterward, "It didn't hurt. It wasn't meant to, was it, doctor?" He was to reflect on those words for the rest of his life. A second fundamental experience was personal. After a nurse helped him to relax following a painful injury in World War I, he studied yoga and relaxation while he was stationed in India. That these isolated experiences would form the basis for a leap in scientific thought is truly remarkable. Equally remarkable is the fact that Dick-Read's theories have been borne out by contemporary research.

In analyzing the mechanism of contractions, Dick-Read began by pointing out that the uterus has three layers of muscle: an outer layer that is basically vertical fibers, a middle layer that is a mesh, and an inner layer that is horizontal fibers. The cervix is largely made up of horizontal fibers that encircle the opening, while the vagina has both circular and vertical fibers. Dick-Read cited research that showed that sympathetic (fight-or-flight) nerves make the horizontal fibers contract and the vertical ones relax. Thus stimulation of these nerves tends to prevent cervical dilatation, as well as stretching of the vaginal and perineal muscles. Such contractions tend to squeeze the baby but not expel it. Stimulation of the parasympathetic (relaxation response) nerves, on the other hand, produces just the opposite effects. It makes the circular fibers relax, allowing cervical dilatation and vaginal stretching to take place. Dick-Read believed that relaxation, not contractions, was the most important factor in dilating the cervix. This would explain why mothers don't notice the dilatation that precedes labor and why mothers sometimes dilate very rapidly with relatively few contractions. Most important, parasympathetic stimulation makes the vertical fibers contract, pushing the baby down and out.

Grantly Dick-Read theorized that stimulation of the parasympathetic nerves would tend to produce effective contractions with little or no discomfort, whereas stimulation of the sympathetic nerves would tend to produce painful, ineffective contractions. He pointed out that the parasympathetic system *permits* organs and smooth muscle tissue to work by themselves and simply fine-tunes their responses. The sympathetic system, by contrast, is a more powerful, body-wide response that can readily interrupt the regular functioning of all the smooth-muscle organs. Finally, Dick-Read observed that pain and fear are powerful arousers of the sympathetic nervous system, as they are meant to be in times of danger. Thus he believed that if one can break the fear-tension-pain cycle and get the mother to relax, her labor will proceed naturally and her experience of birth will be physically and mentally entirely different than if she is tense and frightened.

Uterine Contractions

The millions of smooth muscle cells in the uterus are not interconnected by a network of motor nerves. In fact, they are not even fired by an impulse from a motor drive, as the voluntary muscles are. Rather, uterine muscles cells are what might be called *irritable* cells, and they contract by themselves. Each contraction seems to start when a cell or a group of cells near the top of the uterus becomes "hyperirritable" and tenses. Researchers think that any cells near the top of the uterus can initiate a contraction.

Generally the areas where the fallopian tubes enter the uterus are most likely to start a contraction. Cells around the initial group are stimulated by their activity and contract in turn. Thus a contraction spreads out from cell to cell like a wave. Contractions proceed from

Each contraction begins when cells near the top of the uterus become irritable, tense up, and shorten. Contractions start at the top of the uterus and spread to adjacent cells in a downward wave.

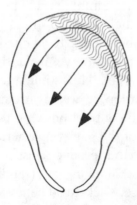 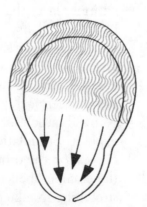 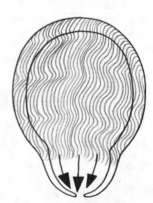

the top down, growing progressively weaker as they reach the bottom of the uterus. This directional orientation is very important in terms of pushing the baby through the birth canal.

Contractions are cyclical; between contractions there is an essential rest period, which the uterus, like other muscles, needs in order to recharge itself biochemically so it can contract again. Before a new contraction can take place, calcium must be pumped out of each muscle cell, the cell has to relax, and the cell membrane must discharge electrically. The rest between contractions also enables the baby to receive more oxygen. During a contraction blood flow to the placenta naturally slows, diminishing the amount of oxygen the baby gets. Normally this isn't dangerous for a healthy baby, even at the height of labor (see p. 358). But without any rest periods at all, the baby would not get sufficient oxygen.

Each contraction has three phases. In the initial *increment* phase the contraction begins to build up as more and more muscle cells become tense. In *acme*, the middle phase, the contraction reaches the point of greatest force. In *decrement*, the final phase, the contraction drops off. The first phase is longest, the second shortest. By placing a hand on the mother's abdomen, the doctor or midwife (or even the mother) can feel a contraction begin long before the mother feels it as a sensation.

Contractions start out being weak, infrequent, and short in duration. At the beginning of labor, contractions take place every 30 minutes or so and only last for 15 to 30 seconds. As labor progresses, contractions increase in frequency until they are only 2 or 3 minutes apart and last 60 to 90 seconds. Contractions also increase in strength or intensity as labor goes on. At the onset, contractions usually increase uterine pressure by about 30 millimeters of mercury. Late in labor the average pressure reaches 50 millimeters and may go as high as 80 to 100. Surprisingly, the highest pressure is reached when the placenta is expelled; pressure then reaches as high as 250 millimeters. During the resting phase between contractions, uterine pressure drops back to 5 to 10 millimeters.

Contractions focus on the *fundus*, the upper part of the uterus, which is referred to as the *active segment*. Each time uterine muscle fibers contract, they shorten. Following a contraction, they do not return to their previous length but remain slightly shorter. Thus the fundus becomes progressively thicker and thicker. As the top of the uterus tightens, it presses harder and harder on the baby, who is squeezed downward by the process. As a result of the top of the uterus contracting and the baby being pushed down, the bottom of the uterus, which is called the *lower uterine segment*, is passively stretched. With each contraction the fibers of the lower segment lengthen and remain longer. Thus as labor proceeds, the whole lower segment expands greatly.

As labor progresses, the top or active segment of the uterus becomes shorter and thicker, pushing the baby down and out. At the same time the passive lower segment of the uterus and the cervix stretch and thin, allowing the baby to pass through.

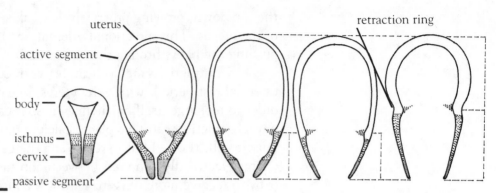

The difference between the active and passive segments is critical to the birth process. Were the uterus to contract equally all over, the baby would merely be squeezed, not pushed out. Instead, the upper and lower parts work together: the lower part lengthens and expands only to the extent that the upper part shortens and contracts. The action of the two parts is so distinct that an indendation forms in the middle of the uterus between the segments. This ring can be felt during labor by placing a hand on the mother's abdomen.

The shortening of the upper segment and the lengthening of the lower segment transform the shape of the uterus, causing it to become longer and narrower as labor progresses. This change tends to straighten the baby's back if it is in a head-down position. When its back is straight, the baby is pushed directly down, centering all the force of the contractions on the lower uterine segment and the cervix. As opposed to the uterus, most of the cervix is made of fibrous connective tissue, not muscle. Toward the end of pregnancy, the collagen fibers holding the cervix closed are dissolved by enzymes, making dilatation easier. The force of the baby's head pressing on the cervix gradually causes it to thin and stretch. This is what the work of the first stage of labor is all about.

Dilatation and Effacement

Doctors and midwives have long been aware that labor naturally divides into several stages. The first stage begins when the contractions have enough intensity, duration, and frequency to begin actively to alter the shape of the cervix. At the beginning of labor the uterus is an almost closed pouch; at most the cervix is open from 1 to 2 centimeters (about the diameter of a dime), but the tube is still 1 to 2 centimeters long. During the first stage of labor the cervix shortens to nothing and simultaneously widens to 10 centimeters (about the size of a wide-mouth jar). The shortening process is called *effacement*, and the widening is called *dilatation*.

Effacement can be visualized by blowing up a balloon: as the balloon gets bigger, the neck actually stretches, shortens, and becomes incorporated into the body of the balloon. In the uterus these changes are made possible by the fact that the cervix is made up of pleated muscle fibers that gradually unfold and lengthen as they are drawn up around the baby. Doctors and midwives measure effacement in terms of percentages: no effacement is called 0 percent, full effacement is 100 percent. Many women, because of Braxton Hicks contractions, are as much as 50 percent effaced when they begin labor; that is, the cervical tube has already shortened from 2 centimeters to 1.

During dilatation the opening of the cervix enlarges enough for the baby to emerge. Dilatation is measured in centimeters, ranging from 0 to 10. The widest part of a baby, the head, averages about 9.5 centimeters when it passes through the birth canal in a tucked position. Like effacement, this process is made possible by the anatomical structure of the cervix. The process can be visualized by watching

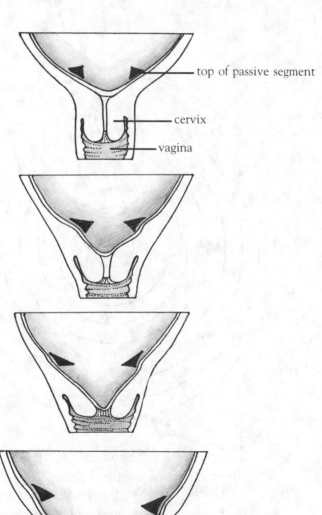

Effacement is the process by which the tube of the cervix slowly shortens and thins in preparation for delivery. *Dilatation* is the process by which the cervical opening widens enough to permit the baby's head to pass through. The two processes overlap and work together, although effacement tends to precede dilatation.

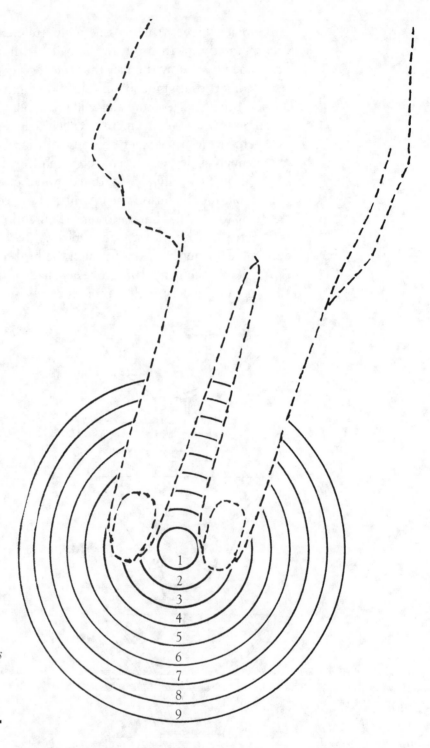

Dilatation is measured in centimeters from 0 to 10. Generally dilatation proceeds very slowly for a long time and then speeds up. Rings shown are actual size.

someone put on a tight turtleneck sweater: the neck of the sweater actually stretches as the head passes through.

The first stage of labor ends when effacement and dilatation are complete. On the average the first stage takes about 12 to 14 hours with a first delivery and 4 to 6 hours with subsequent deliveries. The second stage, which is by far the most momentous and exciting, goes from total dilatation to delivery. The baby finishes its descent and emerges into the world. This stage is much shorter than the first—usually about 50 minutes with a first delivery and only about 20 minutes with subsequent deliveries, although it can be longer. The third stage of labor begins with delivery and ends with expulsion of the placenta. This stage usually averages a mere 5 to 10 minutes but can take longer. The final stage begins with delivery of the placenta and lasts for about an hour. During this stage the uterus continues to contract, clamping down uterine blood vessels, especially around the site where the placenta was attached.

The Friedman Curves for Labor

In the last twenty years a useful new model for labor has been developed by Emanuel Friedman, a professor at Harvard Medical School. It evolved from Dr. Friedman's belief that the old model didn't assist the mother or doctor in dealing with wide variations encountered in labor, especially in the first stage. He felt that the previous description of stages was vague, that one stage often overlapped another, and that labor did not progress in a linear fashion. Based on his own experience with patients, Friedman also felt that the strength, duration, and timing of contractions didn't necessarily give a clear picture of how labor was really progressing. For example, some women are ready to deliver after seemingly poor contractions, while other women are far from ready after a long period of strong contractions.

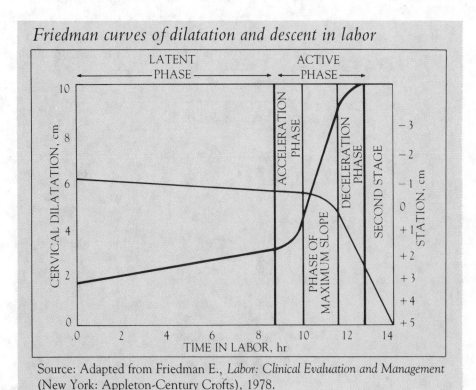

Friedman curves of dilatation and descent in labor

Source: Adapted from Friedman E., *Labor: Clinical Evaluation and Management* (New York: Appleton-Century Crofts), 1978.

Friedman decided to graph dilatation of the cervix and descent of the baby through the birth canal, and study the results. Surprisingly, little work had been done earlier to evaluate the progress of labor in terms of such easily measurable factors. Friedman found that neither dilatation nor descent proceeded at a steady rate, and that dilatation was not completed before descent began, as the old model had implied. His studies showed that both dilatation and descent generally progress rather slowly for a long time and then suddenly speed up, culminating relatively quickly in birth.

Based on the information yielded by his time curves, Friedman postulated that what had formerly been considered the first stage of labor actually separated into two phases, which he called the *latent phase* and the *active phase*. The initial or latent phase is by far the longest part of the first stage. It averages 6½ hours with a first birth and around 5 with subsequent births, with a maximum of 20 hours for some first-time mothers and 14 for women who've had vaginal deliveries before.

In addition to the great variability in the actual length of labor, individual practitioners and hospitals define "normal" labor times differently, mainly because they do not use the same criteria to assess the beginning of labor. Some doctors start timing labor with the first contractions, some with admittance to the hospital, some with the onset of contractions that cause a change in dilatation.

What Friedman calls the latent phase begins with active uterine contractions and continues until the point at which the mother's cervix suddenly begins to dilate more quickly. Contractions in the

Friedman's management recommendations for labor

	RECOMMENDED	EXCEPTIONS
Long latent phase	rest	oxytocin
Long active phase	optimism and support	cesarean section when mother's pelvis is too small
Failure to progress at all in active phase—mother's pelvis too small	cesarean section	no exceptions
Failure to progress at all in active phase, but mother's pelvis adequate	oxytocin	rest

Source: Adapted from Friedman E. *Labor: Clinical Evaluation and Management* (New York: Appleton-Century Crofts), 1978.

latent phase start out 10 to 20 minutes apart and lasting 15 to 20 seconds, and slowly progress to 5 to 7 minutes apart and lasting 30 to 40 seconds. *Throughout the entire latent phase little dilatation actually takes place.* By the end of this phase a woman is only 3 or 4 centimeters dilated. This means that if she was 1 or 2 centimeters when first checked, as is common, then she only dilates 1 or 2 centimeters during the whole of the latent phase.

Friedman believes that this phase is simply a time of preparation, during which uterine muscle fibers learn to work together to produce a smooth, coordinated, wavelike contraction. At the same time biochemical changes are taking place within the cervix, readying it for the phase of rapid dilatation that follows. One of the most significant facts for mothers to be aware of is Friedman's observation that *there is no correlation between either dilatation or duration of the latent phase and the length, discomfort, or outcome of the rest of labor.* Mothers should not become discouraged about lack of progress in the early part of labor; slow progress is *normal* at this point. Friedman points out that the latent phase of labor is the one most susceptible to outside influences, both positive and negative. In particular, sedation, painkillers, stimulants, and stress can all slow labor at this stage (see p. 277).

Since no adverse effects on the baby or mother have been correlated with the length of the latent phase, some doctors and midwives question calling labor abnormal when the latent phase goes outside the Friedman curves. They feel that since labor times generally vary so greatly, it is not useful to define as abnormal the 10 percent of labors that go past the Friedman time curves but that otherwise have no indications of a problem. Some doctors and midwives feel that the average times quoted by Friedman are fast and inflexible. In reality, many mothers do not perform as punctually. As a result, if the Friedman times are adhered to rigidly, they can be the cause of pitocin induction and even cesarean sections performed due to lack of progress in labor. Strict adherence to the times may put pressure on a mother, defeating her efforts to relax and work with her instinctual feelings.

The active phase, the end of the first stage of labor, begins when the mother finally starts to dilate more rapidly and lasts until her cervix is fully dilated and effaced. Friedman notes that when dilatation is complete, the cervix is drawn back so that it merges with the top of the vagina and the lower part of the uterus. The entire active phase takes an average of about 4 hours in a first delivery but can range from under 1 hour to over 12. In subsequent deliveries the active phase averages 2 hours, varying from a matter of minutes to 5 hours.

Based on his analysis of the time curves, Friedman breaks the active phase of labor into three parts: the *acceleration phase,* the *phase of maximum slope,* and the *deceleration phase.* During the acceleration phase the cervix gradually but noticeably begins to dilate at a faster rate. This phase is short and variable, and, unlike the latent phase, often gives the mother and the practitioner an indication of how the rest of labor will proceed. If the acceleration phase is rapid, the rest of labor tends to be shorter; if the acceleration phase is slow, labor tends to be longer.

The *phase of maximum slope* is the period when the most dilatation takes place and when it takes place most rapidly. This is the only stage of labor when dilatation proceeds at a rather constant rate. The average rate is 3 centimeters per hour with a first delivery and almost 6 centimeters an hour with subsequent deliveries. Compared to the 1 or 2 centimeters the mother dilated during the latent phase, this is astonishing and exciting progress. Friedman points out that the rate at this stage is a good index of how efficiently the uterus is working to dilate the cervix. By the end of the maximum slope phase the mother is about 8 centimeters dilated.

Friedman calls the final phase of active labor *deceleration*, a somewhat misleading name because labor is not slowing; neither are the contractions weakening. In fact, they are getting stronger and more frequent. Deceleration refers to the fact that the cervix no longer seems to be dilating quite as rapidly. This apparent slowdown is the result of the cervix being retracted or pulled back over the baby's head. Up to this point the cervix has been dilating in a horizontal plane, from side to side across the baby's head. Now, as the baby begins to descend into the birth canal, the cervix starts to be pulled upward around the head as well as sideways. Thus if only the diameter of the cervix is measured, it appears that dilatation has slowed. Deceleration marks the end of the first stage of labor, the point the traditional model referred to as *transition*. Friedman calls this *turning the corner*.

During the active phase the mother's contractions have become more frequent, longer, and stronger. By the end of this phase they are 2 to 3 minutes apart and last a full 60 seconds. Up to this point all the work of labor has been passively dilating and effacing the cervix and initiating the baby's descent, and the mother has been urged not to push. Now the mother's work becomes actively pushing the baby out.

Pushing does not help to dilate the cervix. In fact, forcefully pushing the baby against the cervix before it is sufficiently dilated can bruise the cervix and slow dilatation. Once the baby's head reaches the pelvic floor (see p. 28), pushing becomes a reflex action that is triggered at the beginning of each contraction. The experience of pushing is similar to that of having a bowel movement, but much more powerful. In fact, at this point women sometimes feel as if they have to have a bowel movement, because the reflex is so similar.

The baby's delivery is not just the result of the mother's contractions, although they play an important role and are remarkably intense at this point. The major factor that causes the baby to descend is the mother's pushing. When the mother squeezes her abdominal muscles, pressure in her abdominal cavity rises, forcing the baby down and out. Pushing becomes most effective when it takes place at the same time as a contraction.

Descent

There are two basic variables that are used to judge the baby's progress toward birth. In the last section we dealt with one variable, dilatation of the cervix. Here we will deal with the second, the baby's descent through the birth canal.

Although the baby is becoming increasingly crowded in the uterus by the beginning of the ninth month, it is still carried high in the abdomen and is "floating free." In mothers who have had previous deliveries, the baby remains high up until sometime after labor begins, but in first-time mothers, descent begins several weeks prior to delivery. This process, called lightening or dropping, was discussed earlier in the chapter.

In the initial stage of descent the baby's head drops down within the circle of the pelvic bones. Once the widest part of the baby's head passes through the *inlet,* the place where the pelvic opening narrows, the baby is said to be *engaged.* The inlet corresponds to an imaginary line that goes from just below the top of the pubic bone in the front of the mother's body to the spot where the sacrum makes a bend in the back. The inlet is sometimes referred to as the *pelvic brim.*

Doctors measure the baby's descent through the birth canal in terms of the *station* or point it has reached. There are eleven imaginary stations, measured in centimeters, along the birth canal. These stations are measured upward and downward from an arbitrary point at about the middle of the pelvis. That point corresponds to a line

The baby is said to be engaged *when the widest part of its head reaches the mother's* inlet, *the point where her pelvis first narrows. At this stage the top of the baby's head just reaches the level of the ischial spines and is said to be at* station 0. *Both station and degree of engagement are measures of how far labor has progressed and the baby has descended.*

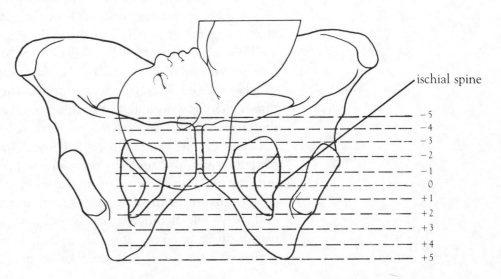

ischial spine

-5
-4
-3
-2
-1
0
+1
+2
+3
+4
+5

between the ischial spines, the little bumps on the sides of the birth canal (see pp. 28–29). It is assigned the number 0. The five stations above are referred to in minus numbers (-5, -4, -3, -2, -1), because at these stations the top of the baby's head (or whatever part comes first) hasn't yet reached the midpoint; the five stations below are referred to in positive numbers ($+1$, $+2$, $+3$, $+4$, $+5$), because the leading part has passed the midpoint.

As the baby starts to enter the pelvis it is considered to be at station -5. It is said to be engaged when the widest part of its head reaches the brim of the pelvis and the top of its head reaches station 0. Just before the moment of birth, when the baby's head reaches the vaginal opening, it's said to be at station $+5$. The last few stations are generally academic because everyone becomes caught up in the imminence of birth, but the earlier stations are useful references for both mother and practitioner because they convey graphically where the baby is and how much further it has to go.

Because the stations are such a valuable indicator of the progress of labor and delivery, Friedman graphed station versus time for a large group of mothers, as he had done with dilatation. When the two graphs are put together, they show a beautiful complementary relationship. The *latent period of dilatation*, during which little widening of the cervix takes place, is matched by a *latent period of descent*, in which the baby makes little downward progress. Like the rate of dilatation, the rate of descent speeds up late in the first stage of labor. With a first delivery the rate of descent increases rapidly during the period of maximum dilatation, but achieves the greatest speed as the cervix is pulled back around the baby's head during deceleration. This speed of descent is maintained until the baby is born. With subsequent deliveries descent doesn't begin *until* the deceleration phase of dilatation, but then it proceeds in much the same way. In this case descent rapidly reaches a maximum speed once dilatation is complete, and continues at this speed until birth takes place.

One of the major points brought out by Friedman's graphs is that descent doesn't begin with the second stage of labor. Rather, it is well under way toward the end of the first stage, while the mother is still actively dilating—especially in first deliveries. The earlier model of labor viewed descent purely as part of the second stage of labor rather than as a normal part of dilatation between 8 and 10 centimeters, when the rate appears to decrease as the cervix starts to draw back. Often first-time mothers become agitated by the new and unexpected sensations caused by the early part of descent and by the apparent slowing of dilatation during the most intense contractions.

Given the distinct phases he found in the first stage of labor and the problems inherent in the old model, Friedman evolved a new way of dividing labor. The old model fails to differentiate the long period of little visible progress that occurs at the beginning of labor.

This failure caused many mothers to become discouraged and anxious early in labor. Friedman believes that this oversight was also the cause of many cesarean sections being done because of lack of progress in the first stage of labor. Moreover, the old theory that descent did not begin until dilatation was complete is at odds with the sensations that mothers experience during the last few centimeters of dilatation, making it more difficult for them to deal with the most intense contractions.

Friedman's model is based on what is actually happening to the mother. We think it tends to be reassuring and thus is worth presenting, even though it is not used by all doctors and midwives. Friedman's model divides labor functionally into three categories: the *preparatory division,* the *dilatational division,* and the *pelvic division.*

The preparatory division starts with the onset of regular contractions and continues until the end of the acceleration phase, when dilatation has begun to speed up. This division is a lengthy period of relatively few external changes but great biochemical changes within the cervix and uterus, anticipating the events to come. It is followed by the dilatational division, a much shorter period during which virtually all the dilatation takes place in a fairly linear fashion, and descent gradually begins as the stage draws to a close. The final and shortest part of labor is the pelvic division, which begins with the deceleration phase when dilatation finishes and retraction takes place. Most important, this is the time when descent reaches its maximum speed and the baby makes its way through the bony pelvic canal by executing a remarkably choreographed series of twists and turns, presenting the narrowest parts of itself to the narrowest parts of the mother's pelvis. The third division ends with the birth of the baby.

The Baby's Position During Labor

The baby's position in the uterus as it starts to descend has far-reaching effects on the kind of labor the mother experiences and on how the doctor or midwife manages her labor. Throughout the early and middle months of pregnancy the baby floats freely in the uterus. As the baby becomes bigger, it becomes more confined, and by the eighth month it takes up a position in which it has the most room. During the last prenatal visits the doctor or midwife determines what the baby's position is through a series of special hand maneuvers (see pp. 230–31).

Several terms are used to define how the baby is situated in the uterus. The *lie* refers to whether the baby is facing up, down, or sideways. Well over 99 percent of all babies are vertical; only a few are sideways. *Presentation* refers to the part of the baby that is nearest the opening of the birth canal. Babies may present with the back of the

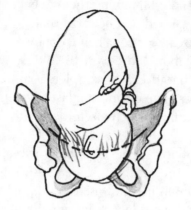

right occiput anterior

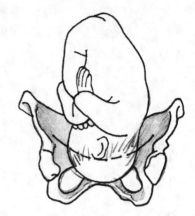

left occiput anterior

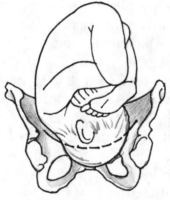

right occiput transverse

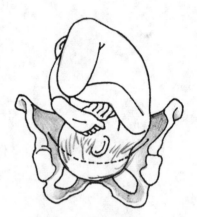

left occiput transverse

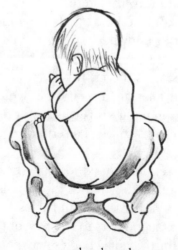

complete breech

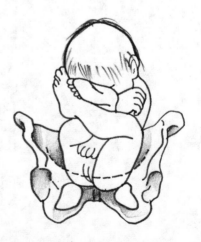

frank breech

head, feet, face, or shoulder first. Of all babies, 96 percent are head down when labor starts. In the second most common position, called *breech*, the baby's rump or foot is nearest the cervix. This accounts for only 3.5 percent of all babies. Doctors speculate that the head, which is compact, usually tends to lie at the bottom of the uterus, and the feet and buttocks tend to lie at the top because they take up more room.

The last and most inclusive term practitioners use is *position*, referring to the relationship of the presenting part to the four directions of the pelvis: left, right, front (*anterior*), back (*posterior*), or sideways (*transverse*). The most common position is called *left occiput transverse* (LOT). Occiput means that the back of the baby's head (the occiput) is nearest the birth canal; left means the occiput is toward the mother's left side; and transverse means that the baby's head is facing side to side. The mirror image of this, *right occiput transverse* (ROT), is the second most common position.

In all the usual head-down, face-backward positions like those just given, labor proceeds in much the same way. Generally if a baby is head down but face forward, it will rotate during labor and be born with its face aimed backward. Among the remaining positions, which are relatively uncommon—breech, face, or shoulder first—labor proceeds differently and is handled differently by the doctor or midwife (see p. 372). Also the mother will experience diverse sensations in labor, or be more aware of them, depending on the baby's position.

Delivery: The Baby's Passage Through the Birth Canal

Doctors refer to the baby's movements through the birth canal as the *cardinal movements*. Although these movements have been accomplished by babies since the beginning of the species, they were not analyzed and described until the eighteenth century. The classic sequence of movements, in which the baby emerges head first, is dictated by the anatomy of the mother's pelvis and the anatomy of the baby's head and shoulders.

Both the baby's head and the opening in the mother's pelvis have an oval rather than a round shape, so they are wider in one direction than the other. Since the oval of the mother's pelvis is only slightly larger than that of the baby's head, the baby can only fit through if the widest diameter of its head is perfectly aligned with the widest diameter of the mother's pelvis, in much the same way as a block can only fit through a shape-sorting box in one position. Fortunately the birth canal is not cylindrical but funnel-shaped, with the widest part of the funnel facing upward.

The muscles lining the canal form walls that guide the baby's

The baby's position in the uterus is defined by the relationship between the mother's pelvis and the part of the baby that is closest to the birth canal. For example, if the baby's head (occiput) is nearest to the birth canal and the back of the head is facing the left side of the mother's pelvis and pointing toward the front (anterior), the baby is said to be left occiput anterior (LOA). The head can also be pointing toward the mother's back (posterior) or directly to the side (transverse). If the baby's rump is closest to the birth canal, the baby is said to be breech. When there are twins, each is in a different position.

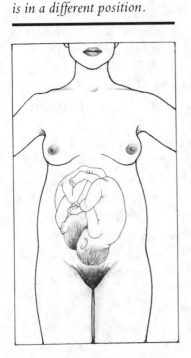

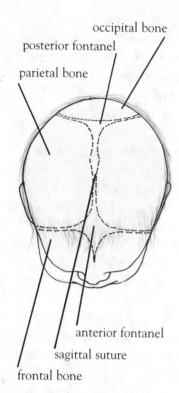

occipital bone

posterior fontanel

parietal bone

anterior fontanel

sagittal suture

frontal bone

The baby's skull is made of compressible bony plates that meet along lines called sutures. The area where several sutures meet is called a fontanel; it is soft to the touch. The anterior fontanel in the front is larger than the posterior fontanel in the back.

head into the correct position. As the head starts to enter the birth canal, the mother's pelvis is wider from side to side (13.5 centimeters) than from front to back (11 centimeters). But as the baby passes through the pelvis, the opening becomes much wider from front to back (12 centimeters) than sideways (10.5 centimeters). Thus the baby's head naturally turns to fit the canal as it descends.

The narrowest part of the baby's head is from side to side—a distance that averages 9.25 centimeters. The second narrowest distance is from front to back when the head is tipped forward, that is, from the soft spot in front to the base of the skull in the back. This distance averages 9.5 centimeters. The widest parts of the baby's head are the distance from just above the eyes to the back of the head—approximately 11.5 centimeters—and the distance from the chin to posterior soft spot—approximately 13.5 centimeters.

The baby's descent is aided by the fact that its skull is made of five thin, bony plates that are actually compressible. These plates are held together at the edges by fibrous membranes. The lines they form are called *sutures.* The areas where several sutures come together are soft spots called *fontanels.* The larger one toward the front is called the *anterior* fontanel; the smaller one to the rear is called the *posterior* fontanel. During labor the doctor can determine which way the baby is facing by doing an internal exam to feel the fontanels and sutures. As the baby descends through the birth canal, the plates often slide slightly over or under one another, depending on how tightly they are squeezed. This process, called *molding,* can make the baby's head ½ to 1 centimeter narrower and helps to accommodate the baby's passage through the canal.

The baby performs eight cardinal movements during delivery. For the sake of clarity they are discussed separately, but they are really part of one long movement in which the baby passes through the birth canal and emerges from the shelter of its mother's womb. The timing of some of the movements varies tremendously depending on several factors, including the anatomy of the individual mother and baby, the direction the baby is facing in the uterus, and whether or not it is the mother's first vaginal birth.

The first two cardinal movements have been discussed already. The initial movement, which is *engagement* (lightening), takes place when the greatest side-to-side diameter of the baby's head reaches the the top of the birth canal, the *inlet.* As we've mentioned, engagement occurs several weeks before labor in first births, whereas it occurs sometime during the first part of labor in subsequent births. The second movement is *descent,* which is initially caused by the downward pressure of uterine contractions and subsequently by the mother's pushing efforts as well.

In the third movement, called *flexion,* the baby's head bends further forward until the chin is tightly tucked against its chest. Tipping the head forward presents a much narrower aspect of the head (9.5 versus 12 centimeters) to the tightening birth canal. The baby often has its head in this position even as it engages, but if it doesn't, the head is tucked down by the walls of the birth canal at the point where the cervix ends and the pelvic bones narrow (station 0), or when the head reaches the *pelvic floor* (station +3) and the muscles around the anus and vaginal opening give the head resistance.

In the fourth movement, called *internal rotation,* the baby's head, which has been slightly sideways, now turns so that its face is pointing directly at the mother's spine. Internal rotation lines up the widest diameter of the baby's head, which is front-to-back, with the widest diameter of the pelvic outlet, which is also front-to-back. The baby's head naturally assumes this position as the mother's pelvis narrows from side to side. This is probably the most important turn the baby makes during descent, because this is the narrowest point in the birth canal. Without this rotation only the smallest babies could be born. The movement takes place at some point between the time the top of the baby's head gets to the ischial spines (station 0) and when it reaches the pelvic floor at the bottom of the birth canal (station +4). Only the baby's head is turned to the mother's back at this point; its shoulders remain slightly sideways because they are still in the wider space at the top of the pelvis.

The fifth movement, called *extension,* involves the baby's head bending backward as its chin untucks and lifts off its chest. This movement is dictated by the fact that the birth canal bends sharply forward and upward at the bottom: the mother's spine curves forward at the base, and also the vaginal opening lies in front of the anus. Extension occurs when the baby's head meets resistance from the mother's spine and the muscles of the pelvic floor.

As extension begins, the perineal area around the anus and vagina bulges more and more, then the vaginal opening begins to dilate and the top of the baby's head first becomes visible. With each contraction that follows, the vagina continues to stretch and more of the head appears. The baby is said to be *crowning* at the instant the vagina stretches around the entire head. The process of extension becomes even more obvious as the forehead, nose, mouth, and chin emerge from the bottom of the vagina. This is the true beginning of birth and it brings with it mingled emotions of joy, wonder, relief, and renewed energy for the mother and those helping her.

The baby's subsequent movements occur rapidly and with seeming ease. The sixth movement, *restitution,* automatically takes place as the last of the baby's head emerges from the vagina. Free of the birth canal, the head "untwists," turning slightly toward the mother's right side and thereby realigning itself with the shoulders, which have been sideways in the birth canal up to this point.

The seventh movement is called *external rotation.* In this move-

This series of drawings shows the descending movements that a baby in one of the common presenting positions (left occiput anterior) automatically makes as it passes through the birth canal. These movements are dictated by the oval shape of the pelvis and the sharp bend that the birth canal makes due to the position of the vaginal opening. To the right of each drawing is an inset that shows the baby's head in relation to the bones of the pelvis. The soft spots are dotted in on the baby's head to show graphically how the head turns during delivery.

(a) Initially, before its head becomes engaged, the baby floats freely in the uterus.

(b) As the head descends and becomes engaged, the baby's chin tucks down toward its chest (flexion), presenting the widest part of the head to the widest part of the birth canal.

(c) As the baby descends further, its face begins to turn toward the mother's spine, presenting the widest part of its head to the widest part of the lower pelvis (internal rotation).

(d) In order to emerge from the birth canal, the baby's face turns completely toward the mother's spine (complete rotation) and its head begins to bend backward, lifting its chin off its chest (beginning extension).

(e) As the baby crowns, beginning to emerge from the birth canal, its head bends

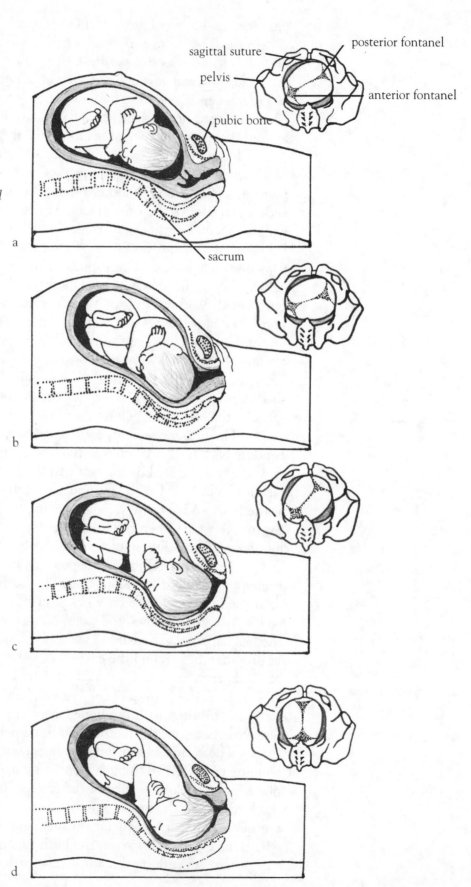

sagittal suture

posterior fontanel

pelvis

anterior fontanel

pubic bone

sacrum

a

b

c

d

further back (complete extension).

(f) As the baby's head emerges fully from the vagina, it turns sideways, aligning itself with the shoulders, which have turned sideways in passing through the narrowest part of the mother's pelvis (external rotation).

(g) The baby's head bends downward, allowing the anterior *or top shoulder to emerge from under the pubic bone.*

(h) The baby bends upward, allowing the posterior *or bottom shoulder to emerge next. The rest of the baby's body slips out easily without any turns.*

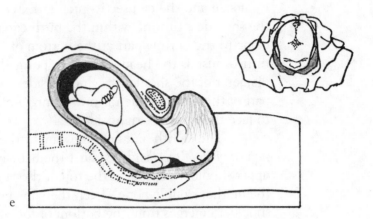

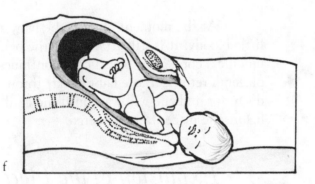

e

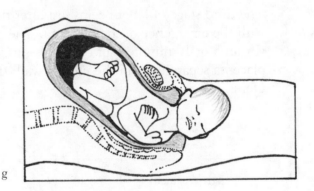

f

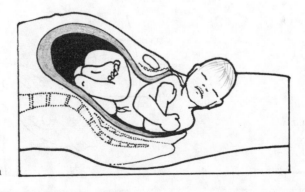

g

h

ment the head turns even further until it is directly facing the mother's right side and she can see its profile. External rotation is the result of the shoulders turning within the birth canal. As the shoulders finally come to the narrow part at the bottom of the pelvis, they are firmly turned, just as the head was at this point. In order for the widest diameter of the shoulders, which is side-to-side, to fit across the widest part of the pelvis, which is now front-to-back, the baby's chest turns to face the mother's right side.

The eighth and final movement the baby makes is called *expulsion* or *birth of the shoulders*. First the baby bends downward, and the upper shoulder appears at the top of the vagina, emerging from under the mother's pubic bone. Then the baby bends upward, and the lower shoulder emerges from the bottom of the vagina. The rest of the body slides out quickly with no further turns and little effort on the mother's part.

At the moment of birth the baby appears wet and perhaps a little bloody. It is still attached to the placenta by the long, ropy umbilical cord. This bluish cord continues to pulse as blood from the placenta returns to the baby's body through its navel. Generally the doctor or midwife will wait until the cord stops pulsing, but then cut it before the placenta is delivered.

Expulsion of the Placenta

The third stage of labor begins just after the baby is born and ends with the emergence of the placenta. The placenta is usually delivered within 5 or 10 minutes but often takes as long as a half-hour. First the placenta separates from the uterine wall; then it is expelled from the uterus.

At the time of delivery the birth canal is one smooth curvilinear passage with a sharp bend at the end. By this stage in labor the active segment of the uterus has shortened, causing the lower segment to stretch, and the cervix has thinned and dilated so that it is continuous with the stretched wall of the vagina (see drawing of uterine segments, p. 282).

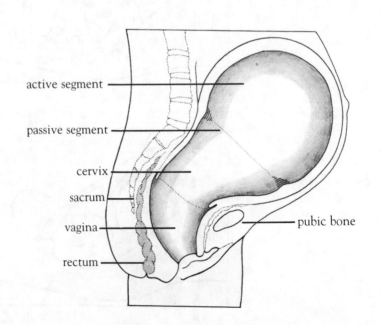

active segment

passive segment

cervix

sacrum

vagina

rectum

pubic bone

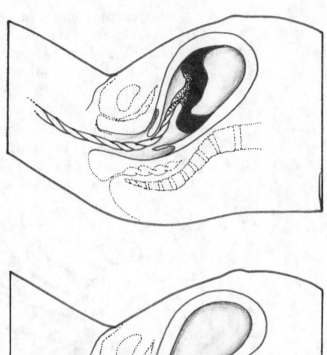

The contractions that follow the delivery of the baby cause the top of the uterus to tighten even more, shearing the uterine wall away from the placenta, which does not contract. Once the placenta has sheared away from the uterine wall, it is rapidly expelled from the uterus along with about 2 cups of blood from the implantation site *where the placenta was attached.*

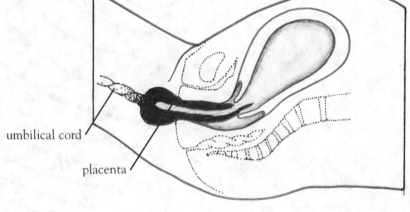

umbilical cord

placenta

Immediately after birth the uterus experiences a lull in contractions that lasts for about 3 to 5 minutes. Then the contractions begin again. The muscle fibers of the uterus are able to contract even more strongly without the baby inside. Although third-stage contractions generate two to five times as much pressure inside the uterus as the earlier ones, they are not particularly uncomfortable for the mother.

With each contraction the uterus shrinks further in size. The placenta, on the other hand, does not shrink because it is made of nonmuscular tissue. It buckles and folds as it is squeezed by the uterus. Since the placenta is not continuous with the uterus but is simply attached at many points, this buckling motion causes the placenta to shear away from the uterine wall, much as paper rips along a perforated line. The weight of the placenta itself (about 1½ pounds) assists the shearing process. Once the placenta has separated, it is expelled by a combination of uterine contractions and the mother actively pushing.

The placenta separates in one of two ways. It may separate at the center first and then at the sides. This is the most common manner and is referred to as a *Schultz.* Alternately, the placenta may separate at the edges first and then at the center, which is called a *Duncan.* With a Schultz the shiny, gray side of the placenta that was unattached appears first. It is followed by a small pool of blood that was dammed behind it. With a Duncan the pool of blood comes first and is followed by the placenta, which emerges inside out, with the rough side that was attached to the uterus appearing first.

The separation of the placenta normally tears many tiny blood vessels at the attachment site. These blood vessels run through layers

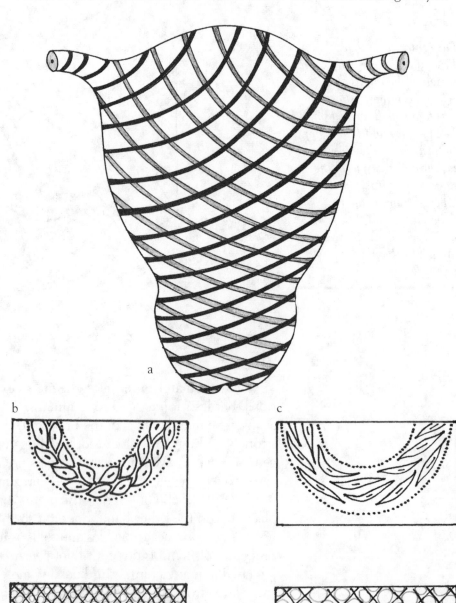

The uterus consists of millions of smooth muscle fibers that are arranged at right angles to each other (a). The blood vessels that lead to the placenta run through these muscle layers (b). After the placenta separates, the muscle fibers in the uterus contract further, clamping off the blood vessels and stopping the bleeding at the implantation site (c). The contraction of the muscle fibers is referred to as a living ligature.

blood vessels

tensed muscle fibers

relaxed muscle fibers

of uterine muscle fibers that lie at right angles to each other. As the uterus contracts, the fibers make tighter and tighter rings around the torn blood vessels until they are clamped off. Doctors refer to the uterine muscle fibers as a *living ligature* or tourniquet.

On the average a mother loses about two cups of blood (600 milliliters) during vaginal delivery and the days following. This represents about half the extra red blood cells she has made during pregnancy. Most of the blood that is lost comes from the separation site or the placenta itself. The rest is blood from the episiotomy (if one was done) and from the normal uterine discharge that follows birth.

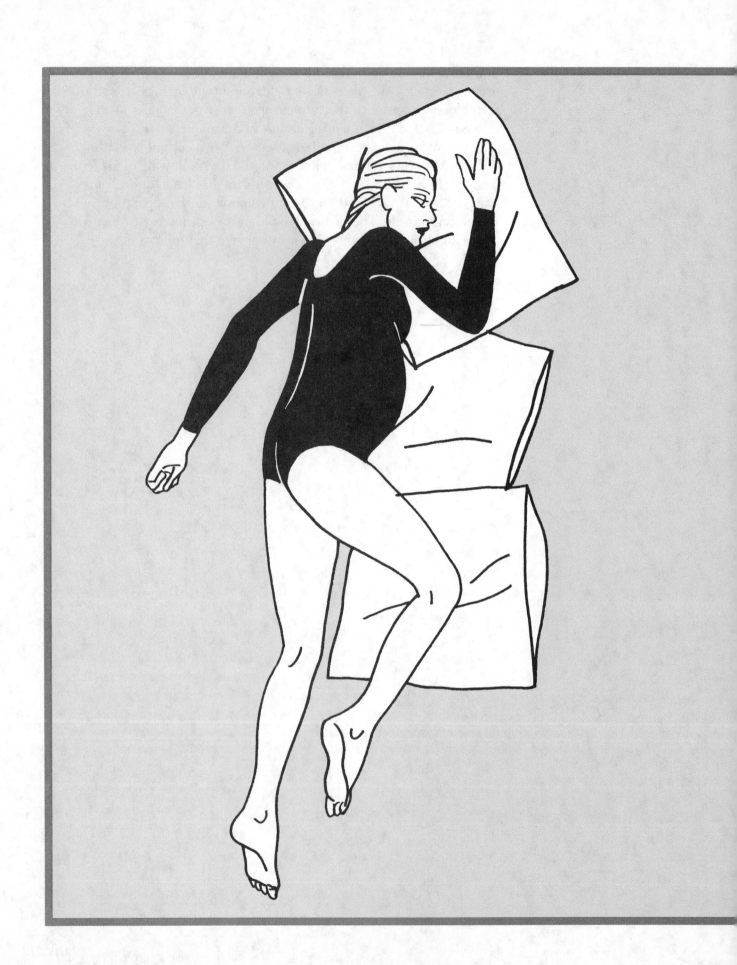

CHAPTER 14

The Mother's Experience of Labor and How It Is Managed

The Mother's Feelings Before Labor

Going into labor is the culmination of months of waiting. Almost always there is a sense of surprise, for this is not an event that the mother schedules like her doctor's appointments. Any special plans have to be altered, and normal routines must be set aside. No one—mother, father, or practitioner—can predict what will happen over the course of the next hours and days. For most people this is a highly unusual situation—very exciting but a bit scary, a little like going on a trip, without plans, to a place you've never been before.

For most mothers, strong and sometimes conflicting feelings are aroused by the beginning of labor. Initially there is often uncertainty as to whether this is really labor, accompanied by a sense of relief that the increasingly annoying symptoms of late pregnancy will soon be over and a sense of joyous anticipation that the baby is about to be born. If labor begins several weeks in advance of the mother's due date, she may feel somewhat dismayed and unprepared physically, emotionally, or practically. She may be overtired, worried that she hasn't practiced her relaxation enough, or upset that she hasn't finished fixing the baby's room or bought enough diapers. This is especially common with first-time mothers, who are about to undergo a profound and mysterious new experience, but it may also apply to second- and third-time mothers who've been very busy in the latter part of pregnancy with their home, job, or other children. On the other hand, if a mother's due date has come and gone and labor still has not commenced, she is likely to be increasingly frustrated, a little concerned, and suddenly unsure of all her expectations about the baby. Certainly she is likely to feel large, ungainly, and uncomfortable. Diverse feelings, both positive and negative, often present themselves as sudden, inexplicable shifts of mood. Shortly before a mother goes into labor she may find herself feeling fine at one moment, then suddenly feeling blue or irritated for no obvious reason. Other people may notice this before the mother even becomes aware of it.

Although few women expect their baby to be born on the very day that the doctor or midwife calculated, most pregnant women, if questioned, would probably say that they expected the delivery to occur within several days of it. The due date is calculated as 280 days after the *first* day of the last normal menstrual period. But since women often are not totally regular in their menstrual cycles, and since the exact time of ovulation is not necessarily 14 days after the start of menstruation, the due date is really an estimation, not an exact measure of the baby's gestational age. The average range for a normal *full-term* infant is two weeks to either side of the due date. Only 5 percent of babies are actually born on their due date.

Almost invariably, mothers report that they are tired during the final weeks of pregnancy. Many women have difficulty sleeping

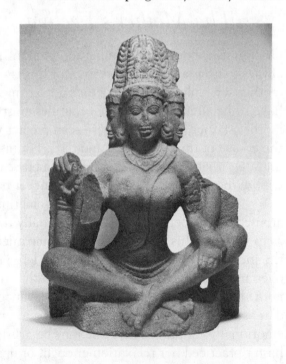

The end of pregnancy is often a time of mixed emotions, of excitement as well as nervousness. In the midst of all these feelings, it's important that an expectant mother try to remain calm and focused. Brahmani, Indian, ninth century. Asian Art Museum of San Francisco. Avery Brundage Collection.

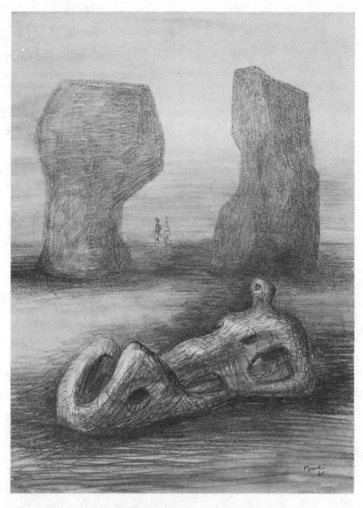

One of the most important labor preparations is to be well rested. As the time of labor and delivery approaches, an expectant mother should take care not to become overtired. Sculpture and Red Rocks, *Henry Moore, 1942. Crayon, wash, pen and ink, 19⅛" x 14¼". Collection, The Museum of Modern Art, New York. Gift of Philip L. Goodwin.*

through the night, either because they can't find a comfortable position or because they have to go to the bathroom more frequently than usual. And they are likely to be keyed up about the impending labor and delivery. Often mothers feel an underlying nervousness and inability to focus their attention, which is certainly understandable. The father frequently shares these feelings. It's as if they have been preparing for nine months to run a marathon—a marathon that is to be held at an unspecified time of day or night during a month-long period. Thus they have to be ready at all times. In a sense they are "on call" just as doctors and midwives are. Preparing for delivery is really a here-and-now situation. The best way to ensure constant readiness is to be like an athlete in training: eat a nutritious diet, get plenty of rest, and exercise regularly, all in a balanced, even manner.

Although the pregnant woman may wonder if it's possible, lapses and excesses of any kind are to be avoided in the last month, as are emotional and physical stresses. More than ever, this is a time for the mother to tune in to her feelings and for friends and family to pamper her. It's common for women to get a sudden burst of energy about a day or two before labor starts. This spurt may be a biological adaptation to help the mother through labor, and it probably has a physiological basis. But if a woman undertakes too much, she may find herself fatigued before labor begins. It's important that mothers realize this and save their energy spurt for labor rather than for madly finishing all the innumerable last-minute chores they can think of.

Some doctors and midwives are very serious about counseling a woman not to become overtired during the last month; they believe that fatigue can make a mother's labor longer and more difficult. Certainly a state of exhaustion would make a marathon more difficult even for the best-conditioned athlete. Often a woman's husband or close friends will realize that she is doing too much before she becomes aware of it, and their concern and help can be invaluable. In fact, fathers should think of this period as the beginning of their role as labor support and coach.

Signs of Impending Labor

True labor may start with the onset of regular contractions, the appearance of the *show* (the bloody mucous plug that has closed the cervix), or, less commonly, the breaking of the bag of waters. The rupture of the membranes that have surrounded the baby for almost nine months allows some of the pale, straw-colored amniotic fluid to escape. The fluid may gush out all at once or leak out more slowly, but it is not accompanied by any discomfort. Although the bag of waters breaks before regular contractions have even begun in 12 percent of all labors, it more frequently occurs at the end of the dilatation phase.

The intact membranes and the fluid behind them help to equalize the pressure on the baby's head and the cord during dilatation. Thus many practitioners now tend not to rupture the membranes to speed labor, as they once did. Unruptured membranes also help to protect the baby and mother against infection because they seal the uterus from the vaginal cavity.

Premature breaking of the bag of waters rarely presents any problems, but doctors and midwives vary widely in the way they handle it. Some are not concerned about the amount of time that elapses before the baby is born because they feel that studies on infection are not conclusive. Others set a fixed period by the end of which they want the baby to be born, and manage labor accordingly. About 80 percent of all mothers will spontaneously go into labor after their membranes rupture; the other 20 percent may require hormonal stimulation to get labor going.

As soon as a mother begins to have contractions on any regular basis, she will probably call her doctor or midwife, who will tell her to time the length of the contractions and the interval between them. The time between contractions is measured from the *beginning* of one contraction to the *beginning* of the next.

As we've mentioned, at first it's difficult to distinguish real labor from false labor (see p. 273), but some characteristics of contractions tend to point to one or the other. False labor contractions tend to be short and not very intense, and they generally don't occur at regular intervals. Real contractions tend to occur on a regular basis and then slowly increase in duration, intensity, and frequency. Whereas walking often tends to make real labor contractions stronger, it doesn't affect false labor contractions or may even relieve them. A mother usually feels that real labor contractions spread from the top of the uterus around to her back, while false labor contractions are mainly felt in the lower abdomen and pelvic area.

Since the two types of labor are difficult to distinguish initially, they can really only be told apart as the contractions speed up. If it becomes clear that a mother is in false labor, she will be told to relax, drink warm tea, enjoy a warm bath, and rest or sleep. If a mother proves to be in real labor, she will be told to do much the same thing. If she is delivering in a hospital or birth center, the mother will be told to remain at home for much of the latency phase of labor unless she lives very far from the hospital, has had previous short labors, or her membranes have ruptured. Each doctor and hospital has slightly different routines to handle this situation.

The practitioner will keep in touch with the mother and examine her when the contractions become regular. If she is to have a hospital or birth-center delivery, she will be told to come in so that she is comfortably situated when the acceleration phase of labor begins. Occasionally the doctor may wish to see the mother right away; other doctors may not want to admit the mother until her contractions are roughly five minutes apart. Unless there is a reason to go

How to distinguish between true and false labor

FALSE LABOR	TRUE LABOR
• Contractions stop.	• Contractions progress.
• Contractions remain irregular.	• Contractions become regular.
• Contractions tend to be short.	• Contractions increase in duration.
• Contractions are not intense.	• Contractions increase in intensity.
• Walking has no effect on contractions or may even stop them.	• Walking increases the intensity of contractions.
• Contractions are felt in the lower part of uterus.	• Contractions are felt in the upper part of uterus.

to the hospital immediately, most doctors and midwives recommend remaining at home during the early phase. Home is a comfortable, familiar environment where it will probably be easiest for the mother to relax. At home the mother can keep herself occupied, walk around, talk to family and friends, and make whatever arrangements are necessary. In the case of a mother who is having a home delivery, she will of course simply remain there and wait for the doctor or midwife to arrive.

Admission to the Hospital or Alternative Birth Center

Once the decision to go to the hospital or birth center is made, many mothers will notice that their contractions slow down or become less regular during the ride or after they arrive. This is not uncommon and is a typical example of how external events can affect labor. If pre-check-in arrangements have been made at the hospital, the father can go directly to the obstetrical area with the mother. If not, before she is admitted the mother will have to sign consent forms for the delivery and possibly for circumcision, and the father will have to fill out financial forms.

The admission procedure, physical layout, and rules of different hospitals and birth centers vary tremendously, so only a few generalizations can be made. First, either the practitioner or a nurse will meet the mother, time her contractions, and do a physical exam. The

By feeling the baby's fontanel on an internal exam, the doctor or midwife can tell which position the baby's head is in. An internal exam also reveals how dilated the mother's cervix is and how far down the baby has descended.

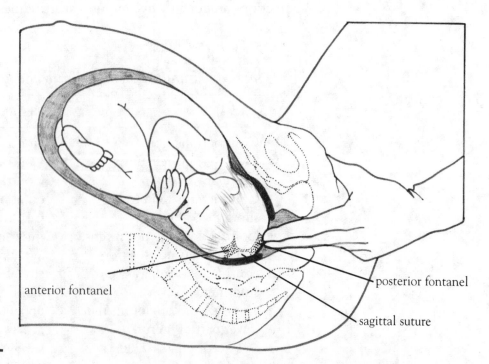

anterior fontanel

posterior fontanel

sagittal suture

mother will then be asked about her medical history, possible drug allergies, onset of contractions, whether the bag of waters has broken, and what she has eaten in the last four hours. Then the person will check the mother's blood pressure and pulse, feel her abdomen to determine what position the baby is in, and listen to the baby's heart rate and evaluate it. Next a pelvic exam will be done to determine how far the mother's cervix is dilated and to verify the baby's position by feeling for the fontanels and suture lines. Then a blood test and urine analysis will probably be done. If the mother has a medical problem or is at high risk, some doctors may also put in an IV line so that she may be given medicines quickly and her fluid levels can be kept up, but this is rarely done routinely.

If the doctor still requires either a shave or an enema, they will be done at this time, though in recent years many medical centers have abandoned these measures as standard procedure. Shaving used to be done to prevent infection and to keep hair from getting in the episiotomy site, but studies have not shown pubic hair to affect the rate of infection, and many babies are now delivered without an episiotomy. Enemas used to be required because it was believed that an empty bowel would allow more room in the birth canal and would assure a clean field around the episiotomy site. It has since been found that only the most severe constipation will narrow the birth canal and infection is not a problem. However, under special circumstances enemas are sometimes given to speed labor because they are known to stimulate uterine contractions.

Many doctors now routinely order the use of a fetal monitor, external or less frequently internal (see p. 355), so that the baby's heartbeat can be followed continuously. During labor the baby's heartbeat averages 120 to 160 beats per minute. Like the uterus, the heart is controlled by the autonomic nervous system; thus when the baby is under stress, its sympathetic nervous system is stimulated and causes its heartbeat to rise. Changes in the mother's position, activity, and contractions also affect the speed at which the baby's heart is beating. If the baby is not getting enough oxygen or is under great stress, its heartbeat will show one of several special patterns. These patterns, as well as the advantages and disadvantages of monitoring, are discussed at length in Chapter 16. This procedure has become so common that the expectant mother needs to educate herself in order to make a thoughtful decision about it.

Whether fetal monitoring should be used routinely with low-risk mothers is one of the great controversies in contemporary obstetrics. It is hoped that the mother will have discussed the routine monitoring practices of her practitioner and the hospital so that she is not surprised by them at the time of delivery. Such surprises can be quite disturbing, interfering with her ability to relax and thereby affecting the tone of her labor.

Early Labor: The Latency Period

During the latency phase in the first part of labor, the mother's cervix is being biochemically readied for the rapid dilatation that will take place in the active phase. Throughout this slow initial stage the mother is also beginning to dilate and efface her cervix. The goals for the mother at this point are to become as relaxed as possible and to get used to the rhythm of labor.

When women realize that they are actually in labor, they are generally excited, happy, a little nervous, and not very troubled by their contractions. They are finally beginning the work that they have been anticipating for so long. Just knowing they are really in labor is a tremendous relief and gives new energy and coping ability. This spurt of energy and excitement can be a little problematic, because a mother who is tired or goes into labor in the middle of the night may find herself too excited to rest or sleep. This is most likely to be true of a first-time mother who doesn't have a realistic sense of the time involved in labor and delivery.

When a mother is tired, sleep is an excellent way to handle early labor. In fact, some doctors recommend that mothers nap if their contractions are not increasing much in strength and frequency. Surprisingly, many women find they are able to doze very satisfactorily, wakening only occasionally with a contraction. First-time mothers can be assured that they won't miss anything; rather, the state of relaxation induced by napping stores energy for the work ahead and allows contractions to take place most efficiently because the mother is not stimulating her sympathetic nervous system with worry or anxiety.

Today many doctors and midwives recommend walking rather than lying down during much of the latency phase and even at the beginning of the active phase. Walking gives the mother something to do, something to concentrate on. It tends to normalize breathing high in the chest and discharge nervous energy. Moreover, walking seems

Although it may seem surprising, napping may be the best way for a mother to handle early labor, particularly if she is very tired or labor is proceeding very slowly.

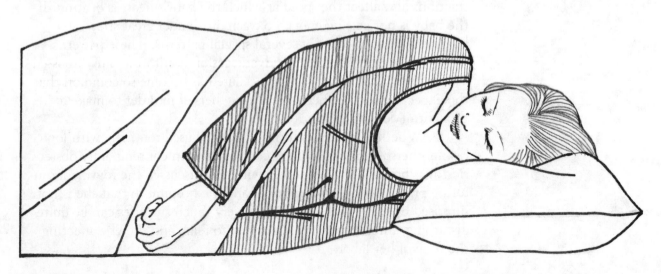

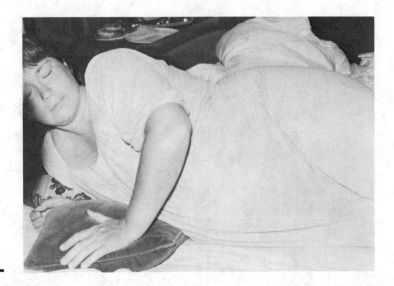

When a mother feels like lying down during labor, she should lie on her side or sit up slightly. Photo by Linda O'Neil.

to be physically exhilarating; it moves the blood around the body, takes pressure off the vena cava which further promotes blood flow, and prevents the abdominal and uterine muscles from tensing. Walking also stimulates uterine contractions and has been used for years as a treatment for weak contractions in early labor.

In a remarkable study of labor Caldeyro-Barcia, a South American pioneer in labor physiology, found that 95 percent of mothers chose a vertical position in the first stage of labor, either walking, standing, or sitting upright, when allowed to choose their position solely on the basis of what was most comfortable. He found that mothers also had more intense, efficient contractions in an upright position than when lying down. In fact, their contractions were almost twice as

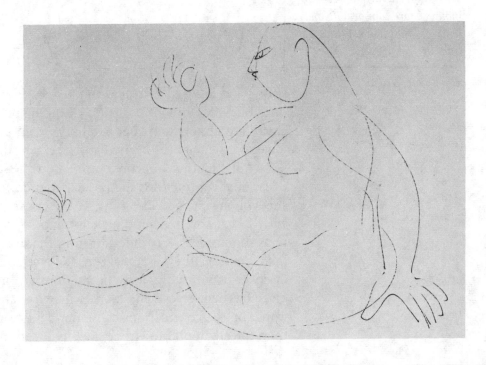

During the early phase of labor the most important thing for the mother to do is to make herself as comfortable as possible. Given the choice, most mothers will choose some kind of upright position, either sitting, standing, or walking.

Nude Figure, Irving Sherman. The Metropolitan Museum of Art. The Elisha Whittelsey Collection.

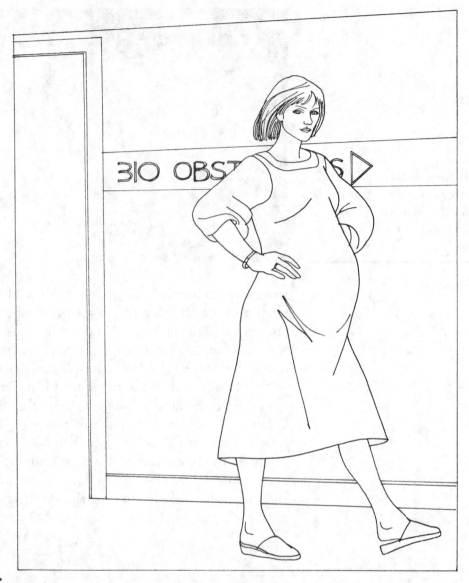

Many doctors and midwives recommend walking rather than sitting or lying down in the early part of labor. Walking generally makes the mother more comfortable and tends to stimulate contractions.

strong and less frequent, and the first stage of labor was shortened by one-third. An upright position, by taking pressure off of the vena cava, also ensured a higher level of oxygen in the mother's blood, lowering the chances of the baby's oxygen supply being compromised.

If a mother has concentrated on the sensations involved in the occasional contractions she has experienced during the last month, she will have a good idea of what the contractions will feel like in early labor. For most mothers contractions during the early latency phase do not feel very different from Braxton Hicks contractions. For many mothers there is a real sense of awe and exhilaration when they discover how easy the first contractions are and realize that they take place by themselves. The mother may feel almost like a spectator, watching the contractions cause her belly to tense in the middle and then spread around to either side. This sense of being an observer is very valuable because it allows the body to do its work with the least possible resistance.

Even though it is the longest part of labor, the latent phase is still just the beginning, and if a woman can continue to ignore the contractions at this point by focusing her attention elsewhere, it will help her to conserve her energy and patience. The slower and longer the labor, the more patience the mother will need and the more she must accept and appreciate the tempo and rhythm of her own body. In addition to walking, listening to music, following a drifting conversation, watching television, or reading are good mental distractions. Mothers may also find it soothing to rub their abdomen or lower back, or have them rubbed by the father or another person.

Positions for the Active Phase of Labor

Toward the end of the latency phase the mother's contractions will start to become more intense. This is the beginning of the active phase, during which her cervix will do most of its dilatation. The contractions become longer, generally stronger, and closer together, giving the mother less time to rest and regroup between them.

As in latency, many women find that they are most comfortable if they can continue to walk during most of the active phase. When labor begins to intensify, mothers may want to stop during a contraction and lean on someone or something. Other mothers may feel more comfortable if they are reclining against pillows or lying on their side. Ironically, the least advisable position is flat on the back, which has been standard hospital procedure for years. As noted, this position slows the mother's return blood flow and tends to diminish the effectiveness of her contractions. Not infrequently a woman may want to be on her knees and elbows, with her chest down. This posture, called the *all-fours position*, takes the weight of the baby off the spine, the pelvic floor, and the rectum. Some women may prefer to sit in a squatting position, but most find they want to move around frequently, changing position as a contraction comes on and again as it subsides. Mothers with fetal monitors will find that their positions and movements are more limited, but they can still be helped to find the most comfortable position.

As their contractions become stronger and closer, most women will find that they need to focus their attention on them totally and will only be able to talk or joke briefly between contractions. Eventually the mother will want all extraneous conversation to cease. Women vary widely in the sensations and amount of discomfort they feel during the active phase. Tremendous pressure may be felt in the lower back, thighs, or the bottom of the cervix. The mother needs to work with the father, the practitioner, or nurse to make herself com-

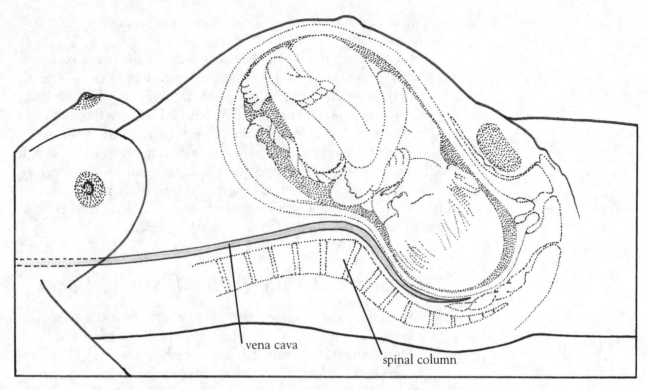

vena cava

spinal column

When a mother lies flat on her back, the baby presses on her vena cava, the major vein that returns blood to the heart from the legs and trunk. Such pressure cuts down on the flow of blood and oxygen to the baby. For this reason doctors no longer advise mothers to lie on their back during labor or delivery.

fortable. These are highly individual questions that, ultimately, the mother herself is best suited to answer. What works best at any one time is likely to change during the course of labor.

As the active phase progresses and her cervix begins to dilate and efface more rapidly, the mother can start using the particular relaxation and/or breathing techniques that she has been taught during her prenatal classes, and she will realize the value and power of them. When the mother feels a contraction begin, she should be silent and concentrate on getting her whole body to feel loose and totally relaxed, as if she were suspended in a pool of warm water. If she has been taught to concentrate on a point (Lamaze), to imagine a relaxing scene, or to visualize her cervix dilating, she should do so now. Methods that concentrate on breathing teach the mother to take one deep breath prior to each contraction. Throughout a contraction the mother should breathe according to the method she has been taught (see chart).

Different ways of handling labor problems

Prolonged or painful latent phase (early first stage)
- Allow the mother to rest or sleep; if necessary, give pain medication to induce sleep.
- Encourage the mother to be patient and trust her body.
- Have mother move as she pleases; encourage her to walk, kneel, sit, stand, lean, or go on her hands and knees.

- Avoid having the mother lie on her back because it is uncomfortable and lowers blood flow to the uterus.
- Offer the mother fruit juice or water with honey or sugar.
- Provide reassurance.
- Provide a continuous caregiver.
- Allow the mother to sit in a warm bath.
- Encourage the mother to practice deep relaxation.
- Rub the mother's back.
- Darken and quiet the room, watch TV, or listen to music at the mother's discretion.
- Have the mother concentrate on the baby or visualize a tranquil scene.
- Avoid pain medication if possible because it may slow down labor.
- In special situations give IV pitocin.

Prolonged or painful second stage
- Provide constant attendance, eye contact, reassurance, and encouragement.
- Avoid having the mother push forcefully or hold her breath while pushing.
- Avoid having the mother pull up on her legs, which uses up her energy.
- Encourage the mother to relax as deeply as possible between contractions.
- Encourage the mother to keep the pelvic floor and all sphincters relaxed during contractions and not to worry about tearing or defecating.
- Encourage the mother to "give in" to contractions and not to fear momentary loss of control or intense sensations.
- Encourage the mother to try different positions, especially squatting, supported squatting, leaning against someone, or lying on her side. Avoid having the mother lie on her back. Having the mother lie on her side helps to slow a rapid delivery. Have the mother get on hands and knees to relieve back pain or to make it easier to rotate the baby from a posterior position. Use a squatting position to widen the pelvic diameter, maximize gravity, and speed delivery.
- Give IV pitocin only in exceptional situations in which the mother's pelvis is considered adequate in size but labor stops progressing totally.
- Use vacuum extraction forceps if the baby is all the way down but the mother's contractions are insufficient to push the baby out.

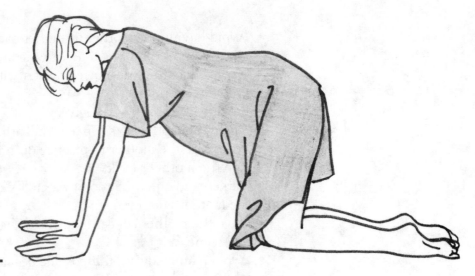

Many women find they are
most comfortable in an all-
fours or squatting position
during the active phase of
labor. Both positions take
pressure off the vena cava,
but the all-fours position also
minimizes pressure on the
mother's back and pelvic
floor.

Supporting the Mother During the Active Phase

At this stage the support person can begin to be of real help to the mother by giving her encouragement and seeing that her needs are met as fully and quickly as possible. For instance, simple requests concerning temperature, light, and noise now become increasingly important to the mother. She should feel free to say whom she wishes to have in the room and to stop conversations that are either distracting or upsetting to her. A mother may become cold and wish to put on socks or a bed jacket; chilling should be avoided because it makes it harder for her to relax. Other women may wish to shower or sponge off, change their gown, or rinse out their mouth. Everything should be done to make the mother as comfortable as possible. Throughout labor she should be encouraged to urinate every few hours, even if she is not aware of any urge to do so. This leaves more space in the pelvis and tends to diminish lower abdominal pain.

As the hard work of labor begins in earnest, a mother may develop a dry mouth and become thirsty because she has been breathing through her mouth. Ice chips tend to be drying, but small amounts of liquids such as water or herb tea (sweetened) or hard candies will help to keep her from becoming parched. The sugar in the candies or tea will also provide energy. Lip balm will keep the mother's lips from becoming dry and cracked.

Solid foods should be avoided because they tend to stay in the stomach and may cause nausea and vomiting. Stomach movement, secretion of digestive juices, and food absorption all drop tremendously in the hours before a woman goes into labor and remain low until after delivery. It is not uncommon for mothers who have had a large meal within several hours of going into labor to throw up, but this invariably makes them more comfortable.

As a rule, obstetricians regard food in labor as unnecessary or unsafe (because of the rare need for general anesthesia), but many midwives experienced with home birth feel otherwise. They believe that in the early stages of labor women who are relaxed and unafraid can tolerate and benefit from food, and that fear is what frequently causes women to become nauseous and vomit. Midwives who feel it's important for mothers to keep their energy and fluid levels high and to keep their blood from becoming acidic (see p. 81) offer women easily digested carbohydrates such as bread, rice, pasta, cheese, or yogurt in the early part of labor. In later labor they give mothers high-calorie liquids such as grape juice, cranberry drink, or honey and water. They avoid citrus drinks or apple juice because those fluids seem more likely to cause vomiting. If a mother does drink fluids, she should make sure that she urinates every hour or two.

Midwives have always felt that good support in labor is as effective as pain medication and can decrease the length of labor by two to three hours, and recent research has shown that the presence of a sympathetic person definitely affects labor. A study by Marshall Klaus in Guatemala found that when one person stayed with the mother throughout labor, she was much more comfortable, her labor was shorter, and fewer medical procedures were needed (see p. 200).

The support of a concerned, knowledgeable person can stop the syndrome of fear, tension, and pain, helping the mother to relax and making her more comfortable. Often reassurance may be expressed through small services such as moving a pillow, answering a question, or timing the contractions and telling the mother when one is halfway or two-thirds over.

By this stage in labor most women will want to have the room totally quiet or have one person who is completely focused on their progress talking to them. Some mothers are encouraged by hearing

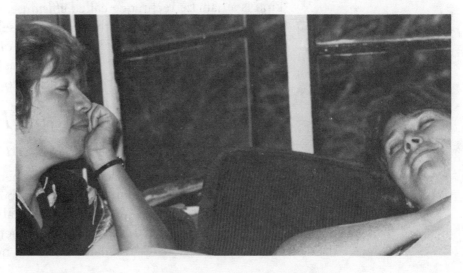

During labor reassurance and support are often more effective than medication. Photo by Linda O'Neil.

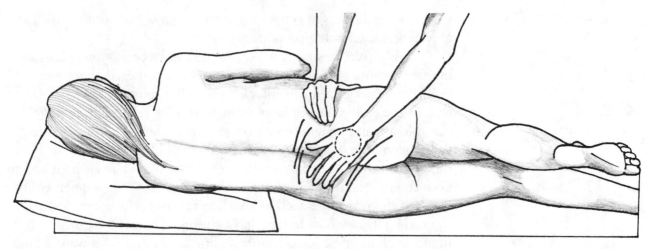

phrases like, "You're doing fine!" or "Terrific, terrific!" repeated over and over again. In addition to encouraging the mother and seeing to her needs, the husband or support person should check for signs of tension such as clenched hands, a grimace, or clenched teeth, and help the mother to relax. Although the mother is really working hard now, the more she tenses her body, the more uncomfortable she is likely to find the contractions.

Women's feelings vary greatly during the active phase of labor. Some mothers may wish to be rubbed or gently massaged; others may not wish to be touched at all. Although a back rub may be helpful, sometimes steady pressure on a specific site in the lower back may be more beneficial, particularly if the baby is in a posterior position and its head is putting pressure on the mother's spine. In this case the support person's palm or a small pillow behind the mother's back can supply counterpressure. This is especially valuable *during* contractions. The amount of pressure should be adjusted according to what feels best to the mother. There are also two types of abdominal massage that mothers sometimes find soothing. One is a general circular pattern of rubbing with most pressure applied to the lower abdomen. The second kind is a Lamaze technique called *effleurage,* which means "feather touch." Using both hands, the mother herself rubs in circles on the left and right sides of her abdomen. Either of these abdominal rubs supplies a pleasant sensation and also acts as a distraction that helps to keep the mother from tensing against the contractions.

The End of the Active Phase and the Beginning of Transition

Around the middle of the active phase, when the contractions have not only increased in length and intensity but have also started to come one after another, the mother will realize that the whole character of labor has changed. Often she will react to this realization with a mixture of emotions, particularly if she has never been in labor before.

On one hand, she will feel both excited and satisfied that at last things are really happening. She will be dilating much more quickly now—an average of 1 centimeter every 15 minutes, or even more, which is astounding progress compared to the 1 centimeter per 4 hours that was average for the latent phase.

Ideally the mother should prepare herself for each successive contraction but mentally step back, separating herself from it as much as possible since she is still not to actively push. However she may find herself fatigued and startled by the heightened force of labor and the new set of physical and emotional sensations that accompany it. If a trained, empathetic person is not available at this point to inspire her and explain what is happening, the mother may become anxious and wonder if she's capable of giving birth naturally after all.

Anxiety is a key problem, because it always causes the mother to tense and strain against the contractions. Paradoxically, this is the time when more than ever the mother needs to stay loose and not fight or bear down. It is the time when the mother needs to concentrate the hardest but keep the most relaxed. Not only do anxiety and tension tend to stimulate the sympathetic nervous system, making contractions less effective and more uncomfortable, they have been shown to lower a person's threshold for pain, which in labor is tremendously influenced by the mother's perception of what is happening.

The change in the intensity of labor at this point is directly linked to changes in physiology. The first stage of labor, the dilatation phase, is nearly complete and is about to finish rather quickly. The majority of women find that the hardest work and the greatest discomfort they experience in labor occurs during the final part of the first stage. The actual delivery or second stage is exhilarating and joyous by comparison. Once a mother realizes how quickly things are progressing now, she is usually able to relax a bit and deal more effectively with the contractions. What might be impossible to handle for another three or four hours becomes tolerable for a half-hour or an hour, which is the average length of the *transition* stage. When the mother's focus shifts to a more imminent goal, her perception of discomfort changes, and the situation becomes a challenge that she again believes she can meet.

When transition begins the mother is about 8 centimeters dilated and her cervix is beginning to retract back over the baby's head, which may result in a sensation of pulling or stretching deep within her pelvis. Friedman refers to this period as *deceleration*, because the rate of dilatation *appears* to slow as the cervix starts to retract. But there is no deceleration in the rhythm of the contractions. During transition the contractions last an average of a minute apiece and occur every 2 to 3 minutes in an absolutely regular rhythm, cresting about two-thirds of the way through and then tapering off, only to begin again without much delay.

Sometimes shortly before and during transition the mother will have digestive symptoms such as hiccuping, burping, or nausea. Vomiting, which will quickly relieve the nausea, may follow. The mother will probably wish to rinse her mouth, either because of a bad taste or thirst. Usually such symptoms are quickly forgotten due to the ongoing progress of labor.

As they enter transition, most mothers will want to get in bed rather than walk, due to the frequency and intensity of their contractions. One of the positions most preferred by mothers at this point is a semi-sitting posture in which they lean back on pillows at about a forty-five-degree angle. Other women prefer to lie on their side or get on all fours and rest their head on pillows. The important thing is for the mother not to be afraid to move and to find the most comfortable position she can.

During the transition period the mother is overwhelmed by incredibly intense sensations throughout her whole body. Perhaps the only other time a woman is so totally and profoundly shaken is during sexual climax. In like manner, her body now completely overtakes her mind and she is caught up in a series of sensations beyond her control. Many women are surprised by the primitiveness and power of these feelings and find themselves less and less concerned with questions of modesty or propriety as they become totally immersed in the experience at hand.

At this point the baby's head will be somewhere between halfway and three-quarters of the way down the birth canal, that is, between station 0 and +3 (see pp. 289–90). The baby is now descending at its maximum speed. The mother may experience a severe low backache that moves as the baby's head begins to descend, passing the ischial spines. This can be eased, if not entirely relieved,

During transition many women are almost overwhelmed by their physical sensations. At some points women may even find themselves becoming disassociated from their own body. Rather than resist this feeling, it may be helpful to concentrate on the idea of floating.

Soaring. *Photo by Michael Samuels.*

Floating Rock. *Photo by Michael Samuels.*

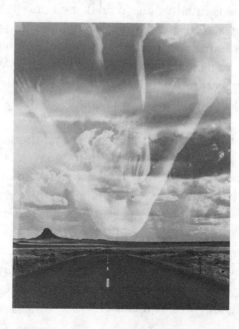

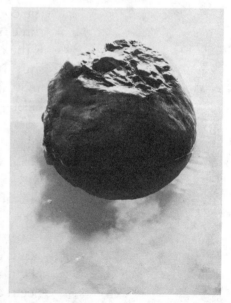

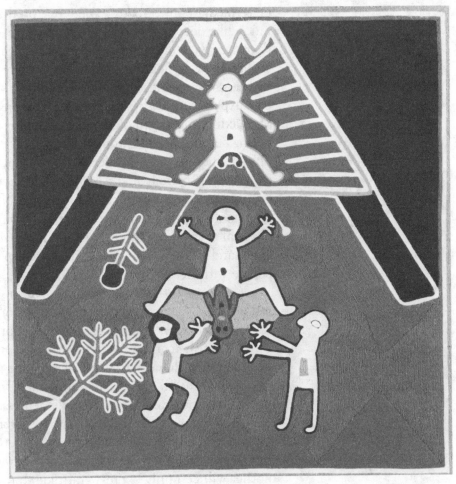

by applying counterpressure, using a hot water bottle, or having the mother kneel on all fours and rock back and forth with the contractions.

Beads of perspiration may break out on the mother's forehead and upper lip, her teeth may chatter, often her legs will shake uncontrollably, and she may even experience cramps in the muscles of her legs and buttocks. These changes probably reflect the extent to which countless nerve receptor sites are being stimulated and are pouring information into the mother's nervous system.

At this point the mother is likely to become inexplicably restless, irritable, exasperated, confused, or forgetful. She may not want to be touched, she may not want to talk or even listen, and she may have trouble comprehending instructions. Between contractions the mother may not only appear exhausted, she may be difficult to arouse. This temporary withdrawal or amnesia is completely natural. It helps to keep the mother focused on what is happening in the present, without thinking about the contraction that just took place or the one that is momentarily to come. She is therefore able to relax profoundly in the brief moments between contractions.

During these moments the mother may experience what might

be termed an out-of-body experience or altered state of consciousness, much like deep meditation or dreaming. Some women actually feel that they have momentarily lost contact with reality, as if their consciousness were floating somewhere outside of their body. Whether this sensation is pleasurable or frightening depends upon the mother's past experience. If she has entered long dreamlike states in the course of relaxing, meditating, exercising, staying awake for long periods, or taking certain drugs, a woman is not likely to be as frightened by this unusual mental state. In fact, not only may she be able to accept the experience, she may find it helpful. However, if the mother should become anxious or frightened by feelings of unreality, those attending her should gently try to reconnect her with reality through talking or physical touch. The mother is in a highly suggestible and sensitive state, and she is likely to be extremely responsive to the mood of the people with her.

It is essential that everyone give the mother positive images and emotional support at this point in labor. With infinite patience, her chosen helpers need to reassure the mother constantly and remind her of what she can do to work with the contractions and make herself most comfortable until delivery actually begins. It is not uncommon for a woman to be emotionally quite labile at this time, doing fine one minute, the next feeling profoundly depressed or angry with everything and everyone. If the mother feels strong, steady, nonjudgmental support, these lapses of good nature will generally be brief and will disappear when the exhilaration of delivery overtakes her. Later the mother will certainly express gratitude to those who helped her and may not even remember the things she said at this point in labor.

The End of Transition

Toward the end of transition, as the baby descends further and further, the mother will experience a whole new set of sensations. Many of these are the result of the baby's head reaching the pelvic floor. As soon as this happens, the mother will begin to feel an overpowering urge to push. Frequently her breathing will become quite noisy: her breath may catch in her throat as she inhales, and she may groan or grunt as she exhales. These noises are a normal part of the mother's intense exertion, just as a person groans when lifting a very heavy object. Although some mothers feel hesitant about making such noises, they may feel better if they do.

During transition mothers often have a feeling of rectal pressure similar to the feeling of having to have a bowel movement. Some mothers even ask for help getting to the bathroom or using a bedpan, although no fecal material will come out. Many midwives believe that walking to the toilet may make the mother more comfortable and may speed labor if it is not moving quickly at this point. But the mother should always be accompanied, because this is generally a time of rapid descent.

If the bag of waters has not yet broken, it probably will do so now. In any case, there is likely to be more bloody show, and if the mother is in a semi-sitting position, she may even notice the perineal area beginning to bulge. All these changes are called *signs of impending second stage,* and they mean that the mother will soon be ready to deliver the baby, although the doctor or midwife may still not want the mother to push because that can cause the cervix to swell if it is not fully dilated (see p. 288).

In order to determine how completely the mother is dilated and how far the baby has descended, the doctor or midwife will do an internal examination. The timing of the exam and the number of checks that are done depend upon the practitioner, the hospital rules, and the speed at which labor is progressing. The exam may be made with the mother lying on her side or on her back. Often mothers will find shifting positions and being examined quite uncomfortable at this point, though they will also be very interested to find out how far the baby has progressed. Generally the exam is done between contractions so as to be least disturbing to the mother, but still, it may help if the mother consciously relaxes, takes a deep breath, and then exhales as the exam is performed. Unless the baby is being continuously monitored, the doctor or midwife will also check the baby's heart rate frequently with a fetoscope an ultrasound devise.

Occasionally near the end of transition the doctor will find that although the mother's cervix is almost completely dilated, the upper rim of the cervix, the *anterior lip,* is lagging behind and has not retracted as far back over the baby's head as the rest of the cervix. It is very important that the mother not begin pushing if this is the case, because pushing will bruise that part of the cervical lip, causing it to swell and slow the progress of labor. Generally the lip is allowed to retract naturally, but sometimes if it becomes swollen the doctor or midwife will gently but firmly push the lip back over the baby's head after a contraction and hold it back during the next contraction. This is uncomfortable for the mother, but it can alleviate the problem and speed transition. An alternative is to have the mother push *gently* at this point, while still breathing in and out evenly. Such gentle pressure may ease the anterior lip over the baby's head.

Breathing Techniques for Transition

Even if a mother is not fully dilated or the anterior lip of her cervix is not fully retracted, she may find it difficult to prevent herself from pushing, which is becoming a stronger and stronger urge. Pushing is a reflex response to the baby's head pressing on the pelvic floor. Once the head reaches a certain level of descent (+ 3), it begins to press on the pelvic floor with each contraction, then slip back a bit between contractions. Thus with each contraction comes a new urge to push.

It's very important during transition that the mother clearly understands what *not* pushing means. She is experiencing many strong sensations now. In addition to feeling an urge to push at the beginning of each contraction, she will also be feeling *continuous* rectal or perineal pressure due to the position of the baby's head. As long as the mother continues to breathe in and out smoothly, without holding her breath or exhaling forcefully, she is not really pushing or *bearing down*. Real pushing involves contracting or squeezing the muscles of the diaphragm, rib cage, and abdomen, either while exhaling slowly and forcefully or while closing the *epiglottis* in the throat, which locks the airway.

Just understanding the physiology of pushing may enable a tense mother to relax again. The goal is to keep her bottom loose, *experiencing* the incredible sensations of downward pressure without adding to them. If the woman starts to bear down, she should consciously breathe out and then in, until the urge to push passes. To keep her breathing steady, it may help if the mother makes her mouth into an O shape. If she still finds herself locking up her breath, she should begin to use one of the breathing techniques she has learned in her prenatal classes. To *pant*, she simply opens her mouth and breathes in and out rapidly and shallowly, concentrating on feeling the air in her throat. She may find it helpful to speed her panting as the contraction peaks, then slow it again as the contraction subsides. In using the *pant-blow technique*, the mother concentrates on relaxing her neck and shoulders and drops her jaw loosely so her mouth is open. As the contraction begins, she breathes in and out rapidly and shallowly through her mouth about 4 or 5 times, then purses her lips and forcefully puffs or blows out through her lips. To get through the entire contraction a mother may need to repeat the pant-blow technique once or twice, or she may need to pant more times in the beginning. Exercise physiologist Elizabeth Noble recommends that the mother keep her breathing below 25 breaths per minute (normal is 12 to 15). In general, these breathing techniques are tiring and should only be done during contractions if the mother has a strong urge to bear down.

With any of the rapid breathing or panting techniques there is a possibility of *hyperventilation*, the symptoms of which are dizziness and tingling around the mouth and fingers. When a woman hyperventilates, she breathes at too rapid a rate or blows too hard or long. As a result, too much carbon dioxide is exhaled from the lungs, which in turn makes the blood become alkaline. The body naturally attempts to reverse this alkalinity by closing down the blood vessels, which causes the mother's symptoms. These symptoms can be counteracted by having the mother slow or stop her panting, or breathe into a paper bag or cupped hands. All these measures return increased amounts of carbon dioxide to the lungs. Between contractions the woman should be encouraged to relax as deeply as possible so as to conserve her energy. Hyperventilation is not dangerous to the mother or baby, but it tends to make the mother lose her focus and control. Because of problems such as hyperventilation and fatigue, many doctors and midwives are de-emphasizing breathing techniques and putting more emphasis on helping the mother relax.

Entering the Second Stage

As transition ends and the second stage of labor becomes imminent, excitement overtakes everyone. Generally the mother's urge to push is irresistible, and it is time for her to do so. The mother often notices a profound lessening of discomfort with her contractions. If she is not delivering in a birthing room, labor bed, or at home, she will be moved into the *delivery room* at this stage. The timing depends upon whether this is a first vaginal birth and on how fast her labor seems to be progressing. With a first baby, the doctor or midwife may have the mother push awhile before moving her, waiting until an inch or two of the baby's head shows between contractions. With subsequent babies, transition and the second stage are likely to move faster, and the mother may be moved to the delivery room before she is even fully dilated.

The second stage begins when the mother is fully dilated and ends with the baby's delivery. This is the most exciting stage of labor and generally the shortest. In a first vaginal delivery the second stage usually lasts an average of 50 minutes or 20 contractions, but it may be considerably shorter. With subsequent deliveries this stage averages only 20 minutes or about 8 contractions. Often the mother is not actively pushing for the first few contractions, so the whole process may seem even shorter to her.

Friedman calls this stage the *pelvic division of labor*, because this is the time when the baby is passing through the birth canal and making the classic twists and bends that are commonly illustrated. At this stage the character of labor once again undergoes a change: the mother no longer has to concentrate on holding back; she is finally able to give in to her overwhelming urge to push. Pushing being easier than not pushing, the mother has a renewed sense of control.

For most women pushing is joyous, satisfying work. They realize that the end of labor is finally in sight and all their efforts will soon be over: they will be able to see and hold their baby. Tired as a woman may be at this point, such knowledge usually brings a new surge of energy. There is progress now with each contraction, and the mother is praised for her efforts rather than being discouraged from doing what her body is telling her to do. For many women the contractions, although no less powerful or frequent, magically seem much easier to deal with. Probably this is partly physical, since the cervix is no longer dilating, and partly psychological, since the mother is able to visualize an end point and participate actively in reaching it.

A few women find that contractions in the second stage are as uncomfortable as those that occur late in the active stage. The explanation for this may be anatomical: a woman's pelvis may be small in relation to her baby, the baby may be presenting in a position that generally tends to make the second stage more uncomfortable, or the mother's cervix may have been bruised during the first stage. But it is often fear that causes the mother to tense and fight the contractions in a new way. Particularly with a first vaginal delivery, the mother may be unprepared for the new sensations she is experiencing.

Now there is an overwhelming sense of not being able to hold back. Many women are surprised and dismayed at how primitive and violent the urge to push actually is. In this way their body is again acting in a manner beyond their control, a fact that may be difficult to accept. It is not uncommon for women to momentarily have doubts as to whether their body can actually open up enough to deliver the baby without being hurt or somehow violated. In particular a number of mothers fear tearing as the baby's head crowns.

It's important that a woman voice such fears whenever she becomes aware of them during labor. Only then will her doctor or midwife, who has the benefit of many other deliveries, be able to help her and explain things to her. As her confidence in her body and her trust in her practitioner overcome her fears, she will often be able to relax again and deal more comfortably with her contractions. Women having their second and third babies seem much less prone to becoming anxious in the second stage because they know their body is capable of giving birth to a baby. Often when the delivery is over mothers will comment on how much less anxious they were the second time, because they had done it before and knew what was happening. Of course, a first-time mother can't know the feeling in advance, but she can develop understanding and faith by learning about other women's experiences.

POSITIONS FOR SECOND-STAGE PUSHING

In the last few years there have been a number of changes in the positions mothers use for pushing during the second stage and delivery. Up until the eighteenth century women pushed their babies out in some kind of upright position: standing, squatting, or sitting on a birth stool, as was the custom in many European countries. But in Europe in the 1770s the birth stool was replaced by having the mother lie on her back in bed. This change of position was introduced by the doctor to

Queen Maria of France, to make it easier for him to use forceps for the delivery. In the 1800s an American obstetrician began having his mothers not only lie on their back but draw up their knees in what came to be called the *lithotomy position.* After the turn of the century hospitals began to use a delivery table with *stirrups* instead of a bed.

The return to the natural position in the United States was started in the 1950s by Forrest Howard, an obstetrician who added a backrest to the conventional delivery table. Since then doctors have experimented with a number of different positions, in response to mothers' demands and the midwifery movement, which has again gained prominence in this country in recent years. Midwives place special emphasis on the mother's comfort and the normalcy of most deliveries, rather than on technical concerns and ease of medical intervention.

The shift away from the lithotomy position has further been prompted by recent studies showing that when the mother lies on her back, the baby and the uterus press on her major veins, slowing blood flow to the heart and oxygen flow to the placenta when the baby is tightly compressed by the birth canal. Studies also verify that pushing is easier and more effective in a squatting position, because the mother can build up greater intrauterine pressure when she squats, and her

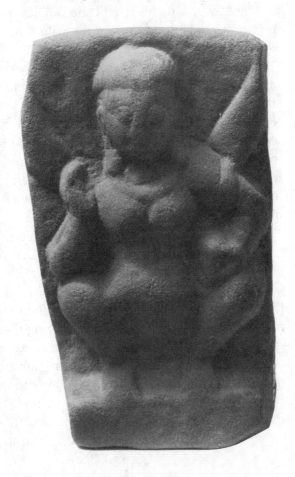

Although squatting has always been the traditional position for pushing in non-industrialized countries, it has just begun to be used again in industrialized countries. Matrika, Indian, third century. The Metropolitan Museum of Art. Rogers Fund.

pelvic joints can actually rotate, allowing the birth canal to widen by as much as 1½ centimeters. The squatting position makes the baby's descent easier because it tilts the pelvis so that the birth canal is straighter. Squatting also means that the mother is pushing *with* gravity, not *against* it, as happens in the last part of delivery when the mother is lying on her back. Finally, in an upright position the muscles around the mother's perineum cannot contract and are kept loose.

Whatever position mother and practitioner choose for pushing, the main task of the second stage is to build enough intra-abdominal pressure to move the baby down the birth canal. Until now the mother's contractions have primarily served to dilate her cervix, moving the baby downward only slightly. Now, when the mother meets a contraction by tensing her upper abdominal muscles and forcefully exhaling, the resulting pressure tends to push the baby out. Each time the baby's head touches the pelvic floor at the beginning of a contraction, the mother feels an irresistible urge to push. This urge is a special reflex: pressure on the pelvic floor always triggers an urge to push, but it doesn't automatically cause the mother to contract her upper abdominal muscles. This means that the mother has some control over pushing. By using breathing techniques, the mother can determine the degree to which she pushes with each contraction. She can either push gently or forcefully, and she is able to stop pushing momentarily in order to help the doctor or midwife slow or control the delivery, especially when the head is crowning.

Currently there is a controversy between those doctors and midwives who tell the mother to push quite forcefully in the second stage and those who tell her to push only as hard and as long as she feels like. Medical personnel used to think that it was best to get the second stage over as quickly as possible, because long periods of intense pressure might have bad effects on the baby or even on the mother. However, although pressure on the baby's head often does affect its heart rate, this has not been shown to be a problem in normal deliveries.

There is a growing trend toward letting the second stage progress at its own rate, paralleling the earlier medical change toward an unhindered first stage of labor. The work of British obstetrician Constance Beynon has influenced this trend toward not pushing too forcefully in the second stage. She found that by not teaching her patients how to push and not instructing them to do so, the second stage became much more peaceful and was only slightly longer. She also found that there were fewer tears and episiotomies and less frequent use of forceps. Beynon believes that the slow stretching caused by an "entirely spontaneous second stage" results in less trauma to the vagina, the perineum, and the uterine supports.

Doctors who believe in strong pushing in the second stage

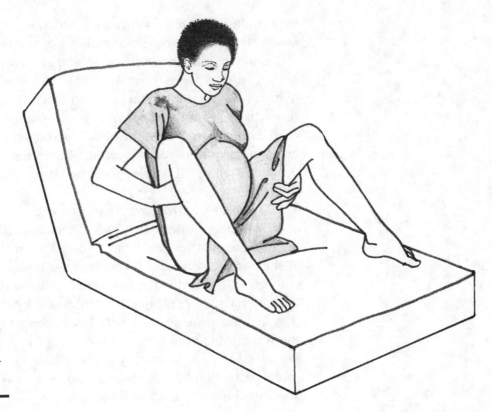

One of the positions most preferred by mothers during transition is semi-sitting. It allows the mother to be supported without putting pressure on the vena cava or her spine.

point out that it makes contractions more effective and shortens labor. If a mother is tired or uncomfortable during the second stage, a shorter labor may be appealing. Doctors who are emphatic about pushing instruct the mother on how to push strongly and effectively, encourage her to start pushing at the beginning of each contraction and to push forcefully throughout the contraction by holding her breath. Doctors who are more moderate only instruct the mother to push more forcefully if her natural efforts are not effective.

Whether or not a woman will be told to push forcefully, it's important for her to know what effective pushing is as well as how to control it during delivery. If a mother is in a semi-reclining position, she will be told to draw her legs up and apart by putting her arms around her knees or thighs. At the same time she will be told to round her back and tuck her head down, touching her chin to her chest. Having her arms, back, and chin in this position tends to maximize the power of the mother's pushing efforts. In the classic sequence the mother is then told to take two deep breaths, *locking up* and holding her breath on the second inhalation. Relaxing her perineum but contracting her upper abdominal muscles, she then pushes down her diaphragm for a count of ten, repeating the maneuver one or two more times before the contraction ends. When this is done correctly the mother will feel the pelvic floor move and her vagina widen.

Sheila Kitzinger, a British childbirth educator, feels that it is very confusing to tell a mother to relax one set of muscles while simultaneously tensing another. She also does not believe in locking up the abdominal muscles because she feels it squeezes the baby rather than pushing it out. She has the mother sit in a semi-reclining position with her back rounded and her chin tucked on her chest, but then she simply has the mother take an easy, deep breath at the beginning of each contraction and hold it. She instructs the mother to visualize pressing down from top to bottom of the uterus, while still remaining otherwise relaxed. Like Beynon, she favors a relaxed, natural second stage.

Most recently some doctors have come to favor a modified form of second stage pushing in which the mother never locks up her breath. The mother may be told to make a grunting noise or to groan as she pushes, because this prevents her from holding her breath. The emphasis is on having the mother keep her perineum relaxed rather than on having her push as forcefully as she can. Generally the mother is in a semi-sitting position with her knees bent and her legs apart, but she is not told to put her arms around her legs and pull. She may be instructed to bear down only as she exhales, or to take in a breath as each contraction begins, exhale, and bear down, squeezing her abdominal muscles for 5 or 6 seconds.

Some studies have shown that pushing for more than 5 seconds causes the baby to get less oxygen and causes its heart rate to drop due to a series of physiological changes that take place in the mother. When a mother holds her breath during a push, the pressure in her chest rises, slowing blood flow to her heart and causing the placenta to get less blood. When these changes occur for more than 6 seconds, the baby starts to get less oxygen. The baby is unaffected if pushing lasts for 5 seconds or less and if the mother does not lock up her breath. Thus many doctors are now recommending that the mother push only when she feels like it, without holding her breath, and that she make each push short.

While the mother is actively pushing, the practitioner or a nurse will keep close track of the baby's heart rate with a fetoscope or a hand-held Doptone ultrasound monitor, unless the baby is being monitored continuously with an electronic monitor. Some doctors or midwives will monitor the heart rate every 15 minutes, others every 5. As crowning approaches, practitioners will often check the heart rate at the end of each contraction. This is standard procedure and is done because the pressure on the baby's head and on the cord is greatest at this point, and the practitioner wants to make sure that the baby is handling it well. The baby's heart rate normally slows slightly with each contraction, then speeds up between contractions.

During the second stage of labor the father's role is not as central as it was during the first stage, but as any mother will attest, the father's presence and support during this stage is no less meaningful.

His continued encouragement and intimate knowledge of the mother are invaluable. From a practical standpoint, he may help by supporting the mother in whatever position she is using to push. If she has a long second stage, the father may continue to press against or rub her back. The father can also assist the mother by timing the contractions, coaching her on breathing techniques, and helping her relax between contractions.

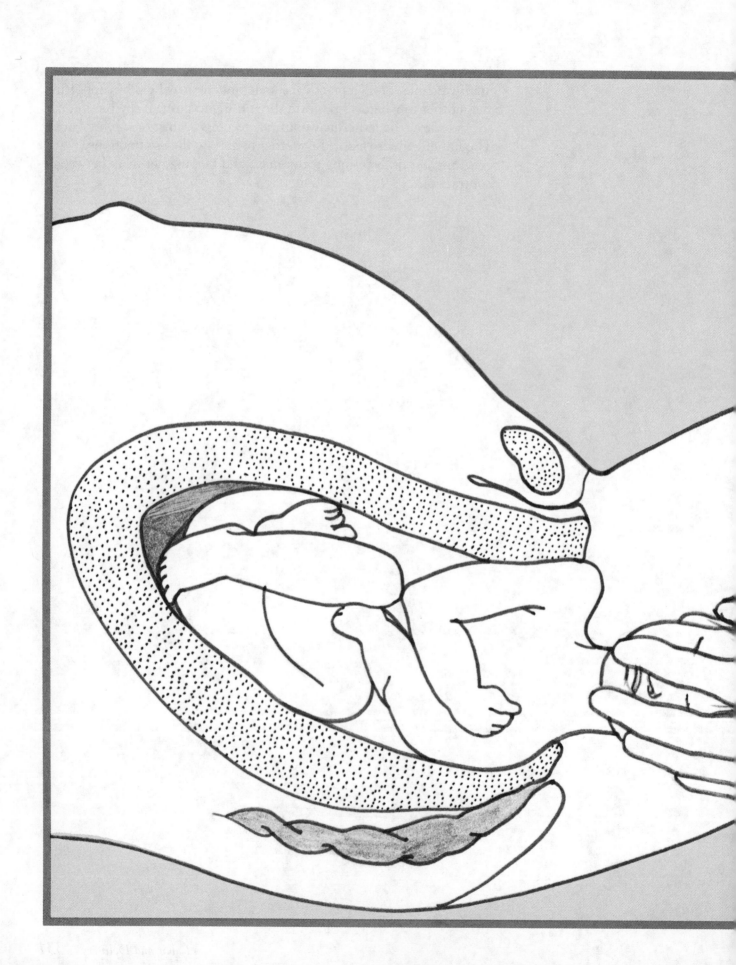

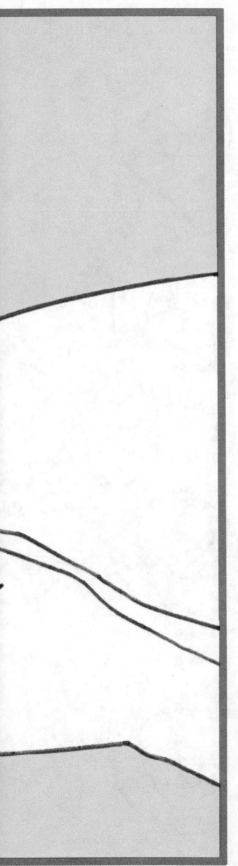

The Mother's Experience of Delivery

The End of the Second Stage of Labor

The delivery itself, which involves the actual expulsion of the baby from the birth canal and its emergence into the outside world, takes a relatively short time. It begins when the baby's head first appears at the opening of the vagina and ends as the baby's feet slip out. Often this interval is a matter of only five or six contractions, but it is filled with new sensations for the mother and an indescribable sense of climax.

As the time of delivery approaches, the baby's head no longer slips back between contractions but continues to inch steadily downward. Many mothers are physically aware of this, and they have a sudden, profound sense that there is no turning back from this point on. With the contractions now come a sense of accomplishment and an impending sense of completion. Often mothers find the contractions easier, even exhilarating at this stage, despite a tremendous feeling of fullness and stretching in the pelvis, as well as continued pressure on the lower back and rectum.

For a number of women the baby's presence in the vagina may even arouse pleasurable sexual feelings. This startles some mothers, but it really isn't surprising considering the number of physiological

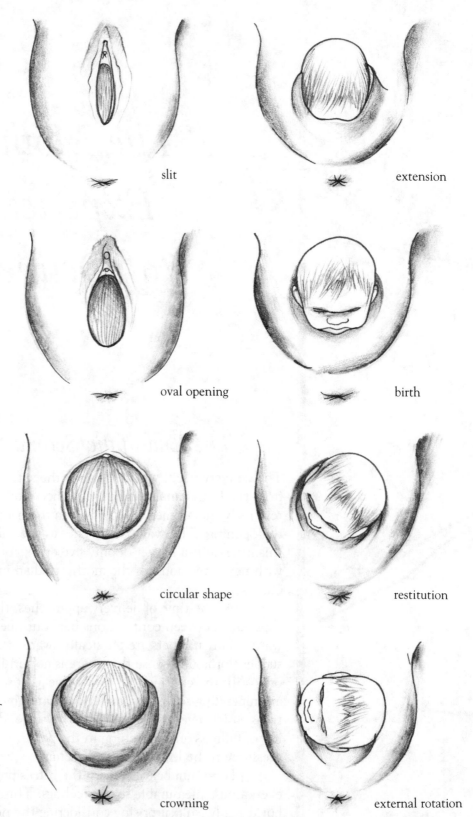

slit

extension

oval opening

birth

circular shape

restitution

As the time of delivery approaches, the baby's head no longer slips back between contractions. The mouth of the vagina widens, changing in shape from a slit to an oval to a circle. As more and more of the baby's head becomes visible, the mother has a tremendous sensation of fullness. It is awe-inspiring for her to watch the baby's head emerge and turn as the rest of its body passes through the birth canal.

crowning

external rotation

parallels that exist. The same hormones are involved, the genital area is similarly engorged with blood, and the many sensory nerves in and around the vagina are stimulated in like manner. As at orgasm, the vagina is wet. A mother may not initially identify feelings of sexual pleasure, because they are mingled with so many other diverse sensations. But the more at ease and confident a mother is at this moment, the more likely she is to become aware of these feelings.

Niles Newton, a well-known birth researcher, has written about the similarities between the experience of childbirth and the experience of orgasm. She cites parallel changes in breathing, utterance of noises, facial expressions, tensing of abdominal muscles, and experiencing of rhythmic contractions of the uterus. During both events women become more uninhibited and tend to enter an altered state of consciousness, from which they emerge with feelings of joy and satisfaction. British born educator Sheila Kitzinger also speaks of the pleasurable sexual sensations that can be aroused by the birth process. She points out that they are most often felt by women who are relaxed during delivery and who are generally sexually open and uninhibited.

Some mothers, especially with a first vaginal birth or a very large baby, have a moment before or during delivery when they fear tearing or splitting open. But it's important that they realize this image is a metaphor rather than a real possibility. The bones of the pelvis are held together with ligaments that can stretch without breaking, while the birth canal and pelvic floor are made of strong muscles and expandable tissue. Although mothers sometimes tear the perineum, this can usually be avoided by a slow, controlled delivery or the use of an episiotomy.

As the baby's head descends further and further, the whole perineal area bulges more and more until the vagina starts to open around the baby's head. *Crowning* occurs when the vagina is spread widest by the emerging head. The tremendous stretching of the vaginal opening at this point produces an intense burning sensation, which often causes the mother to cry out momentarily. This sensation is usually followed by tingling or numbness due to the pressure of the baby's head on the nerves and blood vessels in the area. The larger the head, the more likely the mother is to feel numbness.

Positions for Delivery

Shortly before crowning, if not sooner, the mother will be helped into the position in which she will deliver the baby. Just as with second-stage pushing, several positions have come into use as alternatives to the traditional lithotomy position of having the mother lie on her back with her legs in stirrups. The lithotomy position is less and less

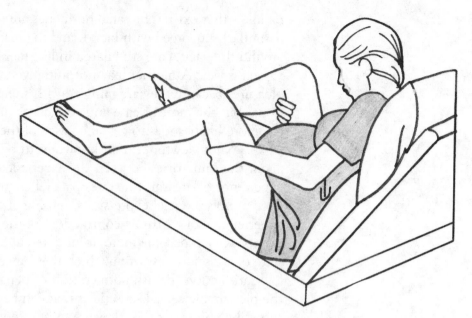

commonly used now because it slows the mother's return blood flow, lowers oxygen to the baby, makes pushing more difficult, and diminishes the effectiveness of contractions. The lithotomy position is also thought to tense the perineum and stretch it in the wrong direction. Finally, if a mother is lying on her back, she can only see the birth in a mirror. However, this position does support the mother's legs and makes it easier for the doctor to see the delivery and do an episiotomy if it is necessary.

The most frequently used new position, called the *dorsal,* has the mother in a semi-sitting posture, leaning against a backrest or pillows. Her legs may be slightly drawn up or, with one of the new delivery chairs, her legs may drop down. Most mothers feel that this is more natural than the lithotomy position and an easier one in which to deliver the baby. Many doctors and midwives prefer the dorsal position because it maximizes the baby's oxygen.

Several other positions are less commonly used in this country. They include having the mother lie on her left side or squat. Lying on the side is the most popular position used in English hospitals because it maximizes blood flow and allows the doctor or midwife a good view of the delivery at the same time. But as in the lithotomy position, the mother can only view the delivery in a mirror. Squatting is the oldest birth position and it remains the most popular one in non-Western cultures. It is also the most commonly used position in Pithiviers, the innovative French hospital known for its pioneering natural childbirth techniques. The squatting position is very effective for pushing, especially when a woman has a narrow pelvis or speed is a consideration. In this posture the mother has immediate access to her baby once it has emerged, and thus many midwives feel it is the most natural position for bonding. However, squatting does not allow the mother or the doctor as good a view of the delivery.

The mother's ability to see the delivery is emphasized not just because it enhances her pleasure. It also helps her work with the doctor or midwife in controlling the delivery. Without being told, she knows exactly how much of the baby has been delivered at any given moment. Before the baby crowns, she is able to view the effectiveness of each contraction in pushing the baby down the birth canal. This awareness of her progress and of how close she is to the moment of delivery gives her a tremendous psychological lift and renewed energy. Some midwives feel that the mother doesn't see the delivery well except by mirror. They often encourage mothers to get feedback on their progress by feeling the baby with their own hands once it has begun to emerge.

After the baby has crowned, watching it advance as it emerges from the birth canal can help the mother to cooperate with the doctor or midwife in slowing the delivery of the head and shoulders, which she does by not pushing during certain contractions, although she may be asked to push *lightly* between contractions. This gives the vaginal opening time to stretch and prevents a hard bulging part of the baby such as the shoulder from catching the vaginal lip and bruising or tearing it. Gradual stretching of the vagina and perineum is especially important if the mother and practitioner choose to deliver the baby without an episiotomy.

In order to restrain herself from pushing, the mother usually needs to use some kind of special breathing technique (see p. 323). She may breathe through an O-shaped mouth, breathe in and out slowly, pant lightly and shallowly, or blow out forcefully if she really has an urge to push. Midwives often call this breathing the baby out. It is very helpful if the mother can consciously relax the area around the perineum at this point.

Episiotomies

An episiotomy is a small incision, about 2 inches long, that is made from the bottom of the vagina down toward the anus or slightly to one side. Twenty years ago in the United States episiotomies were routinely done during childbirth to enlarge the vaginal opening. The procedure became popular in the 1920s, when forceps first came into common use to bring the baby down if labor didn't progress. As of 1980, although forceps were no longer used often, 62 percent of all deliveries in the United States and 90 percent of all first vaginal deliveries had an episiotomy.

Several basic reasons have been given for routinely doing episiotomies. For years it was believed that by enlarging the vaginal opening, an episiotomy tended to prevent stretching of the muscles and ligaments around the perineum, which was assumed to cause weakening of the supports to the bladder, uterus, and/or rectum. Such weakening was thought to result eventually in conditions such as fallen uterus, protruding rectum, or urinary leakage. Although a number of doctors still believe this to be true, most studies have not borne it out.

Other arguments in favor of episiotomies were that a clean surgical incision was easier to repair than an uncontrolled tear, and that large tears were less likely to occur if a mother had an episiotomy, especially with a big baby or a very rapid delivery. For the great majority of mothers the latter considerations do not even apply. Finally, an episiotomy was considered desirable because it shortened the second stage of labor by roughly 15 to 30 minutes, thereby lessening the amount of time the baby's head was pushing against the pelvic floor. This was believed to minimize the chances of brain damage for the baby. Recent studies have shown, however, that in uncomplicated deliveries the length of the second stage does not affect the health of the baby.

Since prepared childbirth became popular in the United States in the late 1960s, routine use of episiotomies has started to decline. Many mothers choosing prepared childbirth have heard that most women in countries such as England and the Netherlands give birth without episiotomies, and they also want to avoid this surgical procedure if possible. Based on this information and their own feelings, mothers have put tremendous consumer pressure on obstetricians to avoid episiotomies as well as to make the entire delivery more natural and less technological.

When obstetricians searched the medical literature and found no unequivocal reason for routinely doing episiotomies, many, like midwives, began to try to avoid them. In birth centers where midwives have primary responsibility, the episiotomy rate runs about 15 percent to 25 percent. Most midwives try to avoid episiotomies because they feel that the recovery is longer and more uncomfortable than with a nonsurgical delivery or even with repair of a tear. They point out that tears are usually much smaller than an episiotomy incision and rarely go through muscle.

Not using an episiotomy involves a much greater degree of cooperation between the mother and the practitioner during the second stage. In order to have a well-controlled delivery, the mother must be able to respond to instructions to refrain from pushing or to push lightly; otherwise she is more likely to tear. Mothers with prepared childbirth training are usually better able to cooperate with the doctor or midwife for several reasons: not only have these mothers been taught special breathing techniques, they have a much better idea of what to expect from childbirth, and they tend to be less upset or frightened than mothers with little or no education about the birth process.

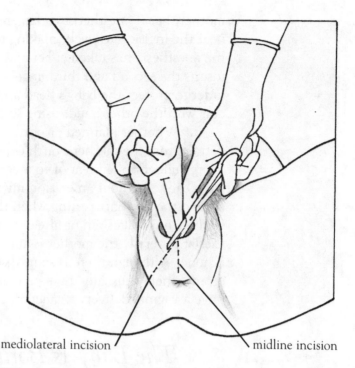

mediolateral incision / \ midline incision

An episiotomy is an incision made from the bottom of the vagina down toward the anus or slightly to one side, to widen the vaginal opening. The decision to do an episiotomy varies with the practitioner, the size of the baby, and the mother's ability to work with the practitioner during contractions.

When they are not planning to do an episiotomy, some doctors and midwives use special techniques to prevent the mother from tearing. At the point of maximum stretching when the baby's head crowns, they massage the mother's perineum with sterile oils, vitamin E oil, or lubricants; some apply heat as well. Many even put slight counterpressure on the perineum until the head has been delivered.

Occasionally, despite all efforts, an episiotomy is necessary when the mother has a difficult time and is unable to work with the doctor or midwife in controlling the delivery. Several other factors may make an episiotomy a desirable option. If the mother has an unusually muscular perineum that does not stretch easily (more common among athletic women), the baby presents in an uncommon position, the baby is very large, the baby is very small so its skull is delicate, or it is important to get the baby out quickly, the practitioner may decide to do an episiotomy. Sometimes the doctor or midwife may choose to do an episiotomy at the last minute if the mother's perineum suddenly shows white stretch marks as crowning begins, indicating that tearing is imminent.

Generally the incision is made between contractions, just before the baby's head crowns. Local anesthesia is almost always given, even though the perineum is often numb from stretching by this time. Xylocaine, a novocainelike anesthesia, can be used for a *pudendal,* which blocks the nerves around the perineum, or it can be injected directly into the area where the incision will be made, which is referred to as a *local infiltration.* In either case the injection takes only a moment and does not affect the baby. The pudendal block, which is given in the vaginal wall, is somewhat more uncomfortable for the mother, but it anesthetizes a larger area and does not cause the tissues near the incision to swell, making the repair somewhat easier. Once the anesthesia has taken effect and the area is numb, the practitioner inserts the second and third fingers of one hand into the vagina in order to protect the baby's head and then rapidly makes one or two cuts with the other hand, using surgical scissors.

Whether planned or not, an episiotomy need not necessarily detract from the mother's birth experience. Certainly it is preferable to a large uncontrolled tear or to a very uncomfortable delivery of a very large baby. Without an episiotomy the mother has a burning sensation around the vaginal opening when the baby crowns. Repair of the episiotomy only takes ten or fifteen minutes and requires no more anesthesia; generally the mother is able to hold the baby while the suturing is done. Although there is some discomfort in the healing of an episiotomy, there is usually some perineal discomfort for most mothers who have a vaginal delivery *without* an episiotomy.

The Baby Is Born

As the moment of delivery approaches, the mother will be able to see the perineum bulge more and more if she is in a semi-sitting position or is viewing the delivery in a mirror. The degree to which the perineum stretches as the top of the baby's head appears is quite remark-

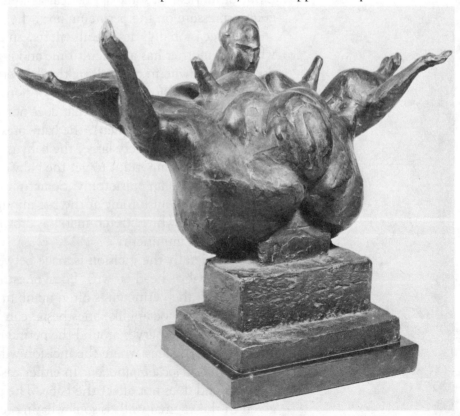

The moment of crowning is one of great joy and exertion for the mother. Dynamo Mother, Gaston Lachaise, 1933. Bronze, 11⅛" x 17¾" x 7½". Collection, The Museum of Modern Art, New York. Gift of Mr. Edward M. M. Warburg.

able. The mouth of the vagina now widens with each contraction, changing in shape from a slit to an oval pointed at the top and bottom. Finally the opening becomes a completely round circle as the baby's head crowns. Looking down, the mother will be able to see the baby's dark, wet hair plastered to the wrinkled skin of its scalp. For most women there is no more miraculous sight: there is exhilaration, joy, wonder, and for first-time mothers especially an almost total sense of disbelief that this event is occurring, that they are actually giving birth after the months of waiting. For many mothers, and for the others in the room, there may be a sudden feeling that they are watching all this happen in slow motion, almost as in a dream.

As the baby's head begins crowning, the doctor or midwife will use both hands to control the delivery of the head. The exact placement of each hand depends on the mother's position and the way the baby is presenting. We will describe the position of the practitioner's hands in the most common situation, with the mother half sitting or lying on her back while the baby emerges from the birth canal head-first, with its chin facing the mother's back (vertex anterior). To prevent the baby's head from emerging too quickly, the doctor or midwife will press lightly but firmly on the baby's head and may also press on the mother's perineum with the other hand. Often the lower hand will be covered with a towel to keep the area clean. Some practitioners control the delivery of the head in a slightly different way. The top hand still presses on the baby's head, but the other hand is pressed behind the mother's anus, up under the baby's chin. Midwives do not tend to use this position because it is more uncomfortable for the mother.

To prevent the baby's head from emerging from the vagina too quickly, the doctor or midwife presses one hand gently but firmly against the baby's head and sometimes presses the other hand on the mother's perineum. At this point the doctor or midwife may also ask the mother to breathe high in her chest so that she does not push.

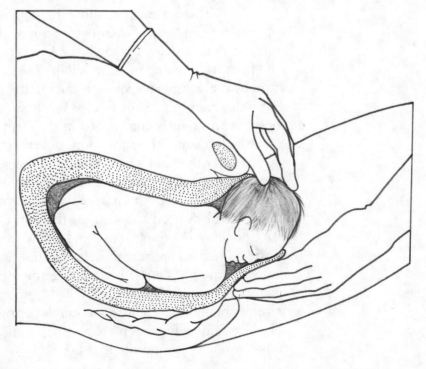

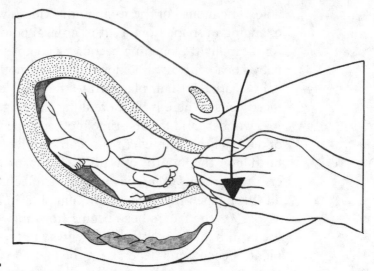

The doctor or midwife gently supports the baby's head once it has emerged and puts light downward pressure on the head to help ease the top shoulder out.

Using one or both hands, the practitioner allows the baby's head to emerge slowly over one or two contractions. During this time the mother may be asked to pant or blow so that she does not actively push. As soon as the baby's head has completely appeared, the doctor or midwife will slide a hand in behind the top of the baby's head to check for the cord. A quarter of the time a loop of the umbilical cord will be around the baby's neck, but this generally isn't a problem because the cord is so loose the practitioner can simply slip the cord over the baby's head or slip it back over the baby's shoulders as they are delivered. In the few cases in which the cord is tight, the practitioner tells the mother to pant, and cuts and clamps the cord immediately.

As the head emerges, amniotic fluid often drains from the baby's mouth and nose. The doctor or midwife will wipe away the amniotic fluid and any blood on the baby's face and gently suction fluid from its nose and mouth. Wiping the baby's face helps to keep it warm by preventing evaporation; suctioning clears the baby's throat so that it does not inhale any fluid as its chest emerges. As long as the chest remains tightly compressed in the birth canal, no air or fluid can enter the lungs and the baby cannot even utter its first cry.

After the baby's head has fully emerged, it spontaneously turns from facedown to sideways (restitution and external rotation, see pp. 295–98). The doctor or midwife does not control this but merely supports the baby's head and watches this part of the delivery. Next the practitioner puts a hand above and below the baby's head and applies gentle downward pressure to help the top shoulder slip easily out from under the mother's pubic bone. Once the top shoulder is clear, the practitioner gently pulls up and out, helping to deliver the lower shoulder by sliding it past the mother's perineum. The delivery of the shoulders generally takes place so quickly and requires so little help from the doctor or midwife that it is really a matter of guiding rather

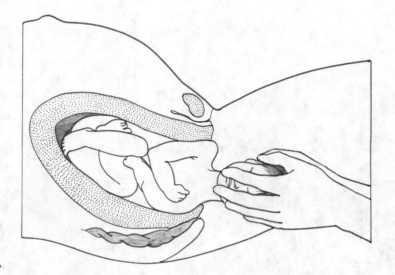

The doctor or midwife gently lifts the baby's head upward to guide the lower shoulder out. The delivery of the shoulders takes place so quickly it appears like one continuous movement.

than pulling the baby out. Once the shoulders emerge, the chest rapidly slides out, quickly followed by the upper and lower arms. Meanwhile the doctor or midwife slides a hand under the baby, both to support its body and to control the delivery of the baby's bottom hand.

Often more fluid comes out as the baby's chest emerges. This helps to clear the baby's airway in preparation for its first breath and is part of the miraculous process the baby's body undergoes in switching from getting oxygen from its mother's blood to supplying its own oxygen by breathing. Up to now the baby's lungs have been filled with *pleural fluid,* but to begin normal breathing the lungs must be cleared of fluid and inflated with air (see p. 451). Once out of the birth canal, the chest expands reflexively, creating a vacuum that causes air to rush into the lungs so that the baby automatically takes its first breath. The baby may utter its first cry at this point, although some healthy babies naturally remain silent, which need not be a cause for concern.

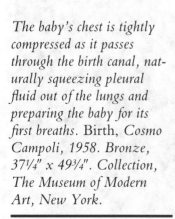

The baby's chest is tightly compressed as it passes through the birth canal, naturally squeezing pleural fluid out of the lungs and preparing the baby for its first breaths. Birth, Cosmo Campoli, 1958. *Bronze, 37¼" x 49¾". Collection, The Museum of Modern Art, New York.*

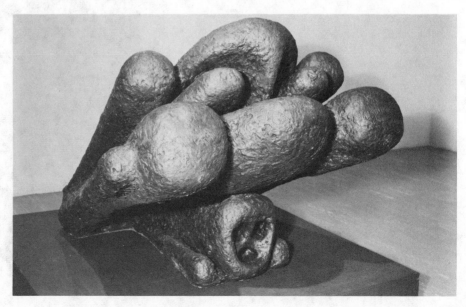

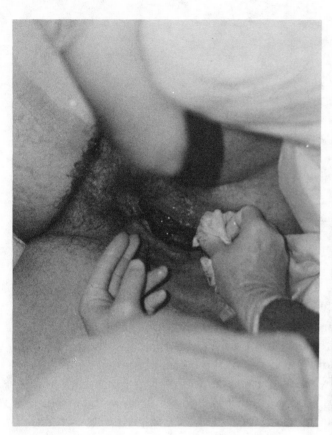

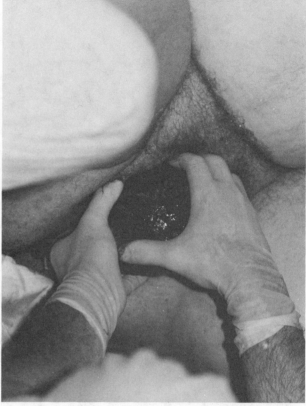

As the baby emerges, it's a new miracle every time. Photos by Linda O'Neil.

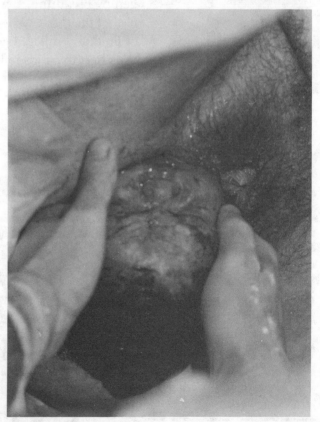

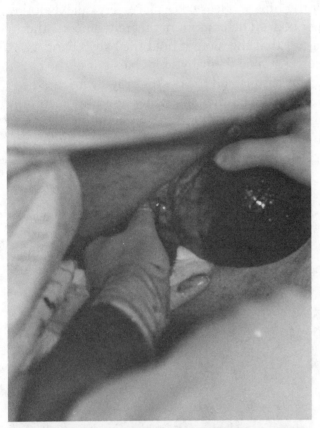

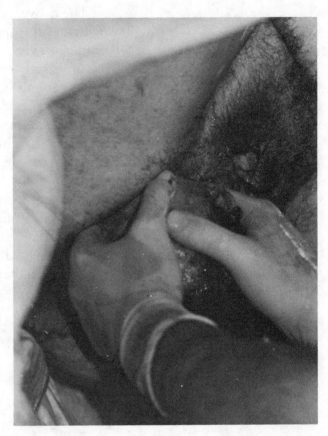

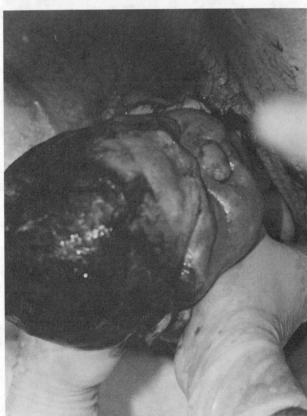

The delivery of the hips and legs takes place very quickly following that of the upper body. The practitioner merely supports the baby and may even suggest that the mother hold the baby's hand as the rest of its body emerges. Once the baby's hips pass out of the vagina, its genitals become visible and the doctor or midwife can distinguish the sex. Sometimes the mother and father find it momentarily difficult to determine because the baby's genitals are quite swollen at the time of birth. This swelling is completely normal and is the result of hormones that are produced in large amounts toward the end of pregnancy.

In order for the baby to take its first breath, the respiratory center in its brain must be stimulated to send signals to the muscles of the chest and diaphragm. If the baby does not immediately begin to breathe or cry out, the doctor or midwife may stimulate the breathing reflex by gently rubbing the baby's back or by tapping the baby's feet.

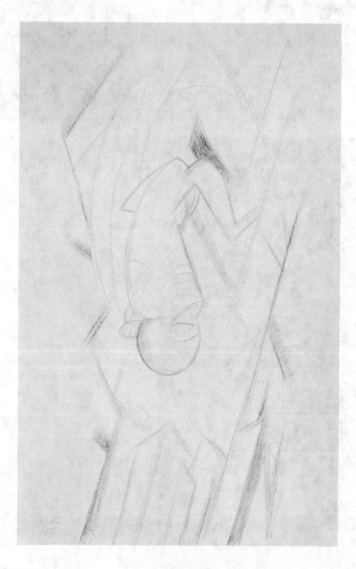

Once the shoulders have emerged, the rest of the baby slips out quickly and easily. Birth, *Jacob Epstein, 1913. Red crayon, 27⅛" x 17⅛". Collection, The Museum of Modern Art, New York. Gift of Mr. and Mrs. Richard Deutsch.*

In the old days doctors and midwives would hold the baby by the ankles, head down, in order to promote drainage from the lungs. They also used to slap the baby's buttocks in order to start the breathing reflex.

Some doctors and midwives, including the French obstetrician Frederick Leboyer, recommend not cutting the umbilical cord for 4 or 5 minutes after the baby is born or until the cord stops pulsing with blood. They feel that this gives the baby the advantage of two ways of oxygenating its blood during the transitional period when it has just started to breathe. The newborn's breathing is normally a little rapid, noisy, and even irregular for about the first half-hour after birth.

After the baby slips all the way out, the doctor or midwife holds the baby's head down, slightly below the level of the mother. This is done for a period of 30 seconds to 3 minutes, or until the cord stops pulsating. During this time 50 to 100 milliliters (approximately ¼ cup to ½ cup) of blood from the cord and placenta flow into the baby. Studies have shown that the maximum amount of blood is transferred in 3 minutes if the baby is held *level* with the mother and in 30 seconds if the baby is held well *below* the mother. In order to prevent blood from draining back into the placenta, the baby will probably not be placed on the mother until the cord has been clamped. The additional blood adds to the baby's iron stores and its blood volume, although it's generally not harmful to the baby if the cord is cut earlier.

The doctor or midwife will usually clamp and cut the umbilical cord once it has stopped pulsating, although there is great variability in the time at which this is done. Two clamps are attached to the cord close to the baby's body, and the cut is made between them. The clamp closest to the body is left on 24 hours, and the stub of the cord dries and falls off naturally. In the past a simple square knot was tied around the cord to prevent it from bleeding.

As delivery nears completion, the mother's and father's attention become focused on whether the baby is whole and well. Once the doctor or midwife puts the baby on the mother's chest, she instinctively begins to examine the baby closely, counting its fingers and toes, touching it all over and often cooing or talking to it in a special tone of voice. Thus the mother greets her baby and begins the process of bonding as she sees the baby face to face for the first time.

For the mother the moment of birth has a sense of sweetness and emotional fullness that can't adequately be expressed in words. Although she has been through so much with this baby, she suddenly senses that this is only the beginning. Her hard work and courageous efforts have brought one of life's greatest journeys to an end, only to open up the vista of the journey to come. For mother and father this is a very special time that will bond them together in a new and deeper way.

The First Minutes After Birth

During the first moments after birth babies are quite strange and marvelous-looking creatures. They are wet with amniotic fluid and may be tinged with blood from the site where the placenta separated from the uterine wall. Their skin is covered with varying amounts of a cheesy-looking substance called the *vernix caseosa*, which has protected them from their immersion in amniotic fluid. It is quite normal for the baby's skin to have a bluish color right after birth. As breathing becomes well established and more oxygen is delivered to the blood, this bluish hue fades and the baby takes on a more natural color except for its fingers and toes, which retain a bluish tint for a longer time.

Parents frequently feel that the baby looks "long," and indeed the baby's head has often been lengthened by molding and may appear quite pointed for a time. This pointedness is a normal occurrence that is due to the soft bones of the skull overriding one another during the tight passage through the birth canal. The process of molding is a

Immediately after birth the baby is placed on its side on the mother's chest in an age-old movement.

Mother and Child, Oceania, nineteenth–twentieth century. The Metropolitan Museum of Art. The Michael C. Rockefeller Memorial Collection.

Mother and Child, Ivory Coast. Lowie Museum of Anthropology, University of California, Berkeley.

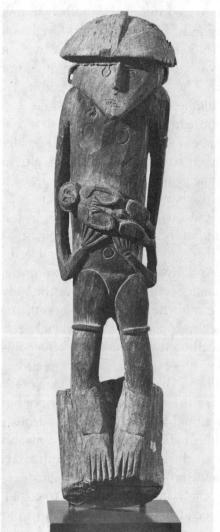
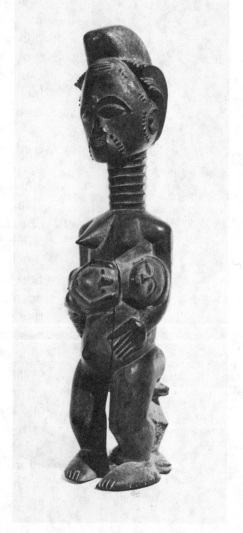

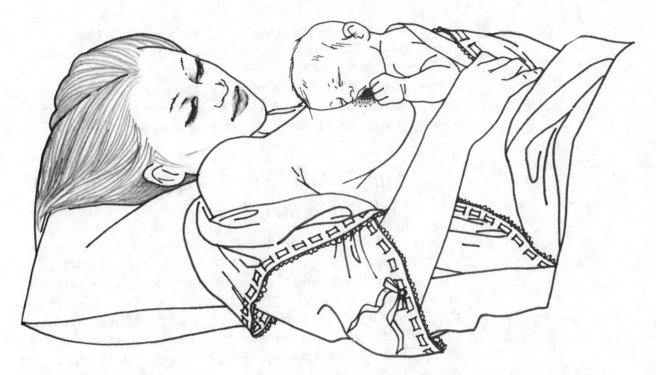

The first hour after birth is a precious and important one. Mother and baby touch, look at, and listen to one another, and the baby will attempt to nurse. The whole process of mother and baby forming an initial attachment is called bonding.

marvelous adaptation of nature that both protects the baby's head from injury and makes the delivery easier for the mother.

In the minutes after birth, perhaps even before the cord is cut, the baby is lightly dried off and then immediately placed on its side on the mother's chest. In this position the baby is able to look into its mother's eyes and begin nursing movements. During the first half-hour or so baby and mother tend to be quite alert and interested in each other. Both have innate curiosity about and ageless patterns of relating to each other. In this first period mother and baby touch, look at, and listen to one another, adding tremendously to their knowledge of each other and laying a foundation for their future relationship. For baby, mother, and the father these first minutes together serve to promote and deepen their attachment to one another. These initial, intimate interactions are referred to as *bonding* (see p. 467).

As unobtrusively as possible, so as not to interfere with the process of bonding, the doctor or midwife will check the baby at one minute after birth and again at five minutes after birth. This is a normal part of good neonatal care. The baby is evaluated for color, muscle tone, reactivity, breathing, and heart rate, an assessment that is known as the *Apgar score.* If the mother has had pain medication near the time of delivery or some types of anesthesia, the baby is not likely to respond as alertly as if the mother had had no medication of any kind. Even local anesthesia may affect the baby slightly, although new types and lower dosages have less effect than in the past.

Within minutes of being placed on the mother's chest, the baby will begin to make sucking movements and will actually nurse if the nipple is guided to its mouth. This instinctual behavior not only seems pleasing to the baby, it stimulates the mother's uterus to contract and clamp down. This is an example of how inborn bioprograms of mother and newborn mesh and work for their mutual benefit.

The Third Stage: Delivering the Placenta

Delivery of the placenta usually goes almost unnoticed by the mother and father because they are so taken up with the baby and each other. The mother's contractions begin again within three to five minutes after the baby is born and continue to occur every 4 or 5 minutes until the placenta is expelled from the uterus. These postdelivery contractions cause the placenta to separate by shrinking the size of the uterus (see p. 298). The third stage usually takes around 5 to 15 minutes but may occasionally take as long as a half-hour and, more rarely, may take place immediately after delivery. As with earlier contractions, these are entirely involuntary, but they feel very different to the mother, more like the contractions of early labor.

During third-stage contractions the doctor or midwife usually rests a hand lightly on the mother's abdomen to feel her uterus. Mid-

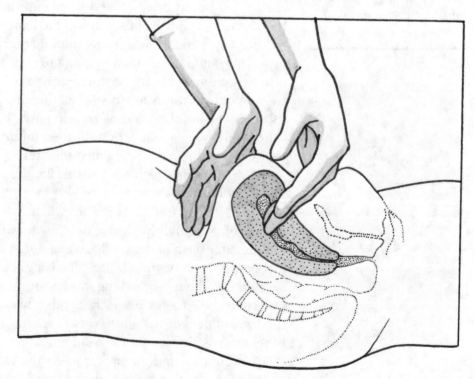

Following the delivery of the placenta, the doctor or midwife may massage the abdomen, supporting the uterus above the pelvic bone with one hand and putting downward pressure on the uterus with the other hand. The mother will be told to do this herself if her uterus becomes soft during the first few hours after birth.

wives call this guarding the uterus. There are two reasons for doing this. First, there should not be any pressure on the uterus until the placenta has naturally separated. Until then massage or pressure can cause incomplete separation. Second, the doctor or midwife can feel how well the uterus is shrinking by the way it changes from soft and flat to firm and round.

The practitioner can tell that the placenta has separated even before it is expelled: the uterus rises higher in the abdomen, while the umbilical cord emerging from the mouth of the vagina becomes noticeably longer, and a gush of blood from the separation site may pass out of the vagina. Once the doctor or midwife is sure that separation is complete, he or she will ask the mother to bear down, creating more pressure in her abdomen, which helps to push the placenta out. To assist the mother and support her uterus at this point, the practitioner may press down on her abdomen and upward toward her navel at the same time. This keeps the uterus tipped back and puts indirect pressure on it to expel the placenta. The practitioner may also exert gentle traction on the umbilical cord, pulling it downward as the placenta passes through the birth canal and then upward out of the vagina.

If the mother is in a semi-sitting or squatting position, delivery of the placenta usually takes place quickly and with little help from the doctor or midwife. The mother feels the expulsion of the placenta as a soft, warm, comforting sensation within her vagina, very different from the intense pressure, stretching, and burning produced by delivery of the baby's head. If little blood preceded the delivery of the placenta, a gush of blood will come out as it is expelled. In either case, this loss of blood is completely normal; the timing is just a matter of whether the placenta initially separated at the center or at the edges (see pp. 299–301). As noted, the mother usually loses about 200 to 500 milliliters (about 1 to 2 cups) of blood, which she can safely afford because of the vast increase in blood volume that has taken place during pregnancy.

After the placenta has emerged, the membranes that surrounded the baby gradually separate on their own (see p. 300). The doctor or midwife then carefully spreads out the placenta and examines it to verify that it is normal and that no part of it has remained attached to the separation site. If it hasn't already been done, the doctor or midwife also takes a sample of blood from the end of the umbilical cord for routine laboratory tests. Many mothers, often to their surprise, find themselves very interested in the placenta and ask to see it. It is indeed a remarkable structure, 5 to 7 inches in diameter and weighing a little over a pound. It is dark red on the side that was attached, shiny gray on the other side, and richly supplied with blood vessels.

The Fourth Stage of Labor

Doctors refer to the hour following the expulsion of the placenta as the fourth stage of delivery. For the mother this is a time of triumphant weariness and becoming acquainted with her baby. For the doctor or midwife this is a time to do any necessary suturing and to monitor the mother's readjustment to a nonpregnant state. Specifically, the practitioner watches to see that the mother's uterus is clamping down properly, which stops the bleeding from the site where the placenta was attached.

If the mother's uterus begins to feel soft and "boggy" as opposed to hard, and/or if the mother continues to bleed, the doctor or midwife will massage her uterus in a special way. With one hand supporting the uterus just above the pelvic bone, the practitioner or nurse will gently massage the top of the mother's uterus with the other hand. Usually the mother will be shown how to check her uterus herself and how to knead it if it becomes soft later. Many doctors also routinely give the mother a shot of oxytocin, ergonovine, or methylergonovine, drugs that cause the uterus to contract. Nursing naturally stimulates the release of oxytocin, thereby helping the uterus clamp down.

After delivery of the placenta and membranes, the doctor or midwife will carefully examine the mother's perineum, lower vagina, and the area around her urethra. If an episiotomy has been done, or if she has torn, the practitioner will do any necessary suturing. When an episiotomy has been done, the area generally remains anesthetized; if not, local anesthesia is given before any stitches are put in. With anesthesia in effect, the mother feels pressure but no pain when the stitches are put in.

Since an episiotomy incision cuts through several layers of tissue, it is repaired in several stages. Each layer is individually sutured with a material that will naturally dissolve after several weeks. A careful repair requires time and patience and generally takes between 5 and 30 minutes. During this time the mother is usually so involved with the baby and her husband that she is only vaguely aware of what the practitioner is doing.

Once any necessary suturing has been done, the mother is washed, helped to change into a fresh gown, and given a pad to absorb the *lochia*, the discharge that normally drains from the uterus for several days after delivery (see p. 408). During the first hour after birth many mothers experience chills, for which they should simply be given blankets or warm clothing. This is perfectly normal, although doctors are still not certain of the cause. It is thought to be a physiological reaction to loss of body fluids and blood.

The new mother will be encouraged to urinate as soon as possible after the delivery, because her bladder tone will still not be normal. A full bladder is not only uncomfortable, it makes it harder for her uterus to clamp down sufficiently. The mother will need some assistance getting to the bathroom if she feels very tired or a little shaky, but walking itself is good for her.

For the first hour or two after delivery, the new mother, father, and baby will want to spend time becoming acquainted, but after a time both mother and baby will find that the exhaustion of all their efforts has caught up with them. Often the mother herself will want to nap when the baby falls asleep for the first time.

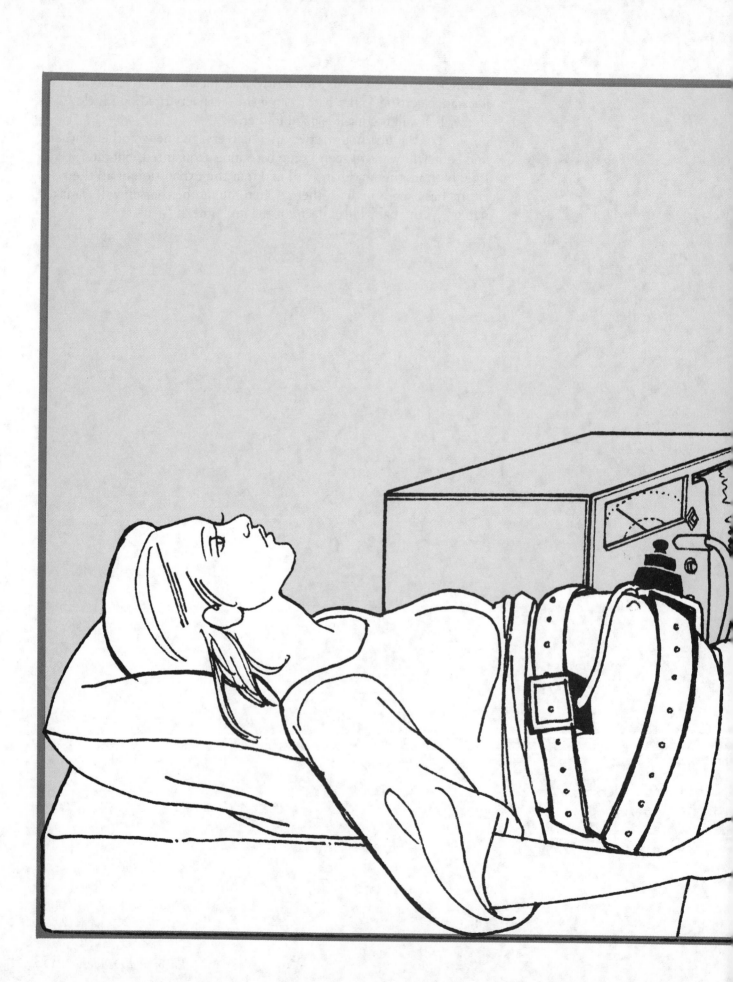

Fetal Monitoring

Types of Monitoring

Like the mother's heartbeat, the baby's gives a general indication of its health. For this reason doctors and midwives listen to the baby's heartbeat when it first becomes audible with a fetoscope or with an ultrasound device and thereafter at every regular prenatal visit or at any time there are indications of a possible problem. During labor the practitioner or a nurse checks the baby's heartbeat at frequent intervals, since labor is a more physically stressful time for the baby than pregnancy.

During each contraction the placenta is compressed, cutting down on the blood flow to the baby, which in turn reduces the baby's oxygen. This temporary decrease in oxygen is of no consequence to the average baby and mother, but it can be a problem if the baby is not optimally healthy or if the mother has certain medical conditions. Babies are considered to be at risk if they are very early or late, very small or large, or if they are likely to have a condition such as respiratory distress syndrome. A baby may also be at risk if the mother has toxemia, diabetes, heart disease, or a prior history of obstetrical complications.

Since the late 1800s it has been known that specific changes in the baby's heart rate are reliable indicators of early fetal distress. At

355

that time doctors used a regular stethoscope to listen to the baby's heartbeat, but in 1910 an American doctor invented a special stethoscope which he called the *fetoscope*. The fetoscope differs from a regular stethoscope in that the listening bell is positioned by moving the head, which allows practitioners to use their hands to determine the baby's position at the same time. The fetoscope has now largely been replaced by a portable ultrasound device, such as the Doptone, which is easier to use and can pick up sounds that may be hard for the ear to distinguish.

In the late 1960s and early 1970s electronic techniques became available to pick up the baby's heartbeat and record it on a graph. These techniques are called *electronic fetal monitoring* or *EFM*. There are two types of electronic fetal monitors: one uses external leads that are taped to the mother's abdomen, the other uses an internal lead that is inserted under the baby's scalp. Both of them provide a continuous record of the baby's heartbeat and can be used in conjunction with an electronic pickup that measures the motion of the uterus during contractions. Used during labor this allows the doctor or midwife to see the effect of each contraction on the baby's heart rate.

The most popular form of electronic fetal monitoring today is external. With this device the fetal heart rate is measured with pulsed ultrasound. Two straps containing electronic transducers are placed around the mother's abdomen: one records the baby's heartbeat, the other measures the strength of her contractions. The transducers are easily affected by movement or being rubbed, so for all practical purposes the mother's movements are fairly restricted while the monitor is in use. When an external monitor is simply used briefly upon admission or occasionally throughout labor, it functions much like an elaborate fetoscope exam, but it provides a continuous reading. Intermittent

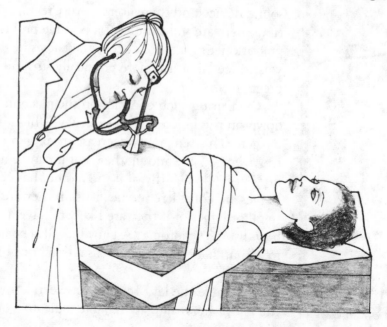

The simplest form of monitoring involves a special stethoscope called the fetoscope, which allows the doctor or midwife to listen to the baby's heart. A small, portable ultrasound machine can be used instead.

use of an external electronic monitor is not that common. It tends to be most frequent in birth-room situations and family-centered obstetrical centers where the mother's free movement in labor is considered important. More typically the external electronic fetal monitor is attached to the mother's abdomen upon admission and is kept in place until after delivery.

By far the most accurate means of monitoring the baby's heart rate—and the one that provides the most information—is *internal monitoring*. The electrode is inserted through the cervix into the baby's scalp. It has a safety feature that prevents it from penetrating more than 2 millimeters. It records the heartbeat by picking up electrical impulses from the baby's heart, like an electrocardiogram (EKG). In addition to the electrode, a transducer is strapped around the mother's abdomen to measure the pressure of the contractions. To insert the electrode under the baby's scalp, the mother's cervix has to be dilated 1 to 2 centimeters and her bag of waters must be ruptured. When the doctor ruptures the membranes, the mother will feel a gush of amniotic fluid, but this procedure is not uncomfortable. Once the leads are in place, they provide a continuous, detailed picture of the baby's heart rate in comparison with the mother's contractions.

External fetal monitors that use ultrasound can be strapped around the mother's abdomen and used continuously or intermittently to monitor the baby's heartbeat. External monitors are currently in common use.

Fetal Heart Rate Patterns

Like an adult's the baby's heart rate is controlled by its autonomic nervous system: the sympathetic branch increases the heart rate, while the parasympathetic branch decreases it (see p. 139). The fetal heart rate rises and falls in response to sound, the mother's emotional-hormonal

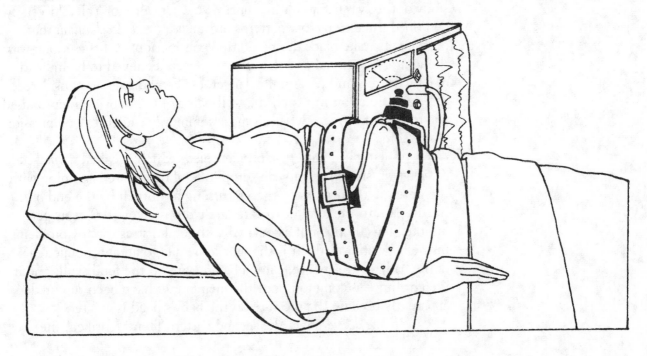

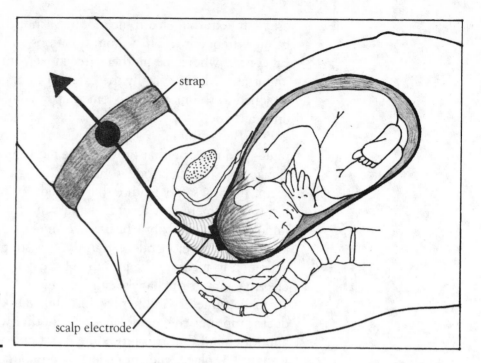

strap

scalp electrode

The most accurate form of monitoring uses a tiny electrode that is inserted just under the baby's skin after the mother's bag of waters has been broken. This device electronically records the baby's heartbeat.

state, the contractions, and changes in the baby's activity. During labor the average range of the baby's heart rate is 120 to 160 beats per minute. It is normal for the heart rate to rapidly increase or decrease by as much as 8 beats per minute. Such shifts show that the baby is reacting to changes in its environment.

Although it has long been known that the baby's heart rate often slows markedly in response to uterine contractions, the first study of this was not published until 1967. Dr. Hon of Yale University described three transitory patterns of *fetal heart rate deceleration* that occasionally take place during uterine contractions. Of these, one was thought to be normal and the other two were believed to be indicative of fetal distress and potentially dangerous. Fetal distress is considered to be any situation in which the well-being of the baby is compromised due to lack of oxygen, which is most commonly caused by compression of the cord.

The typical pattern Hon identified, which is called *normal early deceleration*, shows a significant drop in fetal heart rate beginning with the onset of a contraction, then returning to normal by the end of it. In this pattern the fetal heart rate rarely drops below 100 beats per minute. This drop is not associated with fetal distress or any problems in the baby after birth. It is thought to be due to an autonomic reflex of the baby's vagus nerve, caused by pressure on the fetal skull, and it is eight times as common once the membranes have been ruptured, apparently because the pressure on the baby's head is greater.

In *late deceleration*, the second pattern Hon identified, the baby's heart rate drops after the contraction begins and remains depressed after it has ended. Late deceleration is a pattern that may be associated with lack of oxygen for the baby. It is frequently seen in high-risk pregnancies and may precede having a baby in fetal distress or one born in a neurologically depressed state. However, the late deceleration pattern can often be corrected by having the mother turn on her side. This position takes the pressure off the large vein returning blood to her heart, thereby directly increasing the flow of blood and oxygen to the placenta.

The third pattern Hon identified he called *variable deceleration.* In this pattern the drop in the baby's heart rate is not associated with the contractions in any way. Variable deceleration is also a sign of oxygen insufficiency and is thought to be caused by pressure on the umbilical cord. In most cases it, too, is totally relieved by turning the mother on her side.

In addition to these three patterns, researchers now recognize a number of other patterns that are less common including rises in fetal heartbeat, which are not uncommon and are not significant if they only occur occasionally. Despite the clear categories established by Hon, it is now acknowledged that fetal heart rate patterns are much more complicated than was previously thought. Take, for example, variable decelerations, which are seen in 25 percent to 30 percent of all labors. Although some studies show a relationship between variable decelerations and the newborn's condition right after birth, others show no association at all. In fact, they demonstrate that babies who exhibit this potentially serious deceleration pattern are almost invariably healthy.

Even late decelerations, which occur in less than 10 percent of labors and are considered the earliest sign of fetal distress, do not necessarily correlate with newborn depression. The great majority of late decelerations are caused by management of labor. Both anesthetics and the hormone pitocin, which is given to speed up contractions, are known to be major causes of late deceleration. Another cause is having the mother lie on her back. If these factors are avoided or corrected, the late deceleration pattern is usually altered.

At present electronic monitoring not only picks up 95 percent of those babies who are truly in fetal distress but also many babies who appear to be in distress but are not. Doctors have come to realize that it requires great sophistication to interpret deceleration patterns. A diagnosis of fetal distress cannot be made solely on the basis of monitoring. To confirm the diagnosis of fetal distress, doctors have developed a procedure in which they take a sample of blood from a vein in the baby's scalp and test its pH. An unusually acidic result (less than 7.2) indicates that the baby is low on oxygen and tends to confirm the diagnosis of fetal distress as suggested by a deceleration pattern on the monitor.

The Value of Monitoring

The basic rationale for monitoring is to improve the condition of babies at birth. There is a tremendous drive worldwide to lower perinatal mortality and congenital defects. In the United States this has led to a significant rise in the use of technical procedures. Foremost among them is the use of continuous electronic fetal monitoring.

In 1979 the National Institute of Child Health and Human Development (NICHD) published a report on predictors of fetal distress. Their data showed that 30 percent of stillbirths and neonatal deaths were attributable to events that kept the baby from getting enough oxygen during labor and delivery. About 20 to 40 percent of cerebral palsy, 10 percent of severe mental retardation, and an unknown amount of subtle neurological damage are also thought to be due to lack of oxygen during labor and delivery. Of these babies, most are born to mothers in the high-risk category.

Doctors have thought that if fetal monitoring could identify these babies in distress during labor, they could greatly improve newborn statistics. Although there is no question that fetal monitoring does pick up infants in distress, its effect on newborn illness and mortality rates is questionable, particularly in the case of low-risk mothers.

Generally a new medical procedure is not put into widespread use until carefully controlled studies have demonstrated both its efficacy and its advantages over previous techniques. Electronic fetal monitoring has been widely adopted without large-scale studies primarily because it does not appear dangerous in itself. But it certainly is an intrusive factor that changes the mother's experience of labor, and it may even have added unintentionally to the dramatic rise in cesarean rates that has taken place in the last few years.

A number of factors make it very difficult to assess accurately the effect of electronic fetal monitoring on the health of newborns. First, the percentage of babies born with serious problems is actually very small. At most only two or three babies out of every thousand will experience problems that could be avoided if monitoring were completely successful. Thus to demonstrate a statistically significant improvement from monitoring, a study would have to deal with over 20,000 mothers with diagnosed *high-risk* pregnancies. Second, many social and medical factors, including improved nutrition, more sophisticated prenatal care, and the establishment of intensive care nurseries, are simultaneously tending to improve newborn health statistics. This means that a definitive study would require hundreds of thousands of mothers, carefully matched for age, income level, and obstetrical history, half of whom were randomly chosen to be monitored and half of whom were not. A study of this magnitude would be difficult and expensive, and up to now no such study has been done.

Many small-scale fetal monitoring studies have compared the

difference in newborn statistics before and after monitoring was introduced at a number of hospitals. These studies, which, when combined, dealt with over 100,000 pregnancies, showed a slight decline in newborn mortality and morbidity (illness) after the introduction of monitoring. However, these studies do not prove that monitoring was the cause of the decline, because they do not take into consideration other medical changes that may have taken place in the same time period, such as the establishment of highly specialized neonatal nurseries.

Some studies have attempted to match relatively small groups of mothers and note the difference between a group that was monitored and a control group that was not. Four out of five of these studies showed that electronic fetal monitoring gave *no advantage* over conventional monitoring with a fetoscope. The fifth study showed that electronic monitoring was of benefit only in high-risk patients. Unfortunately, the studies cannot be considered statistically significant, because the mothers were few in number and they were not randomly chosen. The most famous study, by Havercamp, showed that 1 baby in 256 was found to be in fetal distress among a group of high-risk mothers who were checked by fetoscope, whereas sixteen times as many babies were found to be in distress among a group of 463 high-risk mothers who were electronically monitored. In this study all the babies in distress were delivered by cesarean section, and all of them scored well on neurological assessments at birth. No babies in either group experienced significant illness or death. Havercamp concluded that there was as good an outcome for babies in the fetoscope group as for ones in the electronic fetal monitoring (EFM) group, but the EFM group had a much greater cesarean rate.

The largest controlled study, done by Neutra, compared fetoscope monitoring with EFM. It showed even more remarkable results. Out of 16,000 deliveries at Beth Israel Hospital in Boston, over 50 percent of newborn deaths were caused by severe congenital abnormalities or prematurity. Electronic fetal monitoring could not have affected the outcome for these babies in any way. After correcting for these and other risk factors, it was found that, overall, the fetoscope group had 1.4 times the risk of the EFM group. But when the mothers were also divided into high- and low-risk categories, a different picture emerged: statistically, electronic monitoring appeared to save 109 lives per 1,000 babies in the high-risk group, 1.6 times as many as fetoscope monitoring. But among the low-risk group, there was a .6 per 1,000 higher death rate among babies who were electronically monitored. Although the study did not randomly determine who was monitored and who was not, the results suggest that monitoring is of greatest benefit for high-risk mothers and of questionable value for mothers in the low-risk group.

Finally, there have been a number of studies of electronic monitoring that attempted to assess its usefulness in preventing mental retardation and cerebral palsy in the newborn. Based on analysis of these studies, the National Institute of Child Health and Human Development estimates that at the maximum, monitoring *all* mothers would prevent 1 case of severe mental retardation and 1 case of cerebral palsy per 2,000 live births.

Side Effects of Monitoring

Electronic fetal monitoring is basically regarded as a safe procedure, but there are problems and/or complications associated with the use of each type of electronic monitoring. The most common form of external monitor, which is strapped around the mother's abdomen, uses ultrasound, a technique that has not yet been *proved* to be completely safe, particularly for continuous use (see p. 237).

Family-centered birth units and midwives are quick to point out other disadvantages to continuous external monitoring. The straps are somewhat uncomfortable, and they greatly restrict the mother's movements during labor, generally confining her to bed on her back or her side. The mother's movements can displace the electronic pickups, confusing the readouts and requiring frequent readjustment. Ironically, the best monitoring data come when the mother lies relatively still on her back, the position that is most likely to put pressure on the mother's vena cava, slowing blood flow to the placenta and resulting in fetal distress. In addition to keeping the mother from changing positions in a normal manner, the straps often prevent her from receiving valuable, nontechnical comfort measures from the people assisting her.

Internal monitoring has its own set of disadvantages and complications, although it should be noted that there is generally a very low incidence of the latter. Studies have shown that babies monitored internally have a .3 percent to 4.5 percent chance of developing an infection at the site where the electrode was inserted. The great majority of infections recorded were not serious, but most required treatment with local antibiotics.

Researchers are concerned that the internal monitor may also be a factor in some uterine infections, particularly among mothers who had internal monitoring followed by a cesarean. Rupturing the fetal membranes to insert the internal monitor likewise increases the risk of infection for the baby, and it changes the patterns of pressure on both the baby's head and the mother's cervix during labor (see p. 306). An intact bag of water cushions the baby's head, helps to even out pressure on the cervix, and lessens the chances of the baby's umbilical cord being compressed during contractions (a common cause of variable deceleration in the baby's heart rate). However, doctors who use the internal monitor generally consider most complications to be rare, correctable, or less than the potential risks of a fetoscope-monitored delivery, particularly in the case of a high-risk mother.

A number of disadvantages are common to both internal and external electronic monitoring. Many mothers are disturbed by the technical, medical atmosphere that external, and especially internal, monitors bring to labor. For these women monitoring is simply another factor that reduces their control over the birth situation and interferes with creating a supportive, human atmosphere. Such technical equipment may produce negative emotions such as fear and dependency in mothers. As has been noted elsewhere, fear can have deleterious effects on labor, slowing contractions and impairing blood flow to the baby. On the other hand, some mothers are reassured by the potential safety offered by monitoring or feel that being able to predict the onset of each contraction in advance makes it easier for them to deal with labor.

Perhaps most significantly, there is great concern over the fact that almost all studies show that electronic monitoring is associated with higher-than-average cesarean rates (see p. 378). Because monitoring is more frequently used in large medical centers that generally have higher cesarean rates anyway, it is difficult to determine whether the elevated rates are due to monitoring or are simply associated with highly technical care. Three recent studies have shown that the rates of cesareans performed for reasons *other* than fetal distress were also higher among mothers who were continuously monitored than mothers who were not.

The Monitoring Controversy

The advantages of electronic monitoring technology as opposed to the desire of many women for as natural a birth as possible have created another major controversy in modern obstetrics. Strong advocates of the technique feel that it can enhance the likelihood of a healthy outcome for the baby and should be used routinely in all births. More moderate supporters feel that it should basically be used with high-risk mothers. Critics of the technique feel that it offers no advantage over careful fetoscope monitoring in all low-risk pregnancies and even in most high-risk ones. They specifically point out that monitoring interferes with the natural course of labor and can in itself cause problems.

Helen Varney, director of Maternal Nursing at Yale, has said, "Use of the fetal monitors for women with medical and/or obstetrical complications that may compromise the baby is an invaluable aid to the physician in effecting a viable outcome for the fetus. . . . The vast majority of births, however, are normal and uncomplicated. They neither require this advanced technology in order to effect the safe delivery of a healthy baby nor is it desirable. Use of the fetal monitors is intrusive both in its procedure and in its effect on an orientation of family-centered care, quiet work and joy, non-intrusive facilitation of natural processes within the realm of normal, and focus on the woman (as opposed to machines)."[1]

Even academic obstetricians have commented on the unproved nature of electronic fetal monitoring (EFM). In the book *Modern Management of High-Risk Pregnancy*, Robert Goodland has observed that "the history of EFM also includes commercialism and widespread uncritical acceptance of new devices into the armamentarium of obstetric skills. Probably no other technique whose value still is questioned by some investigators, both in high- and low-risk patient care, is as widely accepted by academicians, practicing obstetricians, and patients as is EFM."[2]

The National Institute of Child Health and Development (NICHD) has reviewed all the studies on the effects of monitoring and summarized its conclusions and recommendations. They suggest that with low-risk patients it is sufficient to monitor the mother with a fetoscope every 15 minutes during the first stage and every 5 minutes during the second stage. They state that "the weight of present evidence from prospective and retrospective analyses show no apparent effect of EFM upon perinatal mortality and morbidity in low-risk patients, but they acknowledge that under certain circumstances mothers and physicians may choose to use EFM even if the mothers are low risk. As maternal and fetal risk increases, there is a trend suggesting a beneficial effect of EFM. . . ."[3] The report goes on to state that EFM should be "strongly considered" in high-risk patients.

The NICHD reviewing committee cautions that a diagnosis of fetal distress should not be made on the basis of any single piece of data. In particular, it points out that intermittent or continuous monitoring should be viewed as a *screening* rather than a *diagnostic* technique, because it identifies so many babies as being in distress who prove to be healthy upon delivery. To verify a diagnosis of fetal distress, they recommend the use of a fetal scalp blood pH test.

NIHCD recognizes that pregnant women and their doctors are now confronted with difficult decisions regarding optimum labor care that currently must be based on incomplete information. The report recommends that the proper use of any form of monitoring, in both high- and low-risk patients, "should at the outset include a discussion with the patient of her wishes, concerns, and questions concerning benefits, limitations, and risks of fetal monitoring. Women should have the opportunity to discuss the use of all forms of monitoring during the course of prenatal care, and again upon admission to the labor suite."[4] Finally the report recommends that any form of monitoring should be accompanied by "supportive and knowledgeable personnel who are attentive to the patient's expectations regarding the conduct of her labor."[5] It goes on to say that "maternity services should be encouraged to integrate concepts of family-centered care with care of women who are electronically monitored."[6]

We feel that electronic monitoring is another situation in which informed mothers can and should make choices that take into consideration both their own feelings and the health of their babies. The point is for mothers to choose the alternative that will make them feel optimally reassured and confident during labor. It is important that a woman's doctor or midwife be in basic agreement with the mother's decision and supportive of it. For this reason fetal monitoring is another topic a woman should discuss with her doctor or midwife relatively early in her prenatal care.

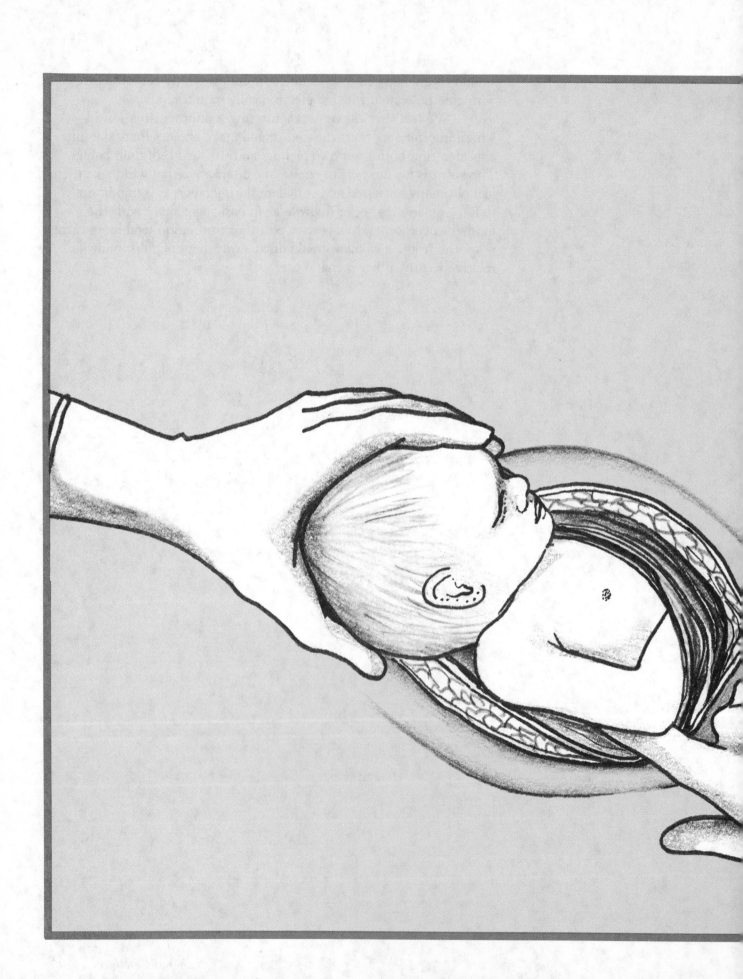

CHAPTER 17

Cesarean Birth

Making Cesareans a Positive Birth Experience

As recently as twenty years ago a cesarean section was an uncommon procedure resorted to only when the life of the mother or baby was in imminent danger. The average woman reading a pregnancy book at that time would not have had to concern herself with cesarean delivery, and indeed it probably would not have been discussed in the book. At the present time the average mother needs to be informed about cesarean birth because it is very much a part of contemporary obstetrics in the United States.

Probably no woman would have a c-section rather than a vaginal birth given the choice, but since 15 to 30 percent of all deliveries are currently by cesarean, it is important expectant mothers understand what is involved. The point is not that all pregnant women should prepare for a cesarean without prior indication but that they should not become so fixated on the *certainty* of a vaginal birth that they find themselves overwhelmingly disheartened if they have to deliver by cesarean.

Because many women who have a c-section find it difficult to come to terms with the experience, we feel it's important to reempha-

367

size the priorities of the birth experience, whether it be vaginal or cesarean: the goal of pregnancy is to become parents of as healthy a child as possible. Birth is a momentous landmark in the development of a family, but it represents only a brief part of parenting. Mothers and fathers are involved in the nurturing experience not only for nine months before the baby is born but for the next twenty or so years afterward.

We believe that parents should visualize a joyous natural birth and do everything they can during pregnancy and labor to make this come true. Such a vision has great significance, and researchers are beginning to find that there are things expectant parents can do to lessen the likelihood of a cesarean section. Nevertheless, we also believe that expectant parents should understand enough about the cesarean experience and the reasons for it so they can accept it and develop a positive attitude about it if it happens.

One of the fundamental characteristics of childbirth, as we have stressed, is that it is an experience an expectant mother and father cannot fully control no matter how much they prepare for it. But they can and should work to affect the outcome of delivery through their actions and their attitudes. Indeed, making the birth experience *positive* was the initial goal of the natural childbirth movement.

The aim of all birth education was and continues to be to make labor and delivery more *pleasurable* for the mother and *healthier* for the baby. To facilitate this, the mother is taught about the whole process of pregnancy and birth, so that she will not be afraid and can meet the many different circumstances of labor and delivery with relaxation, flexibility, and a sense of control.

Acknowledging the recent growing use of cesarean sections to

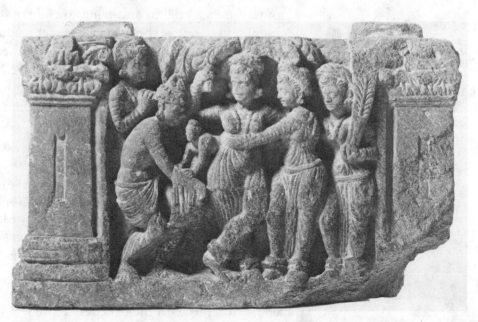

The image of a cesarean birth appears in ancient literature and mythology. Here Maya, surrounded by relatives, attendants, and gods, gives birth to the future Buddha through her right side. Birth of Buddha in the Lumbini Gardens, *Indian, second–third century. Asian Museum of Art, San Francisco. Avery Brundage Collection.*

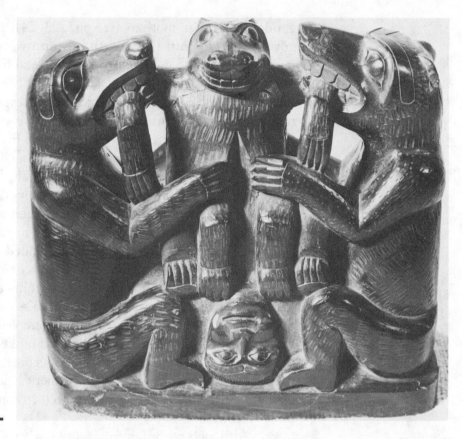

Among the Haida Eskimo, there is a legend that the Bear Mother gave birth to her child by cesarean section, assisted by two grizzly bears. Eskimo carving, 1875. Photograph courtesy of Museum of the American Indian, Heye Foundation.

deal with a variety of labor complications, prenatal classes are now including the study of cesarean birth, so that mothers and fathers can more easily and effectively deal with this experience if necessary. Our goal and the goal of most birth educators is to enable parents to emerge with an affirmative view of their baby's birth whether or not it was by cesarean. When this is achieved the mother feels better, heals faster, bonds more strongly with her baby, and undertakes the tasks of parenting with greater optimism.

The Rise in the Cesarean Birth Rate

Between 1970 and 1978 the United States c-section rate *tripled,* and it is still rising in most communities. In 1970 the average c-section rate was 5.5 percent; by 1978 the rate had reached 15 percent. Today many hospitals have rates of over 20 percent. These rates are fairly uniform throughout the United States. The figures for this country are by far the highest in the world, being higher than Canada, which is second with 13.9 percent, and well above the Netherlands, which has a rate of only 2.7 percent! It is important to note that the Netherlands also has the world's lowest infant mortality and maternal mortality rates. Unlike the United States, its obstetrical care focuses on preventive medicine, with a large number of prenatal visits and early identification of high-risk mothers (see pp. 223–24). Interestingly, its government supports home birth, maternity homes, and nonspecialized obstetrics with general practitioners and midwives doing the majority of the deliveries.

A number of complex social and medical factors have been responsible for the current increase in cesareans in the United States. During the 1960s there was a sharp decline in the birth rate as the use of birth control rose and couples chose to have smaller families. In some cases smaller family size may have been the result of economic necessity, which compelled the mother to work outside the home; in other cases smaller family size may have been a response to the growing desire of women to pursue careers and responsibilities outside. In any case, the decline in family size has tended to put increased emphasis on the health of each baby and the outcome of each pregnancy.

Also during the 1960s infant mortality statistics became recognized as an important measure of a nation's overall quality of health. Surprisingly, the United States did not fare well in comparison to many other Western nations; in fact, we ranked sixteenth in terms of the number of infant deaths per 1,000 recorded births. In an attempt to improve these figures, U.S. government health planners have encouraged the medical community to focus on improving infant mortality statistics.

Although our infant mortality statistics were poor, our technical surgical skills were excellent. Better anesthesia, improved blood transfusion techniques, and the introduction of antibiotics had made cesareans much easier and safer to perform than they were in the 1940s. Thus while a less technically advanced country would have had to concentrate on other means of lowering infant mortality, the United States turned increasingly to cesarean sections as a means of improving newborn health. This decision was supported by studies that had shown that long labors and mid- or high-forceps deliveries were associated with higher rates of cerebral palsy and brain damage. More recently, studies have shown that in the face of some complications, the baby's health and life expectancy were better with a cesarean delivery than a vaginal birth. These complications included premature babies weighing less than 1500 grams (3 pounds 5 ounces), and certain uncommon presentations, such as when the baby is transverse or brow or face first.

In an attempt to improve our overall infant mortality statistics, doctors began to do cesarean sections with premature deliveries instead of doing difficult forceps deliveries, and rather than allowing mother and baby to withstand a very long labor. With the 1970s came the advent of electronic fetal monitors, which were designed to detect early signs of fetal distress. As a result, a number of babies who probably would not previously have been identified as being in distress were diagnosed as such and were also delivered by c-section.

Moreover, until very recently it was believed that once a woman had a cesarean delivery, all her future deliveries would have to be by cesarean to prevent the uterine scar from rupturing due to the force of contractions. Thus all mothers who had a cesarean, regardless of the initial reason, automatically had a repeat cesarean on all subsequent births. As a result of all these factors, the number of cesarean deliveries in the United States and most other Western countries soared dramatically during the 1970s.

In addition to purely medical concerns, there are a group of medical-social factors that are difficult to evaluate accurately but that have probably contributed to the rise in number of c-sections. Doctors and sociologists who study the medical system point out that obstetricians today fear that if they deliver a baby who is not "perfect," they will be sued for malpractice. This concern causes them to practice medicine defensively, making certain decisions on the basis of statistical probabilities. To protect themselves they often elect to do a c-section if there is even the slightest possibility of problems with the birth. Such fears are not totally a figment of the doctors' imagination. Lawsuits have been brought against doctors for failing to do a cesarean and even for delaying one. Nevertheless, many critics feel that obstetricians concern themselves too much with the possibility of being sued, especially when there is a question as to whether cesarean section is the only reasonable alternative under the circumstances.

A significant but overlooked reason for the rise in cesareans has to do with medical education. In their residency programs most young obstetricians have been well trained at performing c-sections but have

Reasons for present cesarean rate

1. Dystocia or failure of labor to progress (31% of cesareans): pelvic opening too small for the baby; birth canal too small for the baby; contractions irregular or not intense enough to dilate the cervix.

2. Breech presentation (12% of cesareans): baby emerging feet first.

3. Repeat cesarean (31% of cesareans): mother has previously given birth by cesarean.

4. Fetal distress (5% of cesareans): baby is shown to have abnormal heartbeat pattern with fetal monitoring, and diagnosis is confirmed by fetal scalp blood pH testing.

5. Other (21% of cesareans): maternal illness such as diabetes or heart disease, active herpes, or medical emergencies such as placenta previa or prolapsed cord.

not been as well trained in alternative ways of dealing with certain difficult labor situations. Whereas midwives are traditionally skilled in supportive labor techniques and changing the mother's positions, doctors are generally better trained in surgical techniques and are much less likely to think in terms of nonsurgical solutions. Because medicine has become so complex, doctors often feel they must determine what is the "best" or "safest" procedure, rather than make a joint decision with the patient after carefully describing the situation and the options.

Indications for a Cesarean Section

Almost 80 percent of all cesareans done in this country are performed for one of four reasons: 31 percent are repeat cesareans; another 31 percent are due to *dystocia*, a broad category that includes all labors that fail to progress in a normal way; 12 percent are done because the baby is in a breech position; and 5 percent are performed because the baby is in fetal distress. These are also the categories in which there has been the greatest rise in c-sections since 1970.

The other 21 percent of cesareans are done for a variety of reasons, including maternal diabetes, maternal heart disease, maternal herpes, twins, Rh incompatibility, and medical emergencies such as placenta previa, abruptio placenta, and prolapsed cord. Each of these latter reasons is responsible for a very small percentage of the total number of c-sections. Among this group, maternal illness and medical emergencies have always been indications for cesarean. With the exception of twins and maternal herpes, the rates for these conditions are not rising.

Dystocia

Dystocia, or failure of labor to progress, is a broad and complex condition that can result from a number of factors that are sometimes interrelated. But one of three basic reasons is believed to underly most cases of dystocia. The first is an abnormality in the birth canal, such as an inadequately sized pelvis (see p. 226) or cervix, which makes it difficult or impossible for the mother to deliver vaginally. The problem of a woman's pelvis being inadequate to pass a *particular* baby is referred to as *cephalopelvic disproportion*. The second cause of dystocia is an unusual presentation of the baby, which makes labor difficult or dangerous. Such presentations include transverse, brow, and face presentation (see pp. 292–93). The third cause of dystocia is inadequate or irregular contractions, which prevent the mother from dilating fully in the first stage or prevent the baby from descending in the second stage although the mother has dilated.

The tremendous increase in the diagnosis of dystocia has largely resulted from a change in the way doctors manage *nonprogressing labors*. Twenty years ago a mother might have been allowed to labor for a much longer time, or the doctor might have delivered the baby from below with forceps. Today doctors tend to judge a woman's labor in comparison to average times established according to the *Friedman curves* (see p. 285). The slowest mothers on the curve are considered to be having abnormal labor, based on the fact that some studies have indicated that babies born after long labors are more likely to have neuro-behavioral problems.

Most mothers diagnosed as having dystocia give birth to babies weighing more than 2500 grams, or 5 pounds 8 ounces. The survival rates for these babies have not been shown to increase with cesarean rather than vaginal birth. And the National Institutes of Health (NIH) has stated that there is still insufficient data on whether the cesarean procedure improves the neurological development of dystocia babies, with the possible exception of those who encounter a prolonged second stage. NIH recommends that "in the absence of fetal distress, management of dysfunctional labor may include such measures as patient rest, hydration, ambulation, sedation, and the use of oxytocin, prior to considering cesarean birth."[1] The NIH report also states that there is a need to further examine this category of cesarean in light of the fact that it has *not* been shown to have survival or neurological advantage over vaginal birth.

Although a cesarean may ultimately be necessary to optimize the chances of having a healthy newborn, there are many alternatives during labor that can help to avoid a c-section due to dystocia. Based on their experience, a number of doctors and midwives feel that dystocias can often be converted into normal labors that end in vaginal birth. They suggest that a mother should be encouraged to walk and to assume other positions that are comfortable to her, rather than lying on her back. In addition, IVs and monitors should be avoided if possible, because they hamper a mother's movements and tend to make her uncomfortable. For many women the pressure to deliver by a specific time that falls within the range of "normal" statistics is a terrible burden. Thus in some labor situations helping a mother to sleep (preferably without the use of drugs) may renew her energy and cause strong, steady, effective contractions to be resumed.

In cases of dystocia it is very important to assuage the mother's fears as well as to make her as comfortable as possible. One of the main points we want to emphasize is that fear and tension interfere with contractions, while relaxation and support encourage labor to take place in an unhindered fashion. And we agree with a number of birth educators and researchers who feel that the constant presence of a supportive person or a labor coach (other than the woman's husband) tends to be most effective in reassuring a mother. In their

Guatemalan studies Marshall Klaus and John Kennell found lower c-section rates for mothers attended by a *doula,* a supportive, non-professional woman who remained with the mother continuously throughout labor (see p. 200).

Breech Presentation

Twelve percent of cesareans are done because of a breech presentation. The breech baby lies with head up and bottom down. Although this is a common position for babies at the end of the second trimester, it usually converts to head down sometime before labor begins, so that only 3 percent of all babies are in breech position at the beginning of labor.

There are actually three kinds of breech babies: 65 percent are *frank breech,* which means the baby's legs are bent at the hips, but the knees are straight, and the feet, in a yogalike way, touch the head; 25 percent are *footling* or *incomplete breech,* with one or both of the legs pointing straight down; and only 10 percent are a *full* or *complete breech,* in which the legs are bent at the hips and knees so that the baby assumes a cross-legged posture.

A vaginal breech delivery is more difficult for both mother and baby than if the baby presents headfirst. It is more dangerous for the baby for several reasons. With a breech presentation the head emerges last, so the baby is not able to begin breathing until the very end of the delivery, making it essential that the baby continue to receive oxygen through the umbilical cord. Sometimes, however, the cord becomes compressed while the torso and head are passing through the birth canal, thereby cutting down on the baby's oxygen supply. With a vaginal breech delivery the head doesn't gradually become molded but is abruptly molded with great force, which can be the cause of brain injury. Due to the lack of head molding, the baby's head almost never delivers spontaneously but must be drawn out with great care by the doctor or midwife.

Due to these risks the mortality rate for breech babies is 3.17 percent, as opposed to 0.84 percent for nonbreech babies. All studies show that smaller, more delicate breech babies fare much better with a cesarean delivery. And several studies have shown better survival rates and lower injury rates among all breech babies delivered by cesarean rather than vaginally. However, other studies, while agreeing with the higher injury rates, have not shown a higher mortality rate with vaginal delivery of babies over 5 pounds 8 ounces. Provided there are no other complications, babies in the frank breech position fare as well with a vaginal delivery as with a cesarean. Nevertheless, the studies have led doctors to increase dramatically the number of deliveries of all types of breech babies by cesarean section. As of 1978, 60 percent of all breech babies in this country were delivered by cesarean.

In reviewing all the breech studies, the National Institutes of Health Committee on Cesarean Section has noted that it is often difficult to assess the data because of other complicating factors, such as prematurity or placenta previa. They have stated that no definite conclusions can be drawn until breech births have been studied in more detail. But they do say that vaginal delivery remains an *acceptable* choice with a frank breech presentation if the baby is under 8 pounds, the mother has a normal-size pelvis, and the physician is experienced in breech deliveries. However, due to the potential problems that could arise with a vaginal delivery, they feel that the family should be intimately involved in making the decision.

Because of insufficient data, conflicting studies, and differences in training and experience, doctors and midwives handle various breech situations in different ways. Pregnant women whose baby is in a breech position near term should discuss the way in which their practitioner usually manages breech deliveries. After careful consideration, if they find they are not in agreement with the practitioner, they can seek out another doctor or midwife in the community who is known to deal differently with breech births.

Some doctors and midwives will attempt to turn a breech baby in utero during the last few weeks of pregnancy. Many midwives have the mother assume a tilted position with the feet elevated above the head for 20 minutes four times a day. The mother may also be advised to visualize the baby turning at the same time. More commonly, doctors and midwives will try to turn the baby manually. Placing hands on the mother's abdomen, the practitioner attempts to move the baby higher up in the uterus. Then, grasping the baby's head and rump externally, he or she attempts to rotate the baby slowly until its head faces the bottom of the uterus. The baby is held in this position for 5 minutes. The procedure is not difficult and does not cause the mother much discomfort. Most obstetricians currently perform the procedure in the hospital, using electronic fetal monitoring to make sure the baby is all right. The mother may be sedated and given an IV in case problems should arise. Not infrequently, however, the baby reverts to a breech position and must be turned a second time. Several studies have shown good results in lowering the breech rate with this technique, but other research has indicated that the procedure may cause complications such as beginning labor.

Repeat Cesarean

Due to the increasing number of c-sections done for dystocia and other reasons, repeat cesarean is now the second largest reason (31 percent) for the procedure. As of 1978, 98.9 percent of women who had had a previous c-section were delivered by cesarean with all subsequent births. This policy of repeat c-sections was based on a speech given in

1916 by Edwin Craigin, an eminent New York obstetrician. Ironically, in attempting to dissuade his colleagues from performing cesareans whenever possible, he observed, "The usual rule is, once a cesarean, always a cesarean."

When Craigin made this statement the cesarean rate was under 1 percent and the procedure carried significant risk. At that time the operation was of the *classical* type, that is, a vertical incision was made into the fundus, the upper part of the uterus. The modern operation, which is called a *low segment cesarean*, uses a transverse incision in the lower part of the uterus.

The dictum, *once a cesarean, always a cesarean,* has been one of the most pervasive concepts in obstetrics. It was based on the belief that the scar tissue from a cesarean was inelastic and weak and could rupture without warning during subsequent labors. This notion was supported by the fact that obstetricians had observed visible signs of scar weakness during repeat cesareans when mothers had first been allowed to experience labor. Also, as the operation became safer and easier to do, doctors elected to perform more and more repeat cesareans rather than face the possible consequences of a vaginal delivery following a cesarean. Despite the fact that there were very few studies on the actual risk for such mothers, obstetricians never questioned the dictum for years.

During the same period, however, there was a very small minority of responsible obstetricians in medical centers in Europe and the United States who routinely allowed some mothers to deliver vaginally after a c-section. Based on their work, studies questioning the repeat cesarean rule began to emerge in the 1950s. A landmark study by Dewhurst followed all vaginal deliveries of British mothers who had previously had a cesarean. Of the 2,292 women, 762 had had a classical incision, while 1,530 had had a low transverse incision. Among the classical group, 4.7 percent experienced rupture during labor; among the low transverse group, 1.2 percent experienced rupture during labor. Even more significantly, Dewhurst found that the results of a rupture varied with the type of incision. A rupture of a classical scar had a maternal mortality rate of 5 percent, whereas there was no mortality among women with rupture of a low transverse scar.

A recent review of most previous studies dealing with both types of incision found that out of 20,400 vaginal deliveries after cesarean, only 456 uterine defects (2.2 percent) occurred. There are actually two different types of *uterine defect* or rupture, one of them being much more serious than the other. In the first type, a *true rupture,* the uterine wall actually opens. In the second type there is a *bloodless separation of muscle fibers,* which is of no danger and requires no treatment. Ninety percent of low transverse ruptures are of the bloodless variety. In addition, 90 percent of all uterine ruptures occur in women with classical incisions.

By the 1970s it became clear that true uterine rupture was rare with either type of incision and that a life-threatening rupture after a transverse incision was unheard of. The largest single study, done by Shy in 1981, actually attempted to predict the outcome of 6,623 deliveries in which women gave birth vaginally after a previous low transverse cesarean. Based on all previous studies, Shy estimated that a vaginal delivery would be 1.2 times safer than a repeat c-section. He also predicted that infant mortality would be higher with a repeat c-section, because the mother is rarely allowed to begin labor spontaneously. Delivery is generally scheduled on the basis of the due date, and there is always a risk that the baby will be premature and experience complications due to lung immaturity.

The results of all these studies have led to the first significant change in the management of repeat cesareans since 1916. Increas-

Prerequisites for a safe vaginal birth after a previous cesarean (VBAC)

Common management guidelines
1. Parents have discussed all the pros and cons of a VBAC with their doctor.

2. The present pregnancy has no indications for recommending a cesarean section.

3. A low transverse incision was used in the previous cesarean section.

4. The mother is admitted to the hospital early in labor, so that her progress can be carefully monitored.

5. Backup facilities for an immediate cesarean section are available.

Controversial management guidelines
1. Some doctors will not permit a trial labor if the mother has previously had a cesarean section because of too small a pelvis.

2. Some doctors won't use drugs that stimulate labor if the mother has had a previous cesarean.

3. Some doctors don't recommend regional anesthesia during a vaginal delivery after a cesarean because they believe it could mask rupture problems.

4. Some doctors recommend the routine use of low forceps to shorten labor if the woman has previously had a cesarean.

ingly obstetricians are allowing carefully selected cesarean mothers to undergo a *trial labor* and to deliver vaginally provided there are no problems. Although doctors still vary greatly in how they manage this situation, certain guidelines are widely adhered to. Basically, the mother has to have had a previous low transverse incision and no present indications for a c-section. During labor the mother must be followed closely, and the hospital must be available and prepared to do a c-section should the need arise.

Other points remain in dispute. These include the routine use of electronic fetal monitoring, the possible use of oxytocin to stimulate contractions, and the use of forceps to shorten labor. Doctors also disagree about the number of vaginal deliveries that can be attempted after a cesarean as well as whether a vaginal delivery should ever be attempted if the cesarean was done because the baby's head was too large for the mother's pelvis (see p. 226).

Out of 3,000 cesarean mothers who were allowed a trial labor, 66 percent successfully gave birth vaginally. Of those women who had had a c-section for reasons other than cephalopelvic disproportion, 70 to 80 percent were successful in delivering vaginally. Although these figures reveal a dramatic shift in obstetrical policy, a number of doctors are still hesitant to attempt trial labor.

A mother who has had a cesarean but wishes to deliver a subsequent baby vaginally must find out the specific reason for her previous cesarean section and the type of incision that was used. She should also check to see whether her doctor feels positively about *vaginal births after a cesarean* (VBACs). If her doctor is not supportive of VBACs, she should seek another opinion from a doctor who is known to be. A mother is much more likely to have a successful VBAC if her doctor is enthusiastic about doing them. Thus even though a mother may have liked the doctor who did her c-section, she might consider switching doctors under these circumstances.

Fetal Distress as a Cause of Cesarean

The diagnosis of fetal distress is now responsible for 5 percent of all cesareans done in the United States and has been responsible for 15 percent of the increase in c-section rates since 1970. Fetal distress occurs either when the baby's oxygen supply is seriously impaired or when the baby is unable to get rid of carbon dioxide quickly enough. A baby in distress used to be very difficult to confirm during labor unless the amniotic fluid showed staining of meconium (early newborn stool) or a drop in the baby's heart rate was picked up during a routine fetoscope exam.

Fetal distress was much less frequently diagnosed before the introduction of electronic fetal monitors, which permit continuous supervision of the baby's heart rate and make it possible to pick up subtle changes whenever they occur. With the use of fetal scalp blood pH testing, the doctor can actually determine if the baby's blood is low on oxygen. These sophisticated techniques can be difficult to interpret and are still not totally accurate, however. As a result, babies are sometimes believed to be in fetal distress when they are not, and vice versa.

Whether fetal monitoring has been the cause of unnecessary c-sections and the tremendous rise in c-sections is one of the sharpest controversies in American obstetrics. A study by Banta for the National Center of Health Sciences Research found that being electronically monitored doubled a woman's chances of a c-section and was indeed a major factor in the rise of c-sections. Concern about this problem led the National Institutes of Health to set up a task force to study the relationship between monitoring and cesareans. NIH concluded that monitoring did contribute to a rise in c-section rates, commenting, however, that the studies were difficult to interpret and tended to be biased. Several recent studies have shown a decline in cesarean rates as medical personnel become used to analyzing monitoring data.

Many midwives and doctors feel that the reclining position that monitors generally force women to adopt during labor is detrimental to the progress of labor and naturally slows blood flow to the baby. Indeed, this fact is so well known that the initial response to an abnormal monitor tracing is to turn the mother on her side. Some doctors and midwives also believe that use of pain relievers, anesthetics, and/or oxytocin during labor increase the likelihood of a cesarean. They feel that these drugs change the rhythm and nature of contractions: oxytocin tends to intensify contractions and speed up their rhythm, pain relievers and anesthetics tend to slow contractions and *may* contribute to situations in which labor fails to progress (see p. 203).

Risks in Cesarean Delivery

Like any operation, a cesarean is not without risk, but the risks to mother and baby are actually very small. At present they are lower than they have ever been in history. The average mortality risk for the mother is only slightly higher for a cesarean than for a vaginal delivery: .08 percent as opposed to .03 percent. Although the mortality risk for a cesarean is approximately three times that of a vaginal delivery, the risk for either kind of delivery is extremely low. The Boston Hospital for Women did over 10,000 cesarean operations between 1968 and 1978 without a single maternal death. In the past the most significant risk in the cesarean procedure was the chance of serious complications resulting from general anesthesia. Since the mother can generally elect to have regional anesthesia, she can usually avoid that risk completely.

A number of medical complications are not uncommon after a cesarean. One study has shown that as many as one-third to one-half of all cesarean mothers have complications following the surgery. Twenty-five to 50 percent run a fever, and a bladder, lung, or wound infection is not infrequent. In fact, infections are frequent enough that some doctors routinely start mothers on broad-spectrum antibiotics before the operation. Other doctors prescribe medication only if an infection develops, since studies have not proved that precautionary antibiotics lower the rate of serious infection, and antibiotics do cross over to the baby in the mother's milk. Other postcesarean complications include incisional bleeding and *thrombophlebitis*, a condition in which blood clots develop in the veins of the legs. Such blood clots are largely avoided by early movement and walking.

Because of the slightly higher mortality rates as well as the increased incidence of complications, doctors do not decide to do a cesarean without medical indication. The benefits of the surgery must outweigh the risks to mother and baby. As with all surgery, the risks of a cesarean are much lower when it is performed by an experienced doctor, anesthesiologist, and medical center. High-risk mothers and mothers who expect to have a repeat cesarean do well to keep this in mind when choosing their obstetrician, in addition to considering the doctor's routines concerning family-centered care and bonding.

Planned and Unplanned Cesareans

From the point of view of timing, there are two kinds of cesareans: planned and unplanned. Planned c-sections are scheduled in advance because of known complications, including repeat cesareans, a proved small pelvis, certain persistent breech presentations, and maternal medical conditions, such as severe diabetes or active herpes lesions.

Unplanned c-sections are done because of unforeseen situations that arise during labor, such as fetal distress or, much more commonly, failure of labor to progress (dystocia). Generally the decision to do an unplanned c-section is made over a period of hours, during which the doctor carefully explains to the parents what is happening and what the alternatives are. If the mother is in the second stage of labor or the baby is in fetal distress, the decision will be made more quickly than if the mother is having inadequate contractions in the active part of the first stage of labor. In some instances a cesarean may not be the only acceptable way to manage the situation, at least initially, and the mother and father may be given some choice in what treatment is instituted.

Currently most childbirth classes include a description of the cesarean operation, the various anesthesias that may be used, and the recovery period. This is done to prepare women who will experience unplanned as well as planned cesareans and to inform them about the choices they will be able to make within the cesarean routine. Preparation has been found to lessen apprehension, facilitate more positive acceptance of the experience, and speed healing.

Determining Gestational Age in a Planned Cesarean

One of the topics that planned cesarean classes cover is the tests that are used to establish fetal maturity. It is important that a baby be full term when it's delivered by cesarean since premature infants often experience respiratory problems because their lungs do not make enough *surfactant*, a substance that keeps the lung tissue from sticking together (see p. 70). So when a cesarean is scheduled in advance, doctors try to ascertain the baby's gestational age as accurately as possible. These tests are not necessary if the mother is allowed to go into labor spontaneously before the cesarean is performed.

The American College of Obstetricians and the American Academy of Pediatrics have issued joint guidelines on determining fetal maturity. The safest, most reliable, and least expensive tests are the practitioner's record of hearing a heartbeat with a fetoscope for 20 weeks, or a period of 33 weeks elapsed since a positive pregnancy test. Another way of establishing age is by measuring the baby's *biparietal head diameter* with an ultrasound test done between 18 and 26 weeks of gestation. The test results are acceptable if the head size calculated corresponds within one week to the size as predicted by menstrual dates. Should there be some question, the test must be repeated by 30 weeks, but no sooner than 3 weeks after the previous test.

If the baby's gestational age has not been positively established by any of these means, the guidelines state that it is a "reasonable option" to allow the mother to go into labor naturally. Otherwise the guidelines recommend *amniocentesis* (see p. 238) late in pregnancy. This allows the doctor to determine the relative amounts of *lecithin* and *sphingomyelin*, chemicals that are secreted by the baby's lungs in about equal concentration until about 34 weeks, when lecithin secretion starts increasing. Delivery can safely be scheduled once there is twice as much lecithin as sphingomyelin in the amniotic fluid, because the baby has a low chance of developing respiratory distress syndrome by this point. A Harvard study done in 1980 showed that there was little to be gained by doing routine amniocentesis in women who were past 38 weeks, as estimated by ultrasound or the record of fetal heart-beat.

The Types of Cesarean Incision

Once a decision has been made to do a cesarean, the doctor will discuss with the mother the kind of incision and anesthesia that will be used. As mentioned, there are two basic types of uterine incision. By far the most common currently is the *low transverse incision,* which is made horizontally across the bottom of the uterus (see illustration). This incision results in the least bleeding, is the easiest to repair, and is least likely to separate or rupture later on. If a mother hopes to have a vaginal delivery in the future, it is absolutely the incision of choice.

The *classical incision,* in which the top of the uterus is cut vertically, is now rarely used except in a few uncommon situations. These include a large baby that is in transverse position with its shoulder down into the birth canal, and the placenta being attached near the bottom of the uterus (*placenta previa,* see p. 261). The classical incision may also be preferred in true emergencies in which time is a factor.

The *uterine* incision should not be confused with the *skin* incision. It is the uterine incision rather than the skin incision that is important in terms of future vaginal births. The most common skin incision is a vertical cut between the navel and the pubic bone. The length of the skin incision varies depending upon the size of the baby's head. The alternative is a transverse cut made just below the pubic

Currently the preferred cesarean skin incision is a transverse cut above the pubic bone; it is rapidly replacing the midline incision (a).
By far the most common uterine incision is the low transverse, which is a horizontal cut in the low segment of the uterus. It is the incision of choice if a mother hopes to have a vaginal delivery sometime in the future (b).

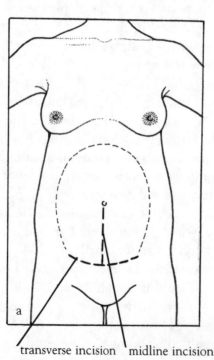

a

transverse incision   midline incision

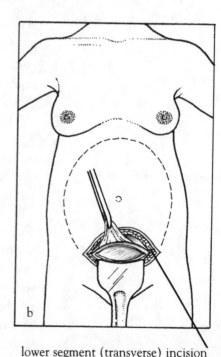

b

lower segment (transverse) incision

hairline. The transverse incision is both better-looking and stronger; the vertical incision is faster and easier to do, particularly in heavier women. Barring specific medical considerations, most doctors will attempt to make both incisions transverse.

The Anesthesia

Several types of anesthesia are commonly used in cesarean operations. First, there is an option of *general* or *regional* anesthetics. With general anesthesia, the mother is put to sleep so that she is unaware of what is happening. During the 1970s general anesthesia was used for 32 to 55 percent of cesarean deliveries in the United States. This figure is dropping, although general anesthesia is still used in certain emergency situations.

The general anesthesia routine begins with IV administration of an anesthetic agent like thiopental, followed by muscle relaxants. The anesthetized state is then maintained by a gas such as nitrous oxide or halothane, plus oxygen and additional muscle relaxants. General anesthesia is given at the last possible moment and is kept light until the baby is born to lessen the effects of the drugs on the baby.

In order to have general anesthesia, the mother must not have had anything to eat or drink for several hours beforehand, to lessen the chances of inhaling food from the stomach into her lungs. This occurrence, called *aspiration*, though very rare, is the most serious risk of the whole operation, but it can be avoided by skilled anesthesiologists. Other side effects of general anesthesia are dry mouth, irritated throat, occasional nausea, and a long period of grogginess after awaking. Of equal importance, the mother misses the delivery of the baby completely and is generally too groggy to bond well with the baby in the first hour after delivery (see pp. 467–79).

Regional anesthesia leaves the mother awake but anesthetizes her from approximately the waist down. Besides leaving the mother able to share in the birth of her baby and to bond with it immediately after delivery, regional anesthesias have other medical advantages. First, they carry no risk of aspiration and have little effect on the baby because they are confined to the mother's spinal canal. Also, since there is little crossover to the baby, the operation can be performed more slowly.

There are two basic types of regional anesthesia: the *spinal saddle block* and the *lumbar epidural*. Both involve the injection of a novocainelike anesthetic into an area of the lower spine. A spinal consists of a single injection between the lumbar vertebrae in the lower part of the spine (see illustration). The anesthetic is injected *into* the spinal fluid beneath the *dura* or surrounding membrane in sufficient quantity

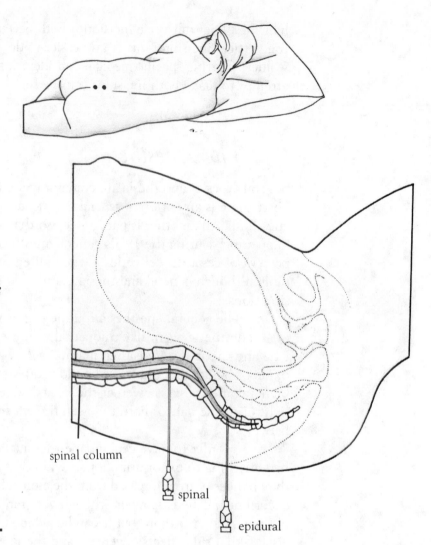

spinal column

spinal

epidural

Two regional anesthesias are commonly used for cesarean deliveries: the spinal saddle-block and the lumbar epidural. With a spinal, a single shot of anesthetic is injected into the spinal fluid. With an epidural, anesthetic is administered continuously into the space around the membrane surrounding the spinal fluid. The epidural has no time limitations and has less effect on the baby.

to numb the large spinal nerves up to the point where the ribs join the breastbone.

In an epidural the anesthetic is injected into the space *outside* the dura rather than into the spinal fluid. This method requires more anesthetic because the nerves are not affected as directly, but the needle can be replaced with a tube and then anesthetic given continuously. An epidural is somewhat more complicated to give than a spinal, but it can be better controlled and administered over a longer period of time; thus most obstetricians consider it the anesthesia of choice. Whereas a spinal produces numbness almost immediately, the epidural requires 15 to 20 minutes to take effect, but it ultimately produces numbness up to the same level as a spinal.

Statistically both types of regional anesthesia are very safe, their most serious risks being a drop in the mother's blood pressure and numbness above the rib cage, both of which are manageable. To avoid a drop in pressure the mother herself or her uterus is tilted slightly to the left to take pressure off the vena cava, just as is now suggested in labor (see p. 312). The mother is also given lots of fluids by IV and, if necessary, drugs to elevate her blood pressure. In the rare instance that the numbing sensations of the anesthesia rise above the mother's rib cage, she should report her sensations to the anesthesiologist. She will then be tilted off her vena cava and given supplementary oxygen to breathe. A spinal used to produce a three- or four-day postsurgical headache in many mothers, but this is much less common now because smaller needles are used. A post anesthesia headache rarely occurs with an epidural.

The first step in administering either general or regional anesthesia is to bring the mother into the delivery room and start an IV in her arm or the back of her hand. The IV helps to maintain her body fluid levels and provides a convenient way to give any drugs that might be necessary. A blood pressure cuff and electrodes for measuring her heartbeat will also be put on. If the mother is to be given general anesthesia, she will be given extra oxygen through a mask, and then the anesthetic will be given through the IV.

If the mother is to receive a spinal or an epidural, she will be helped to lie on her side, pulling her knees up to her chest and tucking her head down. This position opens the spaces between the vertebrae and makes it easier to give the injection. The anesthesiologist will paint the general area with an antiseptic and then probe to feel for just the right site. Usually the anesthesiologist will numb the skin with a small amount of local anesthetic that may sting, then give the actual injection. Most people describe it as feeling no more painful than a regular shot.

With a spinal the mother will rapidly feel tingling and a warm sensation spreading upward from her toes. With an epidural the feelings are the same, but they don't become noticeable for 15 to 20 minutes. In either case the mother will have difficulty moving her legs, because the anesthesia affects motor as well as sensory nerves.

The Operation

Before beginning the operation the doctor will make sure the mother's anesthesia has fully taken effect. Then the doctor will insert a narrow plastic tube called a *catheter* into her bladder to drain any urine, reducing the size of the bladder so that it does not interfere with a low transverse incision. The catheter is generally left in for 12 to 24 hours after the operation.

Next the mother will be washed and draped with sterile sheets. Her arms may be restrained or left free, depending upon the hospital. A low screen is generally put across the mother's chest. It blocks her view of her abdomen and prevents her from breathing on the incision but allows her to watch the doctor and see the baby as soon as it is delivered. In some centers, if the mother wishes, she can ask for a mirror or have the screen taken down so that she can actually see the operation.

If the father is allowed to be present during the birth, he will be seated near the mother at the head of the operating table and will be encouraged to talk to her and hold her hand. This is one of the most important recent trends in cesarean delivery and parallels that of vaginal deliveries almost twenty years ago. More and more, fathers are being brought into the operating room in many hospitals and made part of the process of cesarean birth. The psychological effect of the father's presence on the mother and the new family unit is now considered so important that the National Institutes of Health Committee on Cesarean Childbirth has made a recommendation that hospitals liberalize their policies concerning the option of having the father or someone else attend the cesarean birth.

Studies have shown that allowing fathers in the operating room, as well as not separating the father and baby from the mother afterward, greatly improves the family's response to the cesarean experience. It has also been found that when fathers are present at the cesarean, they have a much greater involvement with their babies. Traditionally doctors have viewed the fathers' presence in the operating room negatively, fearing they might faint or be in the way, but these concerns have not been borne out. Instead it has been found that fathers who participated in delivery had a much more positive attitude toward the birth experience than ones who didn't, and that the mothers had greater satisfaction, less loneliness, and more joy as a result of their husband's support.

Until the baby is born, the anesthesiologist may elect to give the mother extra oxygen through a mask or nasal tube. With a spinal or an epidural the mother will be completely awake during the delivery. She will feel no pain but will be aware of pressure, pulling, and pushing. After making the skin incision, the doctor will proceed to cut carefully through one layer of tissue after another, and the mother will hear the doctor asking for various surgical instruments and clamps to tie off blood vessels that have been cut.

After moving the bladder out of the way, the doctor will make an incision in the uterus and suction out the amniotic fluid. Next he or she will slip a hand under the baby's head and gently lift it out, immediately suctioning out the mouth and nose as in a vaginal birth. The doctor will then pull the baby the rest of the way out, holding it up for mother and father to see and announcing whether it is a boy or girl. As with a vaginal birth, this is a joyful moment, and the excitement and exhilaration are shared by everyone in the room.

As slowly and meticulously as the doctor works, the actual moment of birth comes only 5 to 10 minutes after the start of the

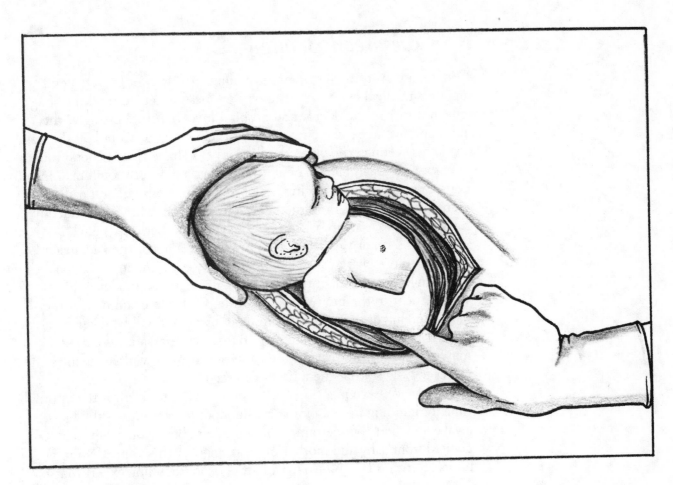

After making the uterine incision, the doctor slips a hand under the baby's head and gently lifts it out. As soon as its nose and mouth have been suctioned out, the baby is presented to the parents. As in a vaginal delivery, the moment the baby emerges is a joyful one.

operation. The rest of the operation takes about a half-hour or so. The doctor clamps the umbilical cord and gives the baby to a pediatrician. Meanwhile the mother will be given oxytocin in her IV line so as to stimulate uterine contractions, which will cause the placenta to separate from the uterine wall. In addition, the doctor will gently massage the uterus. Once the placenta has been removed, the doctor will wipe out the abdomen and thoroughly inspect the uterus. Then the doctor will carefully align and suture the various layers of tissue. If the mother becomes aware of discomfort as opposed to pressure at any point, she should ask the anesthesiologist for additional medication to help her to relax but not sleep.

Once the incision has been closed, the mother will be taken to a recovery room, where she will rest and be closely monitored by the recovery room nurses. They will check her blood pressure, pulse, and IV, as well as make sure that she is passing urine and that her uterus is clamping down. As in a vaginal delivery, her uterus will be massaged if it feels soft. If the mother has had a spinal or an epidural, massaging will not feel uncomfortable for an hour or two, but if the mother has had general anesthesia, she will need pain medication before her uterus can be massaged.

Cesarean Bonding

What happens to the cesarean baby immediately after birth depends upon its medical condition, the type of anesthesia used, and the specific routines of the doctor and hospital involved. Interestingly, the mother may have some choice in what happens, particularly if she has made her feelings known to the doctor beforehand. The general routine for a cesarean baby is one of the things a mother should take into consideration when choosing her obstetrician, hospital, and pediatrician. Obviously it is of most concern to a woman who is scheduled to have a repeat cesarean or who is a high-risk mother (see p. 252).

As soon as the baby's cord has been clamped, the pediatrician will make an Apgar evaluation of the baby, checking its color, pulse, breathing, and movement. Often the baby is placed in a clear plastic warmer next to the mother's head while it is being examined. If the baby is premature or is possibly in fetal distress, it will be taken to an intensive care nursery if necessary. But if the cesarean was done for maternal considerations and the baby is healthy, it will be given to the father to hold so that the mother can see it.

As we have mentioned, the hour right after birth is the optimal time for bonding from a biological standpoint. Not only is the baby awake and alert, but certain profound innate behaviors seem to be elicited from baby and mother more strongly at this point than in the hours afterward (see p. 467). Pediatrician and bonding expert Marshall

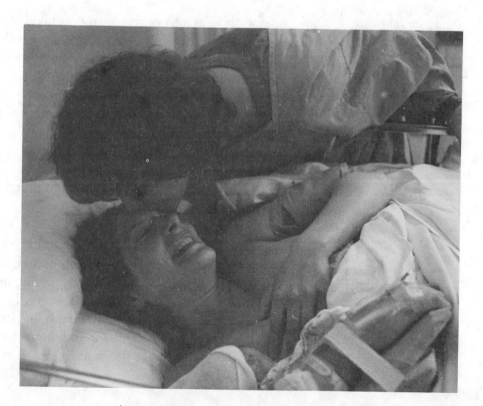

Like a mother who's had a vaginal delivery, a mother who's had a cesarean feels mingled emotions of joy and relief that her baby is healthy.

Patient choices suggested by cesarean support groups

- Allow the mother to forego any preoperative medication.
- Allow the mother to choose regional anesthesia so she can see the baby being born.
- Use epidural anesthesia if a qualified anesthesiologist is attending.
- Use a low transverse skin incision whenever possible for cosmetic reasons.
- Use a low transverse uterine incision to make subsequent vaginal births possible.
- Allow the father to remain with the mother in the delivery room.
- Allow the mother to have her arms free.
- Allow the mother to view the birth without a screen or with a mirror.
- Encourage the doctor to talk reassuringly with the parents during the operation.
- Allow the mother, if possible, or the father to hold the baby immediately after the birth.
- Have the initial routine pediatric exam done where the parents can watch.
- Delay weighing, measuring, and eyedrops until after the initial bonding period.
- Allow the mother, father, and baby to remain together in the recovery room during first hour after birth.
- Allow the mother to nurse the baby as soon as the operation has been completed.
- Allow the mother to have full rooming in as soon as she wishes.
- Allow the mother to have a helper such as her husband or a friend to assist her in caring for the baby.
- Allow siblings to visit the mother and baby daily.
- With repeat cesareans, have preliminary laboratory tests done on an outpatient basis so the mother does not have to be admitted until the day of the surgery.

Klaus has commented, "The power of this attachment is so great that it enables the mother and father to make the unusual sacrifices necessary for the care of their infant day after day, night after night. . . ."[2] Obviously a mother's first moments with her baby are just as important whether the delivery is cesarean or vaginal.

Unfortunately, during the last forty years mother-infant bonding has been seriously interrupted by some of the hospital procedures associated with both vaginal and cesarean deliveries. Typically, newborns have been quickly taken away to the nursery, often before their mothers have really even had a chance to look at them. This routine has changed with respect to vaginal deliveries in recent years. Now it is changing in relation to cesarean deliveries as well, since doctors, medical centers, and expectant parents have become more aware of the importance of the bonding process.

Cesarean bonding routines currently vary tremendously from center to center and doctor to doctor. Based on his research, Marshall Klaus recommends that the cesarean mother be given regional anesthesia and that the father hold the baby next to the mother right after birth. In addition, he advises that mother, father, and baby be moved to a small labor room once the operation is over and the baby be placed next to the mother's chest for at least 15 to 20 minutes and if possible as long as 60 minutes. During this time the mother's pulse, respiration, and uterus should be checked every 10 to 15 minutes, as they would be in the recovery room. If it is naked, the baby should be warmed with a heat panel, but the administration of silver nitrate drops or erythromycin ointment should be delayed for an hour or so because they interfere with the baby's ability to gaze at its mother.

Margaret Spaulding, a family-centered-cesarean advocate, likewise feels that it is crucial to do everything possible to facilitate bonding in the recovery room despite the obvious drawbacks of the IV, catheter, blood-pressure cuff, and drugs. She suggests that the mother should be helped to hold the baby next to her skin right after the delivery and again in the recovery room. If a spinal or epidural was used for the cesarean, the first hour is especially favorable for bonding because the anesthesia has still not worn off and the mother will not yet feel much discomfort around her incision.

Cesarean Recuperation

Once the cesarean mother has been moved from the recovery room to her hospital room, she has the same choices as a noncesarean mother about whether to have the baby room in with her or stay in the nursery except for feedings. But unlike a mother who has had a vaginal delivery, a mother who has had a cesarean is recuperating from abdominal surgery. Despite the remarkable changes in cesarean procedure over the last few years, the fact that it involves major surgery cannot be minimized. It is essential that both mother and father understand this and refrain from placing unrealistic expectations on the mother during the first week.

In addition to the nurses' care, the mother will need all the help, support, and encouragement that the father can give her. This includes seeing that he or some close friend is with her almost con-

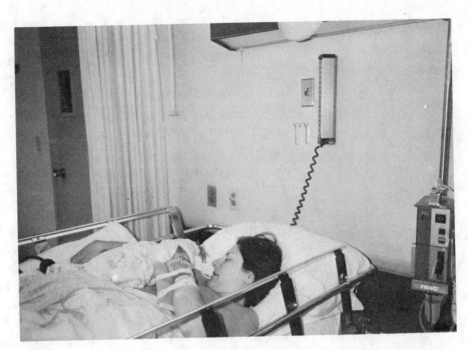

stantly during the first several days. Not all cesarean mothers feel strongly about this, but many do, and sometimes they may not be in an emotional or physical state to make this need clearly known.

Like anyone who has had abdominal surgery, cesarean mothers have a certain amount of postoperative pain, which varies with the ease or difficulty of their labor as well as with their pain tolerance. Once the regional anesthetic has worn off 1 to 3 hours after surgery, the mother will find herself absorbed with the sensations of her own body, and comfort will be one of her primary postpartum concerns. Pain medication is always prescribed after a cesarean, and most mothers find they want it for a day or two. As with any abdominal surgery, the pain tends to be worst for the first day or so, then improves rapidly thereafter.

A mother may experience three types of discomfort: pain around the incision; pain in the uterus, which is accentuated by the oxytocin given to make the uterus clamp down; and pain under the shoulder blades, which can be caused by air being trapped under the diaphragm during the operation. Like mothers who have had vaginal births, cesarean mothers will often notice uterine cramping during nursing, because there is a natural release of oxytocin with the let-down reflex. This discomfort is likely to be more noticeable with second and third babies because the mother's uterus tends to be more stretched and therefore does not shrink back as quickly (see p. 419).

For the cesarean mother taking pain medication is a tradeoff. On one hand, it makes her more comfortable and enables her to move, cough shallowly, nurse, and deal with the baby more easily. In this sense it can help a mother relate to her newborn and her husband in a less distracted manner. On the other hand, too much pain medication can make the mother unresponsive or sleepy and diminish her comunications with the baby and her husband. Margaret Spaulding suggests that the cesarean mother's postpartum pain medicines be carefully measured and timed so as to enhance her interactions with the baby. The goal is to have the mother as alert as possible but still comfortable when the baby needs to nurse or is simply awake and receptive.

In addition to making the mother less alert, pain medication is problematic because it delays the return of normal bladder and bowel function, which usually happens within 24 to 48 hours after surgery. The mother cannot have her IV removed or begin to drink liquids and eat solid foods until she passes gas or has bowel sounds that can be heard with a stethoscope. Both these signs indicate that *peristalsis* or movement has begun again in the digestive system and that the intestines can once more process food.

Many cesarean mothers consider gas cramps to be the most uncomfortable part of their recuperation. Gas cramps tend to peak around the time that normal bowel signs return. They can be lessened and possibly prevented by keeping pain medication to a minimum and by doing postoperative exercises (see following). In particular, the mother can knead her belly while lying on her left side with her knees drawn up. If these measures are not sufficient, the doctor may prescribe rectal suppositories, a small enema, or a rectal tube that will allow the gas to pass.

The mother's urinary catheter is usually removed after 12 to 24 hours, but if the mother continues to require a lot of pain medication and is unable to move about much, she may still have poor bladder tone. Subsequent difficulty in urinating can be a problem for cesarean mothers, just as it occasionally can be for mothers who have had vaginal births. Before a mother is recatheterized there are several remedies that can be tried, such as running water in the mother's hearing or pouring water over the vulva (see p. 421).

Postcesarean Exercise

In the past several decades doctors have become aware that early ambulation after surgery speeds a person's recovery. Walking or simply moving the legs promotes circulation to all parts of the body, which in turn increases wound healing, stimulates bladder tone, and encourages the resumption of peristalsis in the intestines. Early ambulation also lessens the chances of the mother developing postsurgical complications. By stimulating circulation and causing the leg muscles to contract and squeeze blood out of the veins, it makes it unlikely that a mother will develop *thrombophlebitis*, a condition in which blood clots form in the legs. And by encouraging the mother to breathe deeply, it lowers the chances of her developing pneumonia.

While a cesarean mother may accept the value of movement intellectually, she is often uncomfortable enough initially that walking is the last thing she wants to attempt. Nonetheless, the doctor generally leaves orders for her to be gotten out of bed once or twice on the first day, and walked to the bathroom on the second day. Although this may seem superhuman to the mother, with preliminary exercises and the support and encouragement of the nurses, early walking is possible although admittedly somewhat painful at first.

It's important for a mother to realize that moving activities will be uncomfortable *whenever* she first attempts them, but the sooner she accomplishes them, the sooner she will feel better. In fact, the longer the mother waits to walk, the stiffer she will feel and the more painful moving will be. She can be reassured that moving will not affect her stitches. However, for the sake of comfort, during the exercises she can press her hand or a pillow against her incision to support it. Discomfort on first moving can be minimized further by timing it to coincide with the peak of the mother's pain medications. Finally, good nursing techniques and cheerful, firm encouragement from the father will be of great help to the mother.

The current recommendation is for the mother to begin her exercises in the recovery room as soon as the anesthetic begins to wear off. Elizabeth Noble, the well known exercise physiotherapist, suggests a series of exercises for the cesarean mother. First, she recommends that the mother practice *deep abdominal breathing* (see p. 103) to strengthen her abdominal muscles and get air deep into her lungs (see following). Often cesarean mothers have a tendency not to breathe deeply because it can lead to coughing, which hurts after abdominal surgery.

The second exercise Noble and others recommend is called *huffing,* which is a strong exhalation just short of coughing. It consists of quickly and forcefully expelling air from the lungs by contracting the abdominal muscles and pushing upward with the diaphragm. Unlike coughing, huffing doesn't involve shutting the back of the throat, so abdominal pressure doesn't build up as much and it's not as uncomfortable. Huffing is important after a regional anesthetic, but it's *essential* after a general anesthetic because it brings up mucus that has accumulated in the mother's lungs during surgery. In addition to being told to practice huffing, the mother may also be visited by a respiratory therapist who has various machines and devices designed to promote deep breathing and raise excess mucus. Often the equipment has a little ball that graphically demonstrates just how much air the mother is moving with each breath.

Noble suggests that the mother begin doing foot and leg movements next. She can do these with her legs stretched straight out, but it may be more comfortable initially with her knees bent slightly over a pillow. Using either position, the mother wiggles her toes and makes circles with her feet, bending them at the ankle (see pp. 104–07). In a separate exercise she repeatedly tenses the muscles in her thighs and buttocks.

The following exercise is designed to bridge the gap between lying in bed and walking. Noble has the mother lie on her back with one knee bent and the other knee straight, then alternately slide the bent leg down and the straight leg up. In effect, the mother goes through the motions of walking while lying down. All these exercises should be done frequently in the first few hours after the operation. The father can help the mother greatly by encouraging her to do them and helping her to change her position fairly often once she is out of the recovery room.

For most cesarean mothers, it is a challenge to get out of bed the first time. When people get up following major surgery, they often feel weak and dizzy, an effect that is called *postural hypotension.* It is caused by the fact that after lying down for many hours, the body generally becomes less efficient at maintaining blood pressure in the brain. Before the mother attempts to stand, it may be helpful to have her lie with the head of the bed raised for a few minutes.

A nurse should assist the mother in standing and walking the first time and explain to both parents what to do on subsequent walks. The mother's first attempt to stand or at least dangle her feet off the edge of the bed should generally be made 6 to 12 hours after surgery. Usually the nurse will have the mother bend her knees and turn toward the side of the bed while sliding her feet over to the edge. In this position the mother can support her incision while pushing herself up with her lower arm and sliding her feet off the edge of the bed at the same time. There is no need to hurry once she is up. Sitting for a minute or two in this position may make the mother less dizzy as she stands.

When she is ready to get off the bed, the mother should signal

To speed her recovery from anesthesia and prepare for getting up and walking, the cesarean mother should alternately raise one knee and then the other. Although she may find this exercise somewhat uncomfortable, it will facilitate her recuperation.

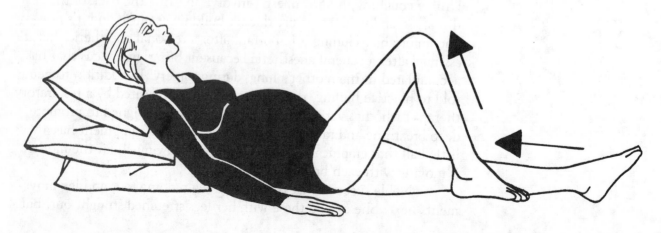

the nurse and the father so that they can support her as she slides her feet down and begins to put weight on them. The mother should stiffen or brace her thighs and abdomen to steady herself. If she pushes herself into a fully upright position, she will find that her abdominal muscles will support the incision and she will be able to take her hand away. If she tends to hunch over and lean forward, she will probably feel that she still needs to support the incision with her hand. Often walking proves to be easier than getting out of bed. The more the mother moves around in the days after her delivery, the better she will tend to feel.

The first few times the mother sits, stands, and walks, she will need support from the nurse or her husband, as well as help to handle her IV pole and urinary bag. These things are a nuisance, but the mother shouldn't let them bother her. The sooner she's up and moving, the sooner the IV and catheter are removed. The mother may notice that when she stands she feels a rush of fluid from her vagina. This discharge is the *lochia,* the same fluid and cells that are sloughed off by the uterus after a vaginal birth (see p. 408). The mother will have been given a belt and pad to absorb the lochia following the operation.

Feelings About Cesarean Delivery

Researchers are becoming increasingly knowledgeable about the emotional effects of a cesarean delivery. A majority of cesarean mothers have strong feelings of disappointment about the birth of their baby. Many circumstances contribute to this feeling. Although the number of cesareans is strongly on the rise, more and more mothers are attending birthing classes that prepare them for a natural vaginal delivery and an immediate period of bonding with their baby. Thus when mothers are confronted with the technical aspects of obstetrics in a cesarean delivery, they often have deeply ambivalent feelings about the experience. Like all mothers, those who've had a cesarean usually feel an enormous sense of relief that their baby is healthy and that they are all right. But feelings of grief, disappointment, and failure at not having a vaginal birth often march alongside these feelings of relief. In addition, there are often feelings of anger and lingering questions as to whether the cesarean was really necessary.

Until very recently cesarean mothers were likely to think they were the only ones who had such feelings. However, studies have shown that many of these feelings are not only shared by other cesarean mothers but to some extent by some mothers who have had vaginal deliveries. In several large studies dealing with mothers' attitudes toward their birth experiences, researchers have found that the most important factor contributing to a positive perception of delivery is the mothers' *sense of control*, the feeling that they participated actively in the decisions that were made and that they were not merely a passive object of care. Thus mothers who have vaginal deliveries in which they receive unexpected, unexplained, or impersonal care may also have feelings of disappointment and dissatisfaction with the birth of their baby. It appears that anytime a woman is forced into a passive, helpless, sick role, she feels a lowered sense of self-esteem. In particular, women who are given significant amounts of drugs (especially general anesthesia) or who are separated from their baby soon after birth often feel that they have been cheated or failed and have questions about their ability to mother.

Research has shown that whenever a birth, either vaginal or cesarean, causes a mother to doubt herself, she is likely to carry this over to her feelings about the baby and her ability to care for it. Studies of postpartum depression indicate that all mothers experience some degree of physical loss and grieving after the birth of their baby. Women often say they miss having the baby inside them because it seemed almost a part of them. Some women also feel keenly that with delivery the focus of attention shifts completely from them to the baby.

The realities of caring for a newborn who must be fed, soothed, and attended to almost constantly are very different from those of

Feelings reported by mothers after cesarean and vaginal births

FEELING	PERCENTAGE OF WOMEN DESCRIBING FEELINGS FOLLOWING	
	CESAREAN BIRTHS	VAGINAL BIRTHS
Sadness	15	0
Anger, resentment	35	6
Fear, worry, anxiety	75	31
Failure or inadequacy	25	6
Pain	50	69
Powerlessness, loss of control	70	25
Abandonment	10	6
Shock, traumatic experience	40	13
Depression, defeat	40	13
Blaming others	30	0
Disappointment	60	13
Fatigue	25	25
Decreased self-esteem	55	0
Crying	15	0

Source: Adapted from Kehoe, C., *The Cesarean Experience* (New York: Appleton-Century-Crofts), 1981, p. 196.

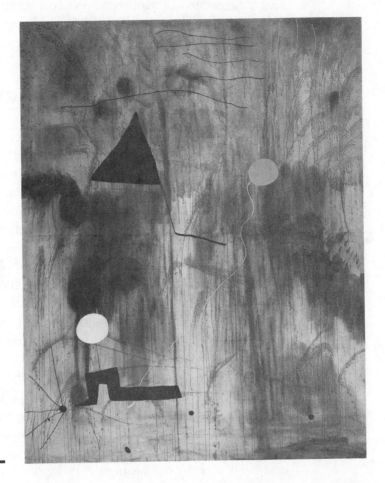

In a cesarean delivery, just as in a vaginal delivery, the moment of birth is the beginning of a new world for mother, father, and baby. Birth of the World, *Joan Miro, 1925. Oil on canvas, 8' 2¾" x 6' 6¾". Collection, The Museum of Modern Art, New York.*

pregnancy. The adjustment can be particularly difficult for a first-time mother who remembers with longing her previous days of freedom (see p. 438). But it appears that among vaginal-delivery mothers, such emotional disappointment has probably lessened somewhat over the last twenty years as the vaginal birth process has been increasingly humanized and mother-infant bonding has been facilitated.

The existence of family-centered cesarean programs with a growing emphasis on bonding is an indication that an enlightened view of cesarean birth is beginning to spread. But no matter how much the cesarean procedure is humanized, several factors remain unalterable. First, cesarean mothers have to experience and recover from major surgery in the midst of becoming a mother. Second, the feelings that a mother brings away from a cesarean depend to a great extent on those she took into the experience, not just on the way the birth was handled.

Studies indicate that cesarean-delivery mothers have a less positive perception of their birth experience than do vaginal-delivery mothers. Following a cesarean delivery, mothers were found to have lowered self-esteem, loss of feelings of femininity, feelings of powerlessness, jealousy of women who've had vaginal deliveries, and difficulty in feeling close to the baby. In addition, all studies of cesarean mothers have reported symptoms indicative of loss and grieving far in excess of those generally reported by vaginal mothers. These feelings include a sense of failure, anger, depression, fear, guilt, pain, self-blame, shame, sadness, fatigue, feeling abnormal, withdrawal, defeat, a tendency to blame others, shock and disbelief, bitterness, abandonment, loneliness, disinterest in one's environment, and helplessness. We include this long list because it is important that cesarean mothers realize that they are not unique or unusual in their feelings. In this regard, it is interesting to note that emergency cesareans engender greater feelings of loss than planned cesareans, with those mothers experiencing greater anger, depression, and need to relive their feelings.

Whether a cesarean is planned or unplanned, the procedure itself is virtually the same. But a mother is likely to feel quite differently about a planned c-section, especially if she has had a previous cesarean delivery. For this reason childbirth educators often hold special classes to help parents deal with the feelings aroused by a planned cesarean and explain what will happen.

The prospect of a repeat cesarean often arouses anxiety about surgery as well as anger and guilt over not being able to deliver vaginally. Like most surgical procedures, cesareans evoke fears of anesthesia, pain, and death. Mothers are frequently concerned with how the anesthesia is given and what they will see and feel. These fears are best dealt with by explaining the procedure in detail to the mother and by answering all her questions, no matter how trivial or irrational they are.

In addition to having the usual concerns about surgery, women who were disappointed over a previous cesarean are likely to find all their earlier unresolved feelings about not having a vaginal birth will

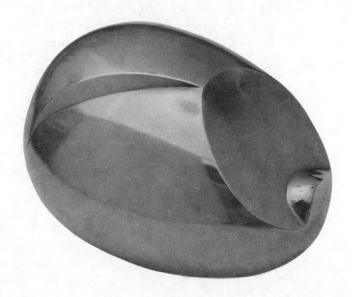

Cesarean babies can look especially beautiful at birth because their heads have not been molded by the birth canal. The Newborn, *Version I, Constantin Brancusi, 1915. Bronze, 5¾" x 8¼". Collection, The Museum of Modern Art, New York. Acquired through the Lillie P. Bliss Bequest.*

reoccur. Such feelings are quite common and are extremely important to deal with. A mother's negative feelings are related to how much education and support she received the previous time, the type of care she had, and how much she counted on a natural delivery.

The more a mother can talk out her feelings with her partner, friends, or other women who have had c-sections, the more likely she will be to deal positively with the upcoming delivery and recovery period. Mothers will find that relaxation and visualization exercises are invaluable, both in terms of getting in touch with old feelings and deliberately creating positive ones about the upcoming delivery (see p. 166).

The Value of Support for Cesarean Mothers

Birth educators, doctors, and nurses find that cesarean-delivery mothers benefit tremendously from help, support, and reassurance. Cesarean mothers need to be with people who can accept and assist them in expressing their feelings. This includes the father, close friends, and understanding medical personnel. Still, it is unlikely that the mother's feelings will be resolved by the time she leaves the hospital. Thus birth educators now recognize a real need for *cesarean support groups,* in which mothers and fathers can talk about their feelings, share their experiences, and come to terms with the delivery. The final goal of the process is for the mother to be able to talk freely and comfortably about the good and bad aspects of the experience and to feel good about herself as a person and a mother.

It's important to reiterate here that the key to increasing the likelihood of a positive cesarean experience is to include the mother in the decision-making process. Factors that tend to enhance a mother's sense of control are regional anesthesia, lack of arm restraints, presence of the father at the delivery, and having a means of viewing the birth. After the actual delivery, the most significant factors are not being separated from the baby or father during the recovery period and having unlimited rooming in during the hospital stay, the option to breast-feed, enough privacy to talk and cry openly, and a roommate (in a semi-private room) who has shared the experience of a cesarean.

Due to the experience of surgery and the normal feelings of grief and adjustment, the cesarean mother needs a great deal of help and support *after* she leaves the hospital as well as before. The support is not unlike that needed by a mother who has had a vaginal delivery, but it is more extensive and essential. In particular, a cesarean-delivery mother needs more rest and physical help. Bending and lifting are difficult for her, and stair climbing will be exhausting for a week or two.

Effects of the Cesarean Experience on the Baby

While it is known that the cesarean experience has profound effects on the mother, not much is known about how the procedure affects the baby because little research has been done in this area. A small but interesting study that evaluated babies on their second day using the Brazelton Newborn Exam showed that cesarean babies were more mature in motor development, had stronger defensive behavior, and less need to be consoled, whereas vaginal babies were more alert, more responsive to visual and auditory stimuli, and more prone to self-quieting. However, this study did not take into account the effect of drugs the mothers had been given.

According to recent studies, the new regional anesthesias and even the general anesthesias used today have much less effect on the baby than did those that were used ten or fifteen years ago. In fact, several large studies have shown that the regional anesthesias, especially the epidural, have *no* measurable effect on the baby, which should be very interesting to concerned cesarean parents.

What *does* affect cesarean babies, and even certain vaginal babies, is the pain medication given to the mother during labor and the postoperative period. Depending on the dosages and timing of medication, the cesarean baby is likely to be sleepy for as long as several days after birth. If pain medication was given early in labor, it may have worn off by the time of delivery, but if the mother has medication late in labor, the baby will probably still be affected by it during the bonding period immediately following birth.

Almost no research has been done on how cesarean birth affects the subtle and complex nature of bonding. It is known from experience with vaginal births that bonding is enhanced by *entrainment*, the process by which mother and baby react to one another, exchanging small gestures and eye movements. Obviously, if the baby or the mother is sleepy or distracted, the intensity of this time is diminished. It is therefore likely that many cesarean mothers have some trouble bonding due to the fact that either they or the baby are not fully alert.

Pain medication interferes with breast-feeding during the first few days, causing the baby to be too sleepy to get on the nipple and suck adequately. The mother's nursing efforts may also be hampered if medication makes her too groggy or fuzzy to do her part in the process. For this reason she may need extra help from the father and/or the nurses. But occasionally pain medication may lower the mother's anxiety about nursing, thereby indirectly facilitating her early endeavors.

Pain medication the mother takes after delivery reaches the baby through her milk. The exact amount that the baby gets will depend upon how much medication the mother receives and the amount of time that elapses between the mother getting her medication and nursing. During the first several days most cesarean babies get some pain medication through the milk because the mother is generally too uncomfortable to nurse without it. The baby will get the *lowest* amount if it nurses either right after the mother receives medication or several hours later, when the medication is beginning to wear off. Medication reaches the milk in highest concentrations about an hour after a pain shot. It's important for the parents to be aware of these facts, not to make them feel guilty if problems arise but to enable both the mother and the father to accept and work with the situation rather than to assign blame or become upset.

Studies following cesarean babies at six months and at one year show no difference in infant development but a striking difference in the family structure. Cesarean fathers were uniformly found to be much more responsive to their babies' signals, spent more time with them, and engaged in more caregiving activities than did fathers of babies who were delivered vaginally. Researchers speculate that this is due to the greater amount of time the fathers spent with the babies in the first days after delivery, while the mothers were coping with their surgical recovery. It would appear that the fathers also felt some of the effects of early intimacy that the mothers were less able to share in.

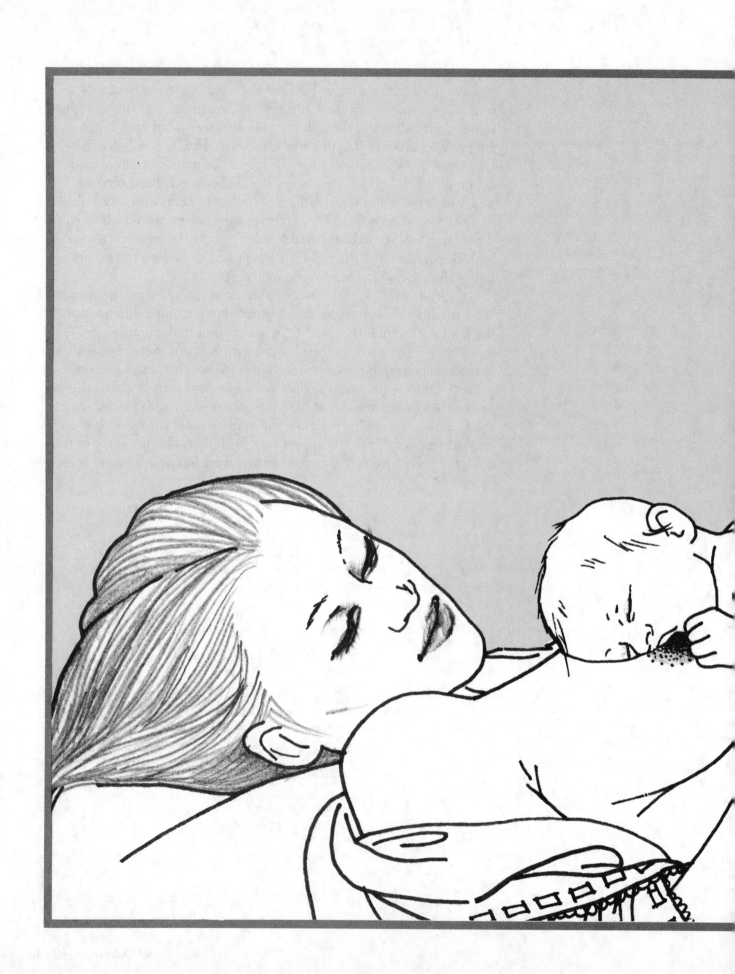

SECTION
IV

*After
the Baby
Is Born*

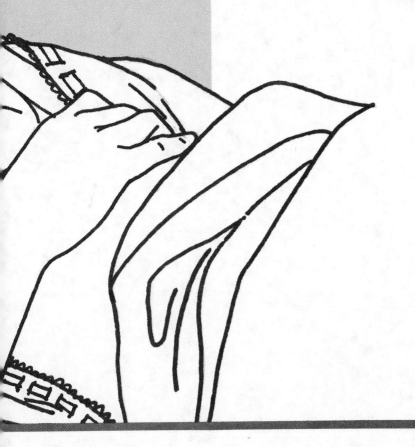

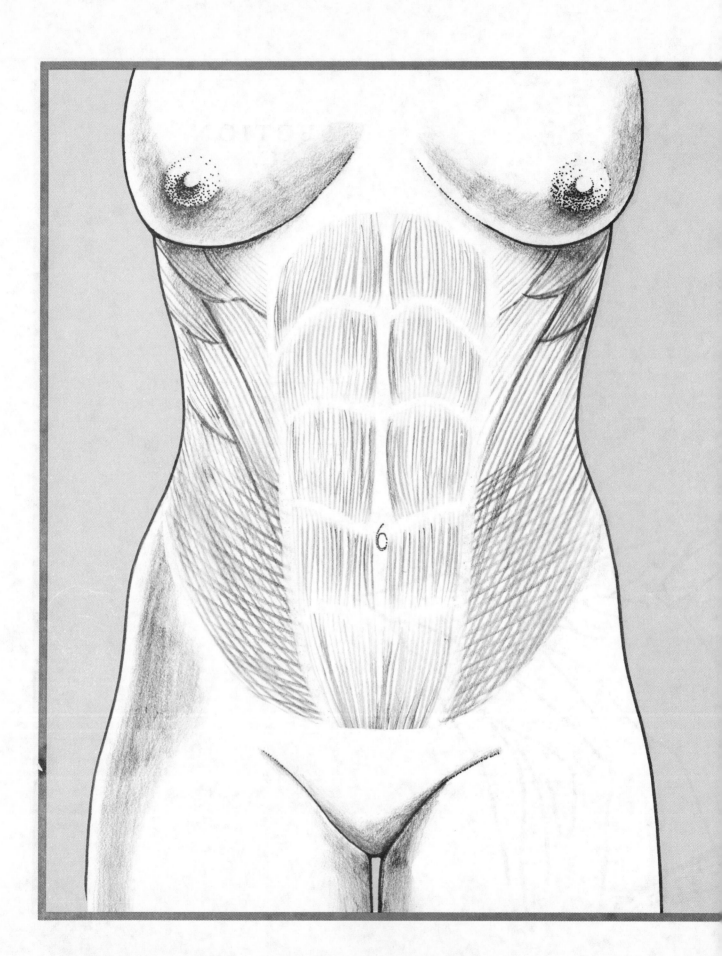

The Mother's Physiology after Childbirth

Returning to the Nonpregnant State

The first weeks after birth are a time of tremendous changes. Suddenly there is a newborn to play with and care for, and many skills to be learned. The baby's daily growth and development take up much of the parents' time and attention. Other than noticing the mother's dramatic change in shape, little thought is generally given to the fact that the mother is no longer pregnant. However, many far-reaching changes are taking place within her body that go unnoticed because they aren't readily visible.

Just as a remarkable series of physiological changes occurred during pregnancy to nurture the baby within the uterus, another series now takes place as the mother's body returns to a nonpregnant state. This process happens gradually over a period of about six weeks and is called the *puerperium*. During this time the remarkable bodily changes associated with nursing occur as well. Many body sensations and even mood changes experienced by the mother in the weeks after the birth are the result of the momentous alterations going on within her body. Understanding the nature of these changes can be both reassuring and useful, helping the mother *and* father adapt to their new roles.

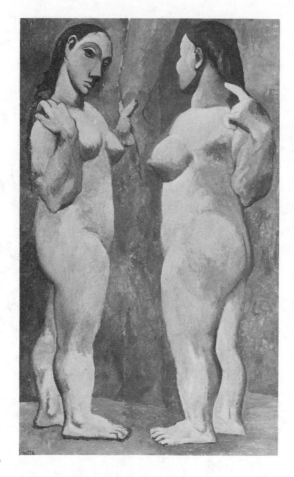

Loss of Weight after Delivery

The most obvious change for new mothers involves their size and weight. The flatness of their stomach directly after birth is stunning in some women, especially first-time mothers; others are dismayed to find that although they are much lighter, they may still appear almost pregnant. Immediately after delivery the mother is about 12 pounds lighter: the baby accounts for an average of 7 to 8 pounds, the placenta 1 to 2 pounds, and the amniotic fluid and lost blood another 1 to 2 pounds. Within the first week the mother generally drops another 5 pounds in excess fluid lost through urination. Throughout pregnancy, high levels of estrogen greatly increase the total amount of body water held between the cells, and the enlarged uterus presses on the *vena cava*, thereby slowing drainage of extracellular fluid as well. Following delivery, the sudden drop in estrogen and the removal of pressure on the vena cava enable the body's fluid levels to return to normal rapidly. Between the second and fifth days after birth, the mother will notice that she urinates much more frequently than usual; almost 3 quarts a day is not uncommon, as opposed to the normal 1½. Loss of fluid in the first week is also due to excessive perspiration.

Further weight loss results from changes that cause the uterus to shrink remarkably. In the first 10 days after birth the top of the uterus decreases from about the height of the navel to about the height of the pubic bone. This parallels a progressive drop in the weight of the uterus from 2.3 pounds at delivery to 1.2 pounds at one week post-delivery, to 11 ounces at two weeks, to 3 ounces at six weeks. By eight weeks the uterus has reached a final, nonpregnant weight of 2 ounces. The total number of cells in the uterus does not decrease; rather the cells shrink to about a tenth of their pregnant size due to a chemical breakdown of the protein within them. This breakdown begins as soon as placental hormones stop circulating and causes low levels of protein to spill into the mother's urine, making it slightly more acidic and possibly causing a burning sensation on urination around the second and third day after delivery.

How the Pelvic Organs Return to Normal

The shrinking of the uterus is called *involution,* and it is accompanied by a profound healing and restructuring of the inner lining. The process is mechanical as well as physiological. As discussed in the chapter on the physiology of labor, the uterus experiences further contractions within minutes of the delivery of the placenta, which causes it to reduce in size and tighten its crisscrossed fibers around the blood vessels that have sheared off at the implantation site (see p. 301). Whereas the pregnant uterus was reddish purple outside because of all the blood it contained, the uterus after delivery turns whitish as blood vessels are clamped down. Inside, the uterus is slightly abraded and rough-looking, especially around the 10-centimeter site where the placenta was embedded in the uterine wall.

After birth, white blood cells move into the uterus by the mil-

In the first ten days after birth the top of the uterus shrinks from the height of the navel to the height of the pubic bone; by eight weeks it has regained its prepregnant size.

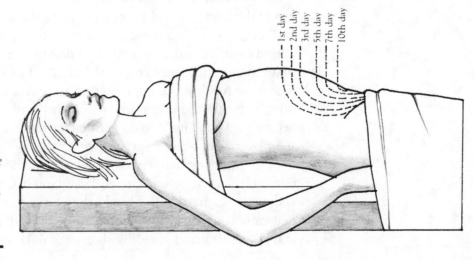

lions and begin the work of restructuring the uterus. The topmost cells, now without a good blood supply, are digested by the white blood cells and sloughed off as the discharge called *lochia.* From the mother's point of view the lochia seems much like a menstrual period, although it goes on for about ten days and produces a heavier flow that varies in color and consistency. For the first two or three days after delivery the discharge is called *lochia rubra* due to its reddish color. It contains mostly blood from the implantation site and cells from the topmost uterine layer. This initial flow is often accompanied by clots, and is so heavy it may cause the mother to feel a flooding sensation when she stands up.

By around the third or fourth day the discharge lessens and becomes paler. It is then called *lochia serosa* because it contains less red blood cells and more clear extracellular fluid, white blood cells, and uterine cells. The lochia serosa continues until about ten days after delivery, gradually altering in color from pinkish to pale pinkish-yellow toward the end. Finally, starting at around the tenth day, the discharge changes to *lochia alba,* a scant creamy white fluid that is made of white blood cells and uterine tissue. By the end of another week or so it disappears altogether.

Lochia has a distinct odor, somewhat like menstrual blood, which tends to be strongest in the serosa phase. Should the mother develop a uterine infection at any point, the lochia will develop an unpleasant odor and the mother will experience lower abdominal pain. While the mother is in the hospital, the doctor or nurse will check the odor of the pads once a day. At home the mother can check it for herself. Infections are relatively uncommon because uterine cells naturally kill bacteria.

While the top layer of the uterus is being broken down and sloughed off, the lower layers are making new cells. By ten days after delivery the whole inner surface of the uterus, except for the implantation site, has been replaced with new epithelial cells; by three weeks it is completely back to normal. Around the implantation site, however, a very different process goes on, healing the area without a scar. New cells begin to grow around the edges of the site, tunneling under the ragged exterior and eventually meeting in the middle. All the old tissue above these new cells is sloughed off in the lochia. The entire process of healing the implantation site takes about six weeks and literally makes the uterus like new. This is of critical importance, because any scarring could eventually interfere with the embedding of the placenta in a future pregnancy.

Following delivery of the placenta, the uterus has a tendency to remain in a contracted state and can be felt through the wall of the abdomen as a hard ball. Should the uterus start to soften, it will automatically trigger a contraction that will clamp down the uterine fibers and prevent further bleeding. For several days after the baby is born the mother will experience occasional contractions, which are referred to as *after-pains*.

During the first twelve hours after delivery the contractions tend to be regular, coordinated, and even more powerful than during labor, though not as noticeable since they are not causing dilatation. After a first delivery uterine muscle tone is generally good, so the uterus doesn't need to contract too often. With subsequent deliveries uterine tone is poorer, so the after-pains tend to be more frequent and intense. Often they occur when the baby starts nursing because its sucking causes the mother's pituitary gland to release *oxytocin,* the hormone that is necessary for milk production (see pp. 411–12) and that also causes the uterus to contract. After-pains take place even in those mothers who choose not to nurse, but they are less frequent.

A full bladder tends to increase after-pains, because as the bladder fills, the uterus is tilted back into a position in which it cannot contract well, so it tends to relax. Thus it's good for the new mother to urinate frequently, especially on the second and third days after delivery, when she is excreting large amounts of the extra fluid that her body has accumulated during pregnancy.

The cervix and the area of the uterus immediately around it also undergo great changes in the days and weeks after birth. At first these tissues are stretched, swollen, and bruised. The cervix itself is usually 3 to 5 centimeters dilated and may have tears around the edges. By the end of the first week the opening narrows to about 1½ centimeters and begins to thicken and take on a tubelike shape again. Return to normal usually occurs by 2 to 4 weeks after delivery, although the opening of the cervix never appears the same once it has been dilated for delivery. In a woman who has never had a baby, the cervical opening looks like a tiny round hole at the end of a tube; in a woman who has delivered vaginally, the opening appears like a line or slit. The lower part of the uterus, which was stretched during delivery to accommodate the baby's head, now shrinks and thickens until it almost disappears. However, the entire uterus remains slightly larger after each baby than it was before.

Directly following delivery the vagina is smooth-walled, swollen, and stretched enough so that it may gape open for a day or two. During the next 3 to 4 weeks the vagina shrinks back, though it also never returns to its predelivery size. Due to the drop in estrogen that occurs after birth, the walls of the vagina tend to remain smooth and somewhat dry. This situation continues for about six months or until menstruation resumes. Not only does the vagina fail to lubricate well, but both the vagina and the labia do not get as much blood flow, so they tend to become engorged much more slowly during sexual arousal. To restore the tone of the muscles surrounding the vagina, which affect both sex and bladder control, special exercises referred to as *Kegels* (see p. 102) must be practiced.

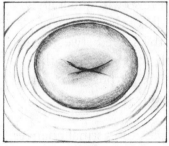

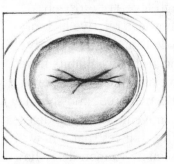

After a vaginal delivery the cervical opening changes in shape from a circle to a slit.

The bladder, like the vagina and uterus, is stretched and flabby right after birth. As a result, it can hold more urine than usual, but it doesn't empty as completely. A new mother may not notice sensations of bladder fullness and may also be apprehensive about urinating due to general perineal tenderness or stitches. These factors, coupled with the need to get rid of extra body fluid, increase the chances of the bladder becoming overly full and distended, which can cause problems with urinating in the first postpartum days. Such a situation is more likely if the mother has been given intravenous fluids and/or oxytocin, but frequent urination will help to avoid it.

Postpartum Changes in the Abdomen

The abdominal wall, like most of the other structures involved in pregnancy, is quite flabby following delivery because the elastic fibers in the skin have been stretched to a remarkable extent. It returns to normal in about a month, except for areas where *stretch marks* had developed. There is no treatment for these marks, which gradually turn silvery white and become less noticeable but never disappear completely.

To regain good abdominal muscle tone, however, the mother must do exercises (see pp. 102–05). This is particularly important in the case of the *rectus abdominus,* a pair of muscles that run in broad bands from the pubic bone to the rib cage. These muscles, which are normally slightly separated, tend to become more so with pregnancy. When the separation is great enough, the middle of the abdomen becomes only skin and fatty tissue. The wider the space between the bands, the longer it takes to regain good muscle tone and close the gap. There is a tendency for the bands to separate further with each pregnancy, especially if the pregnancies are closely spaced or the mother does not do special exercises.

Mothers often experience a number of gastrointestinal changes in the first days after birth. The incredibly high levels of estrogen produced during labor and delivery and the mother's relative lack of movement during labor tend to decrease muscle tone in the digestive system. Moreover, the mother's normal eating and bowel habits have been completely disrupted: she probably hasn't had much to eat or drink in some hours, she's most likely a little dehydrated, and she may have had an enema, which alters the normal movements of the digestive tract. All these factors tend to increase the chances that a new mother will become constipated. In addition, many women delay having a bowel movement due to perineal discomfort, hemorrhoids that developed during pregnancy, or the unwarranted fear that they may break their stitches.

Although the mother is naturally exreting excess fluid, it's essential that she keep up her fluid intake at the same time to make up for the dehydration that often follows labor and delivery and, if she is nursing, to keep up with the dramatic increase in her need for fluids. Large amounts of fruits and foods with fiber, and early regular elimination will help prevent constipation and make bowel movements easier.

Postpartum Changes in Blood, Breathing, and Hormones

During pregnancy the mother's blood volume rises by 1 to 2 liters, but within three weeks of delivery it drops back down to normal. Roughly a third of the loss takes place during delivery; the rest is eliminated by the mother's body. As the excess blood cells naturally die off, they are not replaced. The extra iron from the red blood cells is added to the mother's stores and subsequently passed on to the baby through her milk. The water component of the extra blood is excreted via the kidneys, causing some temporary adjustments in the mother's mineral balance. In the first few hours after delivery and for the next five days or so, the mother's blood clotting ability increases greatly. Enormous amounts of clotting factors, including fibrin threads and sticky platelets, are mobilized in the uterus. In conjunction with blood vessel clampdown this mechanism helps to prevent excessive bleeding and promote healing at the site of placental attachment.

Interestingly, the mother's sudden change in shape after delivery temporarily upsets the amount of air she inhales and exhales. For the first week the amount of air that the mother is able to take in and the overall efficiency with which she breathes drop by almost 10 percent. With more carbon dioxide and less oxygen than normal in her blood, the mother may feel less energetic, especially when she exercises or exerts herself.

In addition to all the other changes the mother undergoes after the birth of her baby, there are rapid endocrine shifts in her body. Following the delivery of the baby and the placenta, the mother experiences a tremendous drop in the levels of estrogen, progesterone, and several other hormones. Within three hours her estrogen level decreases by 90 percent, and progesterone drops similarly. As a result, the mother's smooth muscle tone and metabolic patterns quickly return to their prepregnant state. One of the most interesting metabolic alterations involves the mother's blood sugar levels: during pregnancy the mother's response to her own insulin is lessened; but in the first days after delivery her body actually becomes hyperreactive to insulin, resulting in low blood sugar levels. Still other endocrine changes are brought about by the start of breast-feeding, which stimulates the release of high levels of oxytocin and prolactin.

The sudden dip in some hormones and rise in others make the mother's emotions more labile than usual. Combined with the sweeping changes in her daily patterns, elation over the baby, anxiety over her new responsibilities, and her almost inevitable exhaustion, the hormonal changes help bring about frequent and wide mood swings that are normal between the third to the fifth day after delivery.

The Physiology of Nursing

A complicated interaction among several hormones is responsible for the production of milk in the mammary glands of the mother's breasts (see p. 43). Throughout pregnancy high levels of several hormones have prepared the breasts for nursing: estrogen has caused the growth of ducts and the proliferation of alveoli; progesterone has caused the alveolar milk glands to mature; and prolactin, cortisol, and growth hormone have worked together almost miraculously to turn breast cells into either *secretory cells* that will make milk or *muscle cells* that will squeeze milk down through the ducts.

Once the baby and placenta are delivered, the fetoplacental

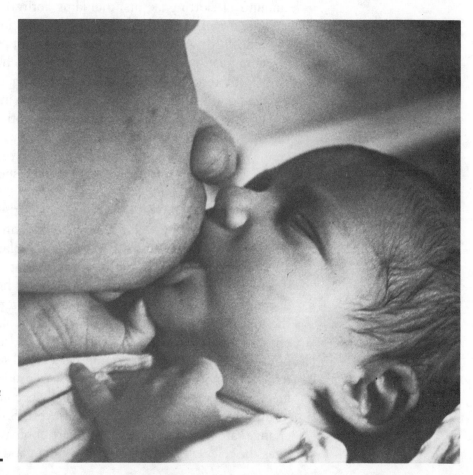

A complicated interaction among several hormones is responsible for the production of breast milk after the baby is born. Photo by Michael Samuels.

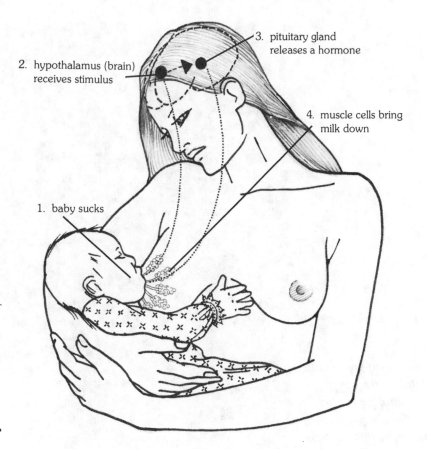

2. hypothalamus (brain)
   receives stimulus

3. pituitary gland
   releases a hormone

4. muscle cells bring
   milk down

1. baby sucks

The mother's breasts don't release milk simply due to suction, but in response to a complicated process called the letdown reflex. The mother's thoughts or the stimulation of the baby's sucking cause the pituitary gland to produce oxytocin, which makes the muscle cells in the milk glands contract and squeeze down the milk.

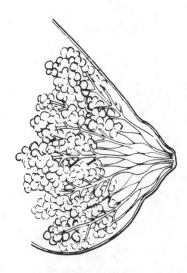

Following delivery the hormone prolactin causes the secretory cells in the mother's breasts to begin to produce milk.

unit no longer maintains the mother's estrogen and progesterone levels. Without high levels of these hormones, prolactin stimulates the mammary glands in the mother's breasts to produce milk. Milk production is not a process that takes place in isolation, however; it does not occur without the baby sucking. Nursing causes the mother's hypothalamus to *stop* producing a *prolactin-inhibiting factor* that normally prevents her from producing milk. When the baby sucks, the inhibiting factor is stopped and the pituitary begins producing prolactin, which stimulates the secretory cells in the breast.

Continued suckling is necessary for continued production of milk. If a mother stops nursing altogether for two or three weeks, prolactin production stops. If a mother nurses twins, she produces twice as much of it. Thus prolactin is produced according to demand. When the mother's breasts are full of milk, her hypothalamus gets messages to secrete prolactin-inhibiting factor to slow milk production. If the baby frequently empties the mother's breasts, the hypothalamus produces less inhibiting factor, so more milk is produced. This complex process enables the mother to adapt to the baby's increasing need for milk, which generally reaches a peak at about three months after birth.

Although prolactin causes the production of milk in the alveoli of the mammary glands, it doesn't cause milk to flow out through the

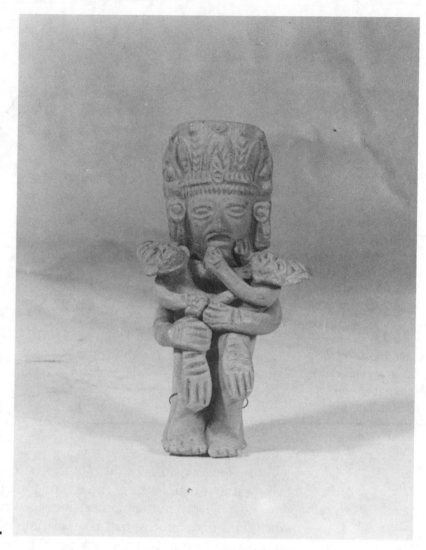

The mother's supply of milk is regulated by the baby's demand. Thus if a mother nurses twins, she produces twice as much prolactin and twice as much milk. Mexican sculpture. Lowie Museum of Anthropology, University of California, Berkeley.

ducts. The baby's sucking only causes a little of the milk to come down. Most milk passes from the alveoli, via the ducts, to the *storage sinuses* around the nipple only when the tiny muscle cells in the breasts actively squeeze the milk down. This is a complicated mechanism, called the *letdown reflex,* which is under the control of the autonomic nervous system and is therefore profoundly affected by the mother's emotional state (see p. 138). The baby's sucking stimulates autonomic sensory nerves in the breast that send messages to the mother's hypothalamus, where they are joined by input from areas of the brain that are affected by thoughts, perceptions, feelings, and emotions. Under the proper conditions, when the hypothalamus receives sucking signals, it causes the pituitary gland to produce oxytocin, which in turn stimulates the muscle cells in the breast to contract.

In order for the hypothalamus to elicit the letdown reflex, the mother must be feeling relaxed and secure. Any stressful situation results in a high level of epinephrine, which decreases blood flow to the breasts, thereby lowering energy for the muscle cells whose job it is to squeeze milk down. Such a tie-in makes sense from an evolutionary point of view: the mother's autonomic nervous system would not tend to activate the letdown reflex in the face of a perceived danger that might arouse the fight-or-flight response. In the modern age fear of being eaten by a saber-toothed tiger has been replaced by job concerns, family pressures, and free-floating anxiety. Sometimes fatigue, overstimulation, or even joyous excitement can interfere with the letdown reflex.

Like many other autonomic reflexes, the letdown reflex is affected by expectation and learning. In the beginning most mothers need a quiet, focused atmosphere and the actual stimulation of the baby's sucking in order to elicit the reflex. In time the reflex may become so practiced that the baby's cry or even the thought of impending nursing will cause the milk to come down.

Milk is being produced in the nursing mother's breasts all the time, but only some of it passes into the ducts where it is readily available to the baby. This initial portion of milk stored in the ducts is called *foremilk*; it is a low-fat, low-protein, "watered-down" milk that contains only small-size molecules that can easily diffuse across the alveolar membranes. Foremilk accounts for approximately a third of the total milk volume of each nursing. The high-fat, high-protein component of the milk remains in the alveolar cells until the mother's letdown reflex is triggered, at which point the alveolar cells are squeezed by surrounding muscle cells. As a result, the milk containing large-size fat globules and protein molecules is squirted into the ducts under pressure. In the ducts this rich milk, called *hindmilk*, mixes with the foremilk. Only if the letdown reflex occurs does the baby get enough rich milk to satisfy its nutritional needs.

The tremendous physiological changes that the mother undergoes after delivery help her body return to its prepregnant state and adapt to the new demands of mothering and nursing. The more the mother understands about the normal body sensations associated with these changes, the less she will worry and the more she will function in harmony with her body. This will enable her to concentrate her energies on the joyful and demanding task of being a new mother.

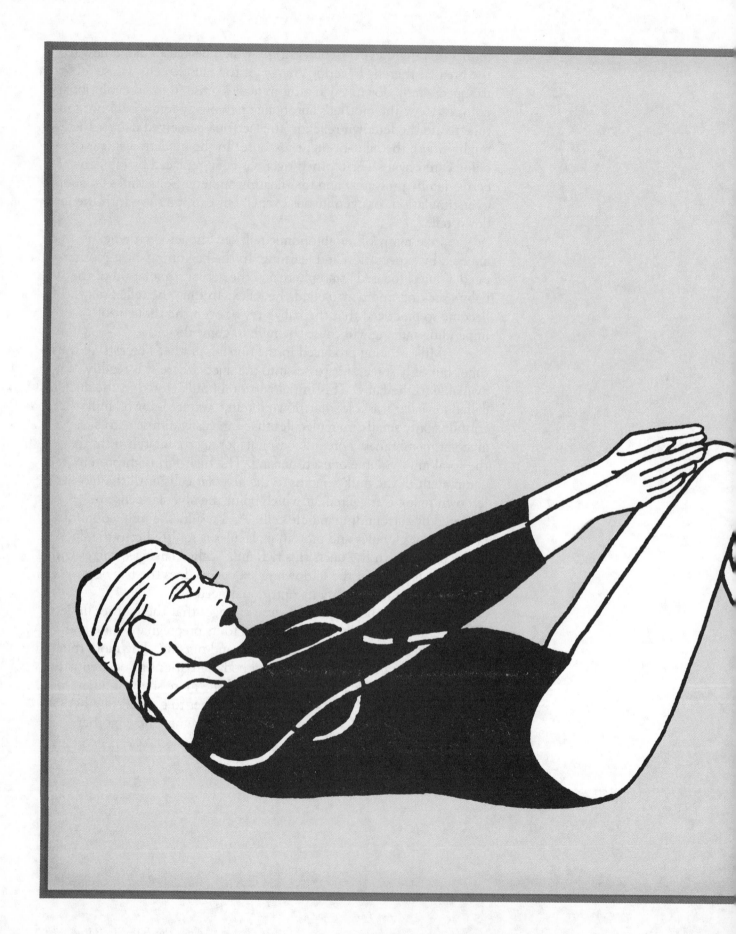

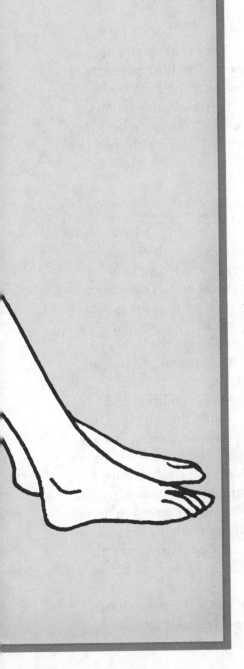

CHAPTER 19

Concerns of the First Few Weeks after Delivery

Birth as a Rite of Passage

Immediately after birth pregnancy slips into the past, and the mother becomes immersed in a whole new set of experiences, sensations, and concerns. Particularly with a first baby, birth is not only an event but a rite of passage in which the mother, father, and baby pass from one set of roles, with its privileges and requirements, to another with new rewards and demands. In fact, there is probably no greater life transformation in modern Western culture that takes places within such a relatively short period of time. One day the expectant parents are a couple filled with anticipation; the next they are a family with a new knowledge of the world, embarked on one of life's most demanding and creative endeavors.

Delivering a baby is an extraordinary experience that involves great preparation, effort, and self-discipline, as well as trust and a willingness to accept forces beyond one's control. Most women who have given birth remember moments of uncertainty, fear, or discomfort during labor and delivery, and they would affirm the idea that birth is a rite of passage. No matter how the situation unfolds, no matter how long or short the mother's labor is, no matter whether she delivers vaginally or by cesarean, she has successfully crossed the bridge into motherhood, an achievement of which she can be very proud.

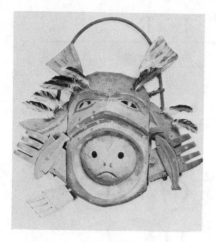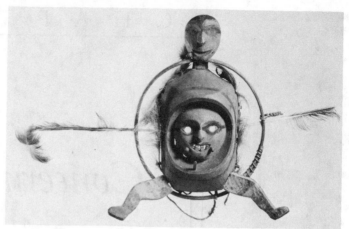

Although the glow of her accomplishment is likely to linger for some days, the mother very quickly becomes involved in the reality of caring for her newborn. Within an hour or so after the birth both mother and baby begin to feel the weariness that inevitably follows such a momentous event, and each will give way to sleep. Where they will nap and whether or not they will be together varies with the place of birth.

Caring for the New Mother

Generally, if a woman gives birth in a hospital, unless she is in a birth room, she will be transferred from the delivery room to a special recovery area or to a regular bed in the obstetrical unit. There she will be checked by the nurses at frequent intervals to see that she is com-fortable and that her uterus remains clamped down. If a woman gives birth at home, the practitioner will remain to observe the mother for the first two hours after birth, monitoring her vital signs and helping to get the household in order.

In the hospital, depending upon the baby's condition and whether the center has rooming in, the baby will either be placed in a bassinet next to the mother or taken to the newborn nursery. Room-ing in does not mean that the mother has sole responsibility for taking care of the baby in the first few hours after birth but that the baby remains in the mother's room so that she is the first to know when the baby wakes or cries. In some hospitals even babies who room in during the day are routinely kept in the nursery during the night. Because such rules can have great emotional impact on the mother and father, they should learn about their particular center's policies long before the baby is born.

Before discharge from the hospital or before the practitioner leaves after a home birth, the mother will be given instructions on how to care for herself and the baby. In particular, the

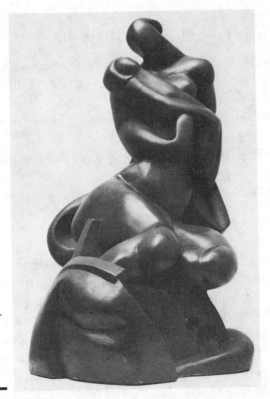

The glow of the new mother's achievement lingers for days. Madonna of the Rocks, Alexander Archipenko, 1912. Painted on plaster, 21" x 13" x 14". Collection, The Museum of Modern Art, New York. Gift of Frances Archipenko and the Perls Galleries.

mother will be shown how to tell if her uterus is clamped down and how to lightly massage it to keep it firm.

The mother will also be instructed on the normal discharge she will have after birth (p. 408). In addition to being told about the usual color changes, she will be told to check the odor of her pad when she changes it. As we mentioned, the lochia usually smells somewhat like menstrual blood; an unpleasant odor could be a sign of infection and should be communicated to the practitioner. While a woman is in the hospital, the nurse will check the pads frequently during the first twenty-four hours after birth, and daily thereafter.

The lochia typically pools in the vagina when the mother is lying down and tends to gush out when she gets up. Bloody, menstruallike clots in the discharge are also normal. Too much physical exertion will tend to prolong bleeding from the placental implantation site, so that the mother is advised to take things easy in the first few days, no matter how well she feels. Tampons are not recommended initially for the lochia because they are uncomfortable while the mother is healing.

Afterbirth Pains

Afterbirth pains begin shortly after the placenta is delivered and feel similar to the contractions experienced in expelling it. They perform an important function in keeping the uterus clamped down and in

- Be reassured that the pains are normal and that they help the body heal by clamping down uterine blood vessels, which stops bleeding.
- Urinate frequently, especially before nursing, to help keep the uterus clamped down.
- Lie on your stomach on a pillow, putting pressure on the uterus.
- Practice relaxation exercises.

clearing the uterus of clots. The pains aren't very uncomfortable with the first baby, but they tend to become stronger and more frequent with subsequent births because the uterus has progressively less muscle tone with delivery and does not clamp down as spontaneously. After-pains are completely normal and generally don't continue for more than three days on the average. As we discussed in the physiology of puerperium, afterpains are often stimulated by the oxytocin released during nursing and can make breast-feeding more difficult for the mother in the early days (see pp. 411–12).

There are several ways to help ease the discomfort of after-pains. The mother should massage her uterus frequently, especially before nursing, because this tends to keep the muscle fibers from relaxing. The harder the uterus, the less likely it is to contract. Sometimes just urinating will relieve the afterpains. In the first postpartum days a full bladder tends to push the still-enlarged uterus backward, making it more difficult for the uterus to clamp down. Moreover, during this period the new mother's fluid levels are in an unnatural state. She is being told to drink lots of liquids to promote milk production, but her body is also trying to rid itself of excess fluid from her cells and extra blood volume.

The mother's bladder is often not sensitive to being full because it has been pushed out of position by the enlarged uterus during the latter part of pregnancy and then sufficiently compressed by the birth process to cause swelling. Bladder distension should be avoided because it increases the likelihood of the mother developing a bladder infection or needing to be catheterized in order to urinate. Even if a mother goes to the bathroom right after birth, her bladder can become full enough within the next twelve hours to make it difficult to urinate a second time. Thus the mother should go to the bathroom more frequently than usual, whether she feels the need or not, particularly before nursing.

When the mother is relaxing or sleeping, it's a good idea for her to lie on her side or stomach with a pillow under her uterus to put continuous pressure on it. If her afterpains are quite severe, initially it will hurt when the mother leans on the pillow, but the pains will subside in a few minutes as the uterus gets hard, and she will become more comfortable. Although it is somewhat awkward, this position can even be used for nursing if the baby is propped up on pillows too.

Another helpful but more general method for coping with afterpains is relaxation. Just as relaxation and breathing exercises were effective during labor, they can be effective now as well. Not only do they help relieve discomfort, but they have the added value of being a nursing aide because they promote the letdown reflex. Relaxing and being reassured that the afterpains will be gone within several days often helps change a mother's perception of the situation and tends to raise her pain threshold.

If sufficient relief cannot be achieved with any of the foregoing methods, the doctor or midwife can prescribe pain medication, but this is to be avoided if possible because the drugs pass to the baby in small amounts through the milk. The most common medications, APC (aspirin-phenacetin-caffeine) with codeine or Darvon, are the same drugs that are given for other discomforts in the first few days after birth. In general, the mother is told to take them about a half-hour before nursing so the baby gets the least effects.

Constipation

Constipation is a very common problem for new mothers during the first days after the baby is born. As we've mentioned, hormonal changes and medication cause intestinal muscle tone to be sluggish

After-birth pains are caused by the uterus naturally clamping down when it becomes too relaxed. The pains can be eased by having the mother lie on her stomach with a pillow underneath; this position puts pressure on the uterus and helps it stay contracted.

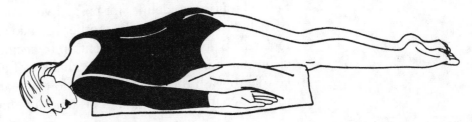

following labor and delivery (see p. 410), and the situation is frequently compounded by lack of food in the mother's digestive tract. Moreover, the mother's abdominal muscles are much less effective at pushing after childbirth because they are so stretched. Women who have had stitches are often hesitant to forcefully expel a bowel movement for fear of tearing their stitches, but they can be reassured that there are several layers of sutures that are made of extremely durable material. The first few bowel movements may be somewhat uncomfortable even for mothers who have not had stitches, because the perineal area may remain tender for a week or so, but a mother shouldn't put off having a bowel movement, since the longer she waits, the larger and harder the stool tends to become.

A mother can do a number of things to promote the return of normal bowel habits. Early walking and a quick return to solid foods are very important. Most women enjoy walking within a few hours after delivery, and many are truly ravenous following the fasting and effort of delivery. If a mother is in a hospital and the kitchen is closed at the time, someone should go out to purchase whatever she wants. Throughout the first week the mother should make sure that she gets plenty of fluids, dried fruit (prunes), and foods that are high in roughage.

Most women do not have their first bowel movement until a day or two after the baby is born. If three or four days go by, a mother is likely to begin to feel uncomfortable. At this point the doctor or midwife will probably prescribe a mild bulk laxative such as Metamucil, a plain laxative such as Milk of Magnesia, a stool softener like Colase, or a suppository like Dulcolax.

Due to all the pushing, stretching, and straining of delivery, mothers who have had hemorrhoids may be troubled by them now. The most effective techniques for hemorrhoidal pain are often the same as those used to soothe the discomfort of stitches (see chart). It is especially important that mothers with hemorrhoids not become constipated, so they are routinely started on stool softeners shortly after delivery. Those few mothers whose hemorrhoids are large enough to protrude after a bowel movement will be taught to push them back inside with a lubricated rubber glove.

Perineal Care

Several routine guidelines for postdelivery care of the perineal area are particularly important if the mother has had an episiotomy or tear repaired. By paying special attention to keeping the perineal area clean, mothers can minimize the chances of infection. Often they will be told to wash their hands both before and after going to the bathroom or changing their pad. This tends to eliminate contamination from external sources and is probably even more important in the hospital than at home.

New mothers are usually given specific instructions designed to prevent stool, which contains bacteria, from coming in contact with the perineal area, the vagina, or the urinary opening, all of which tend to be abraded and therefore more susceptible to infection than usual. If the mother has had an episiotomy or a tear, it is especially important to keep stitches clean. All wiping and cleaning should be done from front to back, from the top of the vagina down past the anus. Many doctors and midwives tell their mothers to wash the perineal area with soap and water or medicated pads each time they go to the bathroom. This not only protects against infection, it generally feels soothing as well.

Almost all new mothers experience some degree of perineal discomfort in the first few days after delivery, whether or not they have stitches. A number of simple remedies may help make the mother more comfortable. Cool or warm tap water can be poured or squirted over the perineal area from top to bottom with a clean pitcher or drugstore squirt bottle. Cool water tends to numb the area; warm water increases local blood circulation, which is healing. Hospitals have *sitz baths* that enable a mother to soak her bottom, and portable ones are available for home use. In addition, many mothers find that gauze pads soaked in witch hazel, or commercial pads like Tucks, are very soothing. Such pads can be used to wipe the perineal area after going to the bathroom or applied to the area when the mother is in bed and left on for up to a half-hour.

Somewhat surprisingly, the exercises called Kegels (see p. 102) are very effective for relieving perineal discomfort. Some midwifery texts suggests starting Kegels within an hour after delivery, because contracting the perineal muscles promotes local circulation and thus stimulates healing. Kegels also tend to lift or pull up these muscles, which makes the mother less uncomfortable when she shifts her position in bed or sits down.

Dealing with perineal discomfort after birth

- Bathe area with cool water from a squirt bottle.
- Sit in a whirlpool bath.
- Do exercises to tighten the pelvic floor (Kegels).
- Apply an ice pack initially.
- Apply dry heat with a lamp after the first day.
- Use anesthetic spray.
- Practice relaxation exercises.

If a mother is very uncomfortable, she can sit on a rubber ring, inflatable swimming tube, or pillow for the first few days, but most doctors and midwives feel that in the long run it's better to sit up tall in a straightback chair. Sitting in this position or sitting tailor-style in lotus position, with the knees bent and the heels drawn up toward the perineum, shifts the mother's weight to the bones of the buttocks, the *ischial tuberosities*, and takes pressure off the perineal area, which makes the mother more comfortable.

If these measures are not effective in dealing with perineal pain, doctors and midwives suggest several other treatments. Some doctors feel that applying ice packs to the perineum shortly after delivery helps avoid discomfort when a mother has had a large episiotomy or repair. Ice numbs the area and reduces swelling by constricting the tiny blood vessels, just as it does with bruises and sprains.

A number of mothers find that dry heat, which increases circulation, makes the perineum more comfortable after the first day. Hospitals have special heat lamps that rest on the mother's legs and direct the light. At home a mother can improvise by using a desk lamp with a 40-watt bulb. Before applying heat, the mother should carefully clean the area of any lochia, cream, or ointment and, if necessary, place a clean pad or absorbent material under her. Care should be taken not to put the lamp too close to the perineum as it can burn, especially if the mother doesn't cleanse the area of any oily substance first. An infrared heat lamp can also be used, but then special precaution must also be taken to avoid burning. With regard to time and distance, the instructions on the heat lamp should be followed closely and the mother should pay attention to how the area feels and adjust the lamp accordingly. In general, dry heat can be applied for 20 or 30 minutes at a time, two or three times a day.

If discomfort is really persistent, the doctor or midwife may suggest the use of a non-prescription topical anesthetic that comes in spray or ointment form, such as Dermoplast spray or Nupercaine ointment. These medicines should be applied according to the instructions, approximately three or four times a day. If such anesthetic medications are not sufficient, the doctor or midwife may prescribe a pain reliever such as APC with codeine, or Darvon. As we've discussed earlier, these drugs do pass through the mother's milk, but not in such large amounts that they should be avoided if a mother is very uncomfortable.

Perineal pain usually reaches its peak on the second or third day and then disappears within another day or so. If a mother has severe or continued pain, either in the hospital or at home, she should inform her practitioner, who will examine her to make sure that the pain is not due to an infection or a *hematoma*, a pool of blood under the skin, although these conditions are uncommon.

Most new mothers are eager to bathe as soon as possible after

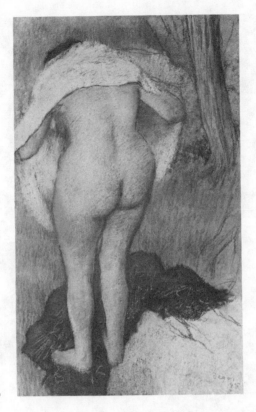

A mother can return to her normal bathing habits shortly after the baby is born. Girl Drying Herself, *Edgar Degas. National Gallery of Art, Washington. Gift of the W. Averell Harriman Foundation.*

the long, hard work of delivery. Perspiration, amniotic fluid, and blood are likely to make the mother feel sticky and dirty, and she may even want to wash her hair, especially if she did not shower during early labor or shortly before. Moreover, a new mother will find that she perspires profusely in the first few days after delivery (see p. 406). In years past there were a number of edicts against early bathing, but today doctors feel that it's fine for a mother to shower as soon as she can get up and walk by herself. If the mother has not stood for some time or feels even a little shaky, she should have someone help her. As of the second day, it's fine for the mother to take a tub bath or swim, even if she has had an episiotomy. By this time there is no longer concern about water getting in the uterus, though most women do not choose to take a bath since they will probably be uncomfortable wearing a tampon for the lochial discharge.

Rest and Recuperation

It cannot be overemphasized how important it is that a mother get sufficient rest in the early days and weeks after the baby is born. Typically both mother and father drastically underestimate their need for sleep, and as a result, the average new mother tends to be very tired, no matter how exhilarated she was after the delivery. Postpartum lack

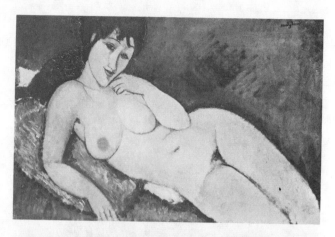

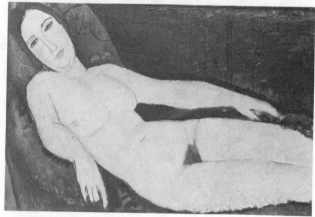

Although a new mother will feel moments of great excitement, she is also likely to feel a profound weariness at times as a result of the birth experience and taking care of the baby.

Nude on a Blue Cushion, *Amedeo Modigliani. National Gallery of Art, Washington. Chester Dale Collection.*

Nude on a Divan, *Amedeo Modigliani. National Gallery of Art, Washington. Chester Dale Collection.*

of sleep is compounded by the fact that often a mother's labor has gone on for a number of hours, especially if she is a first-time mother, and she may be especially exhausted if she went into labor at night or hasn't been sleeping well during the last weeks.

Although nursing is a tremendously rewarding experience, new mothers find that it radically alters their sleep patterns. Babies may nurse almost hourly when allowed to breast-feed entirely on demand, and as a result, new mothers are awakened frequently at night and often find themselves sleep-deprived during the first postpartum days. The new pattern is very different from uninterrupted sleep, and many mothers initially have trouble falling right back to sleep once they have nursed and changed the baby. Sometimes, in immense happiness, parents will talk and play with the baby when it awakens to nurse. As delightful as this time is, it will also add to their fatigue.

Mothers not only tend to get fewer hours of sleep during the night, they get a different kind, because their normal cycles of light sleep, dreaming (REM) sleep, and deep sleep are repeatedly interrupted. Little is known about the effects of frequent awakenings on new mothers, but research has found that it is psychologically upsetting to volunteers in laboratory sleep studies.

New parents have two ways to cope with the problem: go to

bed early, and set aside time for naps. Going to sleep early means assuming a schedule somewhat like an athlete in training. Some nights a mother may become sleepy soon after dinner, but in general, getting to bed by eight or nine will allow both parents to make up for the extra time they will be awake during the night. In self-defense, parents need to tailor their sleep patterns to fit the baby's. If the baby usually sleeps soundly from nine to eleven, then wakes several times before morning, the parents are well advised to adopt the same schedule and forego evening "adult time" until everyone becomes rested and adjusts to the new pattern.

Many new mothers will tell you that they could not have survived the first week physically or emotionally without napping. It doesn't matter if a mother hasn't napped since she was a child herself; this is a time for it. It should be considered part of the requirements of the job of new parenting, just as night workers like nurses, doctors, pilots, and flight attendants accept daytime sleeping as part of their job. If a mother has become accustomed to napping during pregnancy,

Helping new parents avoid fatigue

Most new parents experience considerable fatigue in the first few weeks due to excitement, extra work, extra company, stress, and lack of sleep. In general, the more often the baby wakes at night, the more tired the parents are. Here are suggestions to make things easier:

Take naps during the day *as soon as* the baby goes to sleep.

Go to sleep very early at night to make up for night feedings.

Reduce or eliminate visits—especially ones that are stressful. Set the time and length of the stay in advance.

Make a conscious effort to rest; stay in bed; undertake nothing extra; simplify all household routines, especially meals, cleanup, and baby laundry.

Be alert to early signs of fatigue.

Get help from friends and relatives, especially for household tasks.

Adjust nutrition for increased stress—institute a nursing diet— try taking brewer's yeast or stress vitamins such as B_{12}.

Make use of relaxation exercises, meditation, and visualization.

so much the better. With a new baby, naps often can't be taken according to any fixed schedule or according to the mother's inclinations. Napping, like going to bed at night, has to be adjusted to the baby's sleep cycles. The best way to get a long nap is to go to sleep as soon as the baby does, usually right after it has been diapered and nursed. If a mother spends time talking or doing housework first, she may only get to sleep for a short time before the baby awakens her with hungry cries or happy gurgles.

It's important for new parents to realize that this stressful situation will not last forever, but is worst during the first week and generally much improved after the second week, by which time the mother has regained much of her strength and become more adept at handling nursing and all the other new tasks. Also, by then the baby will probably not be waking quite as often and will have become more skillful at nursing too. During the first few days and weeks both mother and baby are learning to breast-feed and are becoming adjusted to each other's particular style. Even though a second- or third-time mother knows something of what to expect, every mother-baby nursing combination is unique. Occasionally a mother may find breast-feeding more of a challenge with a second or third baby than it was with her first.

Outside Help and Support

In the first few days the mother should free herself to spend as much time as possible getting to know the baby or just resting. These are the two most important tasks for her at this time. The third is to enjoy herself—spending close, relaxed time with her husband, family, and friends. Since there will be more than enough work for several people, these goals are best accomplished if the mother has help. The father can play an extremely important role by seeing that the mother gets the help she needs. The amount of assistance a woman requires is affected by the ease of her delivery, how long she stayed in the hospital, and how demanding the baby is.

For all parents, but especially for first-timers, a new baby brings radical alterations in living habits. Sleeping, eating, working, relaxing, and going out all have to be modified. Adjusting to these changes can be tiring in itself. Even the most positive, joyous life events can be physically and emotionally stressful. In addition, the day-to-day chores of the household are suddenly more time consuming and energy draining than usual.

During the initial postpartum period a mother can often use as much help as she can get. In fact, for most new mothers help is essential for the first week or so after birth. Generally the more support the mother is given at this point, the better she will feel and the sooner she is likely to be able to manage on her own. If help is not forthcoming, a new mother should feel no guilt about asking for it. Often the father will have taken time off from work, or the parents will have a relative, a friend, or someone they have hired staying with them or coming in during the day to do housekeeping tasks. Just doing daily chores is one of the most important "baby presents" that friends and relatives can give new parents.

Helpers are usually invaluable, but occasionally they may turn out to be more of a problem than anything else. A new mother needs to be sure that the person *helps* rather than adds to the work and confusion. Many parents tell hilarious and poignant stories of helpers who insisted on caring for the baby themselves, talked incessantly, criticized everything the mother did, or did nothing. Knowing that such classic situations are all too common doesn't necessarily make them any easier for the new mother or father.

Given the natural lability of her emotions as well as her new responsibilities, the mother may have trouble dealing with such an uncomfortable situation, especially if the helper in question is one of the father's relatives. Whenever possible, it's good if the father handles such situations. If one person isn't helpful or can't do some part of the work, the pragmatic solution is simply to ask someone else.

Using relaxation after the baby is born

The first days after birth are usually joyful and exciting, but they can also be stressful and tiring. Relaxation and visualization are excellent tools for relieving tension and making this the special time the parents have looked forward to. Relaxation is particularly important because the mother is undergoing hormonal changes and adjusting to the new demands of nursing. Complete instructions for relaxation are given on pages 159–64 and for visualization, pages 165–75.

Relax to relieve fatigue.

Relax before nursing, to encourage the letdown reflex.

Relax your whole body, especially the pelvic area, to relieve postdelivery discomfort from the episiotomy and/or vaginal stretching.

Relax to relieve inevitable worries and anxieties about the baby and about being a parent.

Relax when the baby is upset—it will help relax the baby as well.

Relax to help induce sleep.

Although most mothers will take increasing interest in the household tasks that need to be done by the third or fourth day at home, they should be careful not to overdo. A new mother needs to simplify her routines and establish priorities, separating what *has* to be done from what can reasonably be left for a later time. Washing baby clothes and diapers should be delegated specifically to someone capable of getting the job done on a regular basis, so that the mother will not have to worry about it. If washing and drying facilities are poor or unavailable at home, parents should consider using either a diaper service or disposable diapers. Friends can be commissioned to buy any necessities that are missing from the baby's layette.

Housecleaning should be kept to a minimum and done mostly by the father or someone else. It may be a good idea to have a cleaning person in once or twice, even if the mother usually does the housework herself. She should realize that this is not the time for trying to attain superior levels of cleanliness; engaging in compulsive tidying and cleaning will only add to her fatigue, frustration, and tension. On the other hand, it's only natural for the mother to be upset if the house is much more disorganized than usual. Sometimes mothers are concerned about housekeeping as an extension of the nesting instinct, but often they are simply worried about what visitors will think. Actually the mother should be concerned about what visitors can *do*, not what they think, and the truth is that most visitors will be much more interested in the baby and the mother than the house.

Just as this is not a time for housecleaning, neither is it a time for gourmet cooking. The emphasis should be on ease of preparation and good nutrition to meet the demands put on the mother by stress, healing, and milk production. Healthy snacks and plenty of liquids should be available. Casserole-type main dishes that can be heated and reheated are ideal, since a mother often will not be able to finish a meal without being interrupted by a hungry baby. Preparing such dishes is another way for friends to help, and they should be encouraged to do so. Especially in the first few days it may be convenient to order take-out food like pizza, even if the family doesn't do this ordinarily. The main point is that the mother should spend little time in the kitchen initially. Although most new fathers are well meaning, they often do not appreciate how important it is that the mother be relieved of her usual cooking chores. If the father does not want to prepare meals, he should see that someone else takes care of it.

One of the biggest scheduling problems in the first days and weeks is when to have visitors and when not to. In their desire to share their joy and show off their new baby, parents often end up holding open house for friends and relatives. This may be rewarding and fun for both the mother and father when it's happening, but it's likely to result in levels of fatigue that are beyond their expectations. Severe fatigue obviously affects the way the mother relates to the

Using visualization after the baby is born

VISUALIZE	IN ORDER TO	FOR EXAMPLE, VISUALIZE
A strong, healthy baby	Feel good about the baby and relieve inevitable moments of concern	Your baby radiant and beautiful
Positive energy flowing into yourself and the baby	Make yourself and the baby strong	Picture yourself and the baby bathed in warm sunlight
Yourself in happy moments with your young baby	Maximize positive feelings about parenting and relieve moments of tension and doubt	Picture your most enjoyable times with your baby—nursing, falling asleep together, taking walks
Yourself taking care of your baby	Strenthen your confidence—especially in moments of confusion or frustration	Imagine yourself expertly diapering and bathing your baby
Good nursing	Stimulate milk production and the letdown reflex	Imagine the milk coming down from the outer areas of your breast to the nipple; imagine your baby nursing hungrily
The baby being calm and quiet	To help soothe the baby when it is crying or overtired	Visualize the baby feeling drowsy, surrounded by peaceful energy

baby, and can even interfere with the mother's nursing. Parents are advised to limit company to brief daytime periods for the first week and to encourage friends to come at the same time so that the whole day does not get taken up with visiting. Parents should watch for early signs of fatigue and shouldn't hesitate to postpone a scheduled visit if the mother finds herself feeling tense or tired. If a mother is in the hospital, she should feel free to turn away uninvited guests after a very brief visit.

Postpartum Exercise

Just as it's important that the new mother get enough rest in the first few days after delivery, it's also important that she get sufficient exercise, which benefits her in several ways. First, exercise is important in maintaining the mother's overall health and speeding healing. Even the healthiest person is rapidly debilitated by a few days of being immobilized. Exercise not only avoids generalized weakening of muscle and bone, it promotes healing by keeping the uterus clamped down and increasing circulation. Second, it contributes to the mother's emotional well-being (see p. 96). Exercise graphically demonstrates to her how healthy she really is and has a positive psychological effect that has been noted by athletes in training and even by psychiatrists who treat depression. Third, exercise helps a woman return to her prepregnant shape and condition as quickly as possible, as well as preparing her for subsequent pregnancies.

Most doctors and midwives have the mother up and walking within 6 to 8 hours after delivery. Although a mother may feel a little shaky or lightheaded at first, the earlier she walks the better she is likely to feel. In addition to promoting circulation and uterine tone, walking facilitates drainage of the lochia and expulsion of clots that make it harder for the uterus to remain contracted. Early ambulation also stimulates bladder and bowel tone, lowering the chances of constipation or bladder infection.

Frequent walking even helps to prevent *thrombophlebitis*, or blood clots in the veins of the legs. In the hospital nurses will check for warm, tender, or swollen veins in the mother's legs and will instruct her in leg exercises if she is unable to get up due to anesthesia or some other reason. Until a mother feels quite comfortable walking by herself, she should ask for help from her husband, her friends, or the nurses, just as she did during labor.

A group of *specific* exercises are routinely recommended after pregnancy to help the new mother regain her flat stomach and abdominal muscle tone, something that weight loss by itself cannot achieve. For most mothers this is of great psychological as well as physical importance. Strengthening the abdominal muscles is also essential to preventing backache and back problems in later pregnancies. The abdominal muscles support the uterus and keep it from protruding, which in turn keeps the mother's spine from curving forward and creating back conditions.

Postpartum exercises are particularly important for mothers over thirty-five, especially if they have been pregnant before, because they are often not as physically fit as younger mothers. Exercise physiologists believe that older mothers in poor condition are the ones most likely to feel that the pregnancy takes a lot out of them, not because of their age but because of their physical condition.

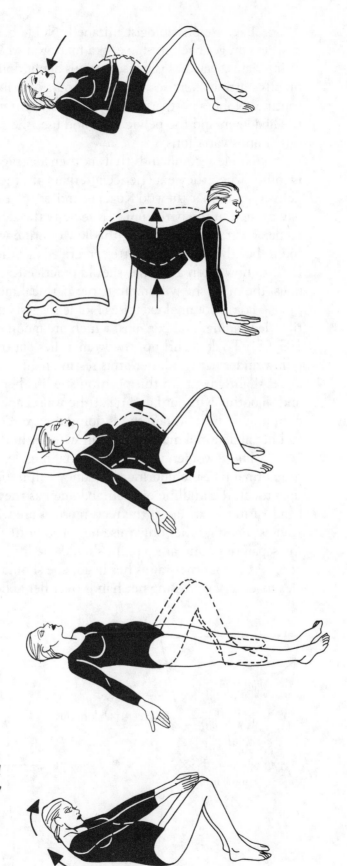

Deep breathing, pelvic tilts, leg slides, and curl-ups are now recommended for keeping fit after birth as well as during pregnancy (p. 100). These exercises are essential in returning a mother's body to its prepregnant condition, particularly if she has had several children or does not get much exercise.

Exercise physiologist Elizabeth Noble believes that a new mother can get back in shape in a matter of weeks if she begins exercising right away and is conscientious about doing it. Noble recommends starting exercises within 24 hours of delivery. Like her prenatal routine, Noble's postpartum regimen concentrates on the muscles of the abdomen and the pelvic floor and uses the same exercises with only minor variations.

Noble recommends that mothers massage their uterus when it is soft or when they experience afterpains in the first few days after delivery, and that they do Kegel exercises (p. 102) at least 20 times a day to tighten the perineum. To review, the sensation of a Kegel can be demonstrated by stopping the flow of urine while going to the bathroom, but the exercise is better practiced at other times. There is no limit to how often a mother should practice Kegels—the more she does, the more she will improve her perineal muscle tone.

For abdominal exercises Noble suggests deep breathing, pelvic tilts, leg sliding, and curl-ups, which are modified sit-ups (pp. 103–05). To do a curl-up, the woman lies flat on her back without a pillow under her head, her arms resting lightly at her sides and her knees slightly bent. In this position she lifts her head and neck slowly and smoothly without bending at the waist, and tries to touch her chin to her chest. When she is doing the exercise correctly, she will feel her abdominal muscles tighten without hurting.

Those women whose abdominal muscles have separated beyond the normal half-inch during pregnancy will notice the separation if they touch the midline of their abdomen as they begin to raise their head during a curl-up. If the recti muscles are widely separated, Noble advises that a mother only raise her head until she can begin to feel the separation, and at no point should she lift her shoulders off the floor. As the mother raises her head, she should actually pull the muscles together by crossing her hands over her abdomen. This exercise

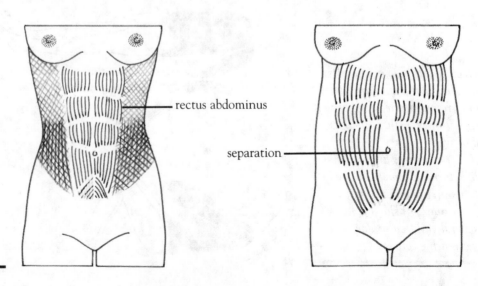

The rectus abdominus, the two broad muscle bands that run from the rib cage to the pubic bone, sometimes become separated during pregnancy. Special abdominal exercises are needed to bring them together again after delivery and restore good muscle tone.

rectus abdominus

separation

should be done up to 50 times a day, but not more than 10 times an hour. If a woman conscientiously performs these modified curl-ups as well as other abdominal exercises, the separation should close within a week or two. Once the muscles have come together, the mother can go on to regular curl-ups.

As soon as possible, the mother should venture outdoors and begin to increase the length of her walks steadily. Generally the baby can accompany her, either in a front pack, carriage, or stroller. Doctors and midwives do not advise, however, that a mother do any kind of stressful exercise during the first several weeks after delivery. Housework that requires bending and stretching should be taken on gradually so as to avoid strain or fatigue. By about two weeks after birth most mothers can begin a complete exercise regimen (p. 100), but it should not be attempted before then.

Postpartum Sex

Women vary widely in their individual responses to sex in the weeks and months after delivery, but certain physiological changes are characteristic following childbirth. Just as there are typical hormonal patterns during pregnancy, there are typical ones in this period too. Regardless of whether or not they breast-feed, all women are *anovulatory* for some time after childbirth, that is, they do not ovulate or menstruate. Breast-feeding tends to extend the immediate postpartum pattern, because the high levels of prolactin that accompany nursing tend to block the pituitary's role in ovulation (see p. 33).

Whether or not a mother nurses, it is impossible to predict the point at which she will begin ovulating and menstruating again. While some mothers do not ovulate until they stop nursing, up to several years after delivery, others begin ovulating as early as 49 days after delivery if they are nursing or 33 days after delivery if they aren't breast-feeding or don't nurse at all feedings. Pregnancy can occur as soon as a woman starts ovulating again.

After delivery the high levels of estrogen that were maintained during pregnancy drop precipitously to below normal. As a result, the vagina neither lubricates very well nor engorges easily, regardless of whether a woman has had a cesarean or a vaginal birth. In the latter case the vagina takes several weeks to recover from the physical changes that took place during the baby's passage through the birth canal. Mothers who have had episiotomies or tears may have anxiety or discomfort from their stitches, and mothers who have had a cesarean have a major abdominal incision to heal. All these factors tend to diminish a new mother's enjoyment of sex. Moreover, women who nurse find it a very sensual experience that sometimes takes the edge off their sexual interest in the early postpartum weeks, particularly in comparison with the peak of sexual arousal they may have enjoyed during the second trimester of pregnancy.

In addition to physiological reasons for decreased sexuality, there are a number of social and emotional factors that may affect a mother's sexual interest. Both parents are often tired and taken up with the tasks of caring for a new baby. The presence of overnight guests or helpers who are not usually part of the family may prove a further distraction. Taken together, these factors often lead to sexual difficulties, or at least adjustments, for couples in the first postpartum weeks.

Most doctors and midwives advise that new mothers abstain from sexual relations for 2 or 3 weeks or until the vagina and uterus have completely healed. Doctors used to advise 6 weeks of abstinence, but shortened this recommendation because so many couples were having sex earlier without contraception. Now practitioners generally speak to mothers about contraception before their follow-up visit. By itself, breast-feeding does not constitute birth control except on a poor statistical basis, especially in Western industrialized countries, possibly because the women may be better nourished. Among nursing mothers who don't use other forms of birth control, 8 percent get pregnant *before* they have a period and 36 percent get pregnant while they are still breast-feeding but their periods have resumed.

Until the follow-up visit at 4 to 6 weeks, most doctors and midwives advise that couples use condoms or foam. If a mother uses a diaphragm, her practitioner will check it at the postpartum visit and advise her if she needs a different size due to changes in the reproductive organs caused by childbirth. Birth control pills are not recommended for nursing mothers because they can decrease milk supply and the hormones pass over to the baby in the milk. A mother who wants to use birth control pills and is not nursing will be started on pills about 4 weeks after delivery. If a woman chooses an IUD for birth control, it will be inserted between 4 to 8 weeks after delivery.

Although some mothers remain relatively uninterested in sex for several months, others find that their interest resumes as soon as they have gotten over the initial period of healing, fatigue, and learning to care for the baby. At that point women usually find that the greatest negative aspect to intercourse is physical discomfort or the fear of it. Elizabeth Bing, a childbirth educator who has written on sexuality during and after pregnancy, suggests that the new mother should initially assume a position on top so that she can control her partner's depth of entry. Bing also points out that the man needs to be very gentle and that both partners must realize that the woman will probably take much longer to become engorged and aroused, and may experience very different sensations than before. Bing recommends that the mother practice Kegels frequently, including during sex, to help get back good muscle tone in the vagina and pelvic floor. Many women

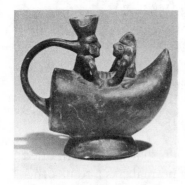

Although some new mothers resume their interest in sex within a few weeks, others find they are content to simply share a physical closeness with their mate. Vessel, Peru. The Fine Arts Museum of San Francisco. Gift of Mr. Drew Chidester.

find their breasts are very erogenous after birth, particularly if they are nursing, although some women have a sense that their breasts should only be handled or suckled by the baby. In order for both partners to enjoy sex, it is likely that they will have to vary their normal routines. Such adjustments are best accomplished when the couple communicate with each other very frankly and accept those changes they cannot control.

Postpartum Emotions

Having a baby is an emotional event as well as a physical occurrence for the mother and father. For many parents birth is a pinnacle unmatched by any other experience in their lives. As with any profound experience, the main participants become totally immersed in a situation that involves great expectations, energy, and concentration.

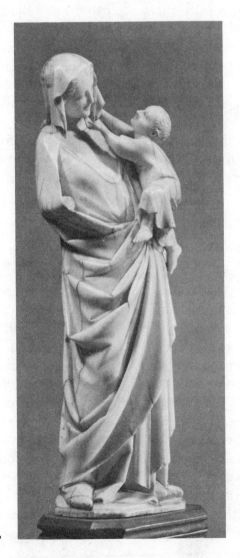

The new mother has a sudden sense of being connected with the elemental forces of life; everyday events take on a new radiance and poignancy. Virgin and Child, French, 1260. The Metropolitan Museum of Art. Gift of J. Pierpont Morgan.

The situation is sharpened and intensified by the fact that the exact outcome can be predicted by neither science nor intuition. Even if birth takes place exactly as the parents have wished for, it still comes as something of a surprise.

This sense of surprise, combined with the sudden all-encompassing needs of the baby, tends to alter dramatically the parents' habits and ways of viewing the world. Faced with so many new situations, parents find themselves relying more on intuition and the advice of others than on logic or knowledge. For most adults these circumstances change their perception of the world, and even the smallest details take on new significance and poignance.

Life becomes redefined in terms of the baby, and the mother's and father's new roles as parents. Suddenly they feel a profound continuity with the whole of life, its endings as well as its beginnings. The baby is born, and the parents are reborn, giving up the child within and becoming parent to themselves as much as the baby. For many people the birth of a child brings a sense of connectedness with other generations, with their own parents as well as with their new baby.

In the first days after delivery most parents are excited and terribly happy. They are grateful for how well things have gone and proud of both the baby and themselves. They want to share the momentous event with everyone and show off the baby. For days the mother and father will recount the story of the birth to family and friends, recalling the difficult parts, the easy parts, and the unexpected parts. In this way they will relive all the circumstances, savoring the wonderful moments and making sense of those that were unsatisfactory or passed too quickly.

DEALING WITH FEELINGS OF DISAPPOINTMENT

All parents dream of a perfect, healthy baby and an easy, ecstatic delivery. Most parents also hope for an all-encompassing bond with a placid, beautiful baby. In a word, they expect to experience instantaneous love, unmarred by any disturbing realities. Whether such expectations are met depends upon how labor and delivery proceed, upon the baby itself, and upon the parents' outlook.

If the labor or delivery was long or difficult, or if an unplanned c-section had to be performed, the mother and father often have feelings of disappointment, failure, guilt, or anger. If the mother anticipated a brief, easy birth and was surprised by what happened, she may feel that she was at fault for not having performed better, or she may even blame the baby. Sometimes new parents feel that the hospital, the practitioner, or the nursing staff has cheated them of the kind of delivery they were expecting. Parents' feelings of dissatisfaction with their delivery experience may or may not be justified from a lay or medical point of view, but the emotions are valid, and they are neither unnatural nor uncommon after a delivery that is less than ideal.

It's important that the mother and father talk between themselves and with others about their feelings. Avoiding these issues only creates problems in the mother-baby and mother-father relationships. By bringing negative feelings out in the open, parents help to defuse them and elicit support and reassurance. Discussing the birth experience with their practitioner or even with knowledgeable friends can often correct misinformation or misconceptions that parents have about the delivery. Understanding the correct and complete reasons for events may dispel lingering feelings of anger and guilt. When parents realize that they are not alone in their feelings and that generally no one is really to blame, they are freed to direct all their energy and attention to the baby.

It is only normal for some parents to feel disappointment with a situation so long awaited and so laden with expectations. Parents should not blame themselves for current medical treatments that are largely out of their control. Neither is there any point in blaming themselves for who they are or the way they react to situations. These factors are a result of lifelong conditioning, and they are unlikely to change during the course of labor and delivery.

Just as the delivery may not have lived up to the parents' expectations, sometimes the baby does not match the image the parents have held throughout the pregnancy either. The most common reason for disappointment with the baby is, of course, its sex. Some parents have their hearts set on a girl, others on a boy. There are many reasons for these feelings, and as with any other sentiment, they have validity of their own. Since there is no changing the sex of the baby, acceptance becomes the goal. In time, love for the baby tends to reconcile most parents' feelings of sadness.

The second most common disappointment with the baby has to do with looks. The newborn's appearance sometimes comes as a great shock to parents, especially with a first baby. Newborn babies do not look like ones in magazines or movies; those babies are usually several weeks to several months old. Babies are actually red and wrinkly just after birth. Their heads are likely to be molded and their skin may have one of many rashes common to newborns (see p. 461). Moreover, parents sometimes find themselves disconcerted because the baby seems so fretful or so unresponsive. Such disappointments frequently are due to lack of knowledge about what newborns are really like. All too often parents have not had much exposure to infants who are only a few days old, and childbirth classes sometimes inadvertently foster this ignorance by focusing on labor and delivery, to the exclusion of newborn information. Once again, frank discussions with medical personnel or experienced mothers will help reassure the new parent.

For most mothers and fathers there is so much joy in the birth of the baby that they are able to handle and accept any of their expectations not being met. The relief of knowing the outcome of delivery is so great, and the reality of the baby is so powerful, that most parents leave the past behind and look to the future with anticipation.

CAUSES OF THE BABY BLUES

Emotions tend to run high in the days following delivery, but eventually the joy, relief, and excitement of the moments just after birth give way to the realities of everyday life and the inevitable problems, adjustments, and fatigue of the first week. Very often around the third day the new mother experiences a sense of emotional letdown. This phenomenon, known as the *postpartum* or *after-baby blues*, has been observed for many years by doctors, midwives, and mothers themselves, both in Europe and America. Its frequency has been estimated at between 50 and 80 percent of new mothers. Typically it occurs between the second and sixth day after birth, with a peak around the third or whenever the mother goes home from the hospital. Baby blues can involve extreme sensitivity, rapid and frequent mood swings, or just sadness, crying, and depression.

Doctors still don't know the exact cause of postpartum blues, but a number of theories have been set forth. Some doctors believe they are the result of the tremendous hormonal changes taking place as the mother's body readjusts to a nonpregnant state (see p. 411). Others think they can be accredited to physiological factors such as fatigue or discomfort from perineal pain or breast engorgement. Still others believe that the blues are caused by emotional or psychological factors such as fears, anxieties, or guilt surrounding the new parental role. Finally, there are theories that attribute the blues to sociological-environmental factors resulting from hospital routines. Most doctors and midwives believe that the after-baby blues are the result of a combination of factors. More importantly, they do not dismiss them as insignificant but think that the mother's feelings should be dealt with in order to help her achieve a truly positive relationship with her new baby in the first weeks.

As we have discussed, during the first several days after delivery, mothers' estrogen and progesterone levels drop off sharply, while the nursing hormones prolactin and oxytocin rise dramatically (see p. 411). There is no question that these hormonal changes also have effects on women's moods and emotions. Other physiological changes after birth are less universal than hormonal changes, and they vary more in intensity, but the majority of women experience some of them. It is only common sense that physical discomforts like perineal pain, breast engorgement, afterpains, and constipation will lessen the mother's enthusiasm to some extent. In particular, breast engorgement and afterpains can affect the mother's nursing and the mood of her

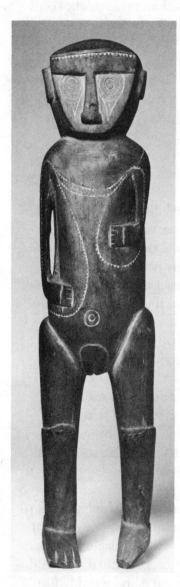

Sometimes around the third day postpartum, the mother experiences a sense of emotional letdown in response to fatigue and the new responsibilities of everyday life. Female figure, Admiralty Island, Melanesia. The Fine Arts Museum of San Francisco, California Midwinter International Exposition.

interactions with the baby. It's probably not a coincidence that baby blues peak on the third day, which is the most common time for the mother's breasts to become engorged with milk. Fatigue is another physiological cause of depression, and its effects cannot be underestimated in evaluating the mother's feelings. Fatigue not only dampens the mother's mood and her sense of humor, it tends to accentuate any physical discomforts she may have.

Psychological factors that affect postpartum depression vary from mother to mother, but they are quite common. Especially with the first baby, many mothers can feel overwhelmed at times by the physical, emotional, and mental demands of their new role and may even yearn for the "simplicity" of being pregnant. By comparison, during pregnancy a mother has relatively few responsibilities, yet she receives a great deal of attention. Then during labor and delivery she is the cental participant in a demanding endeavor. But after birth much of the attention shifts from the mother to the baby, and some mothers feel a sense of anticlimax once the challenge of delivery is over. As the baby's presence becomes a reality, many mothers realize somewhat wistfully that they no longer have as much control over their own schedule and for some time will constantly be at the beck and call of the tiny creature they've given birth to. This point may be particularly upsetting for mothers who have worked right up until delivery.

In addition to all the physical and social changes of the postpartum period, new mothers have a number of skills to master. In particular, they may find themselves anxious and clumsy about performing new tasks like nursing, bathing, or diapering, and they may be chagrined to find that a nurse or their husband is more adept at caring for or soothing the baby. During the first several weeks mothers may regret how little attention they paid to friends with babies or to the child-care instructions in their prenatal classes. Obviously it's not just the diapering or nursing; it's the whole situation. Caring for a new baby is a classic example of a life event that is positive and sought after but is highly stressful in that it requires tremendous adaptation and change that cannot be totally anticipated or prepared for.

The most recent theories about the baby blues speculate that much can be attributed to specific social factors. Hospital routines often separate the mother from the baby and interfere with her natural efforts to bond with the baby. This in itself can be upsetting, because most mothers feel an innate need to hold and touch their babies. In addition, the hospital is an unfamiliar environment that controls when the mother wakes, when and what she eats, and even when she can have visitors. While some mothers react well to enforced rest and lack of responsibility and find the nursing care supportive, others are disturbed by these restrictions. Mothers who enjoy the care and security of the hospital may be upset at first being home alone with their baby.

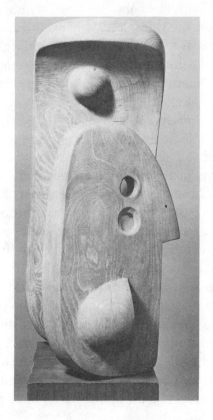

As the mother becomes skill-ful at caring for the newborn and her energy returns, her confidence and optimism will reassert themselves. Mother and Child, *Henry Moore, 1938. Elm wood, 30⅜" x 13⅞" x 15½". Collection, The Museum of Modern Art, New York. Acquired through the Lillie P. Bliss Bequest.*

Having washed, diapered, and nursed the baby, a woman may find herself wondering what she's supposed to do next. Is she to "play" with the baby, is she to do some baby-related task, or is she to begin to pick up the threads of her own life apart from the baby and her husband. The new mother may well experience poignant questions about her own identity amid all the new roles she is playing.

DEALING WITH THE BABY BLUES

The keys to alleviating the baby blues are discussion, information, emotional support, and physical help. The natural tendency is for new mothers to hide their feelings if they are depressed. This is in the nature of depression, and it is intensified by the sense that this should be a happy time and that they should be able to cope with the situation. However, such thoughts are not helpful to themselves or the baby.

The great majority of new mothers feel down or blue at some time or another. Doctors and midwives who deal with this situation all the time are not surprised by these feelings and are generally very supportive. The first step is for the mother to become aware of her feelings and to share them with her family, friends, or practitioner. If a mother's problems are very severe or last more than a few weeks, she should seek professional help.

Because people who are depressed tend to withdraw, it's very important that the father, family members, and friends attend to the mother's moods and draw her out. Not only will talking with the mother help clear up points of misinformation, it will bring forth warmth, reassurance, and help from the people she is close to.

Situations that are problematic for the new mother should be solved one by one. Probably at no other time is the resolution of small problems so meaningful. Each solution, however minor, will contribute to the mother's sense of competence, control, and well-being. In dealing with feelings of emotional letdown, the mother can make good use of the relaxation and visualization skills that she learned during pregnancy (p. 159). Simply relaxing will tend to diminish a mother's anxiety and will help her view her concerns and problems in a more optimistic light. A relaxed state is ideal for getting in touch with her feelings and for becoming more aware of both her positive and negative visualizations about motherhood. As we've discussed earlier, relaxation and support are the two factors research has shown to be most useful in dealing with stressful life situations. The overwhelming majority of intense mood dips that new mothers experience respond readily to attention and concern.

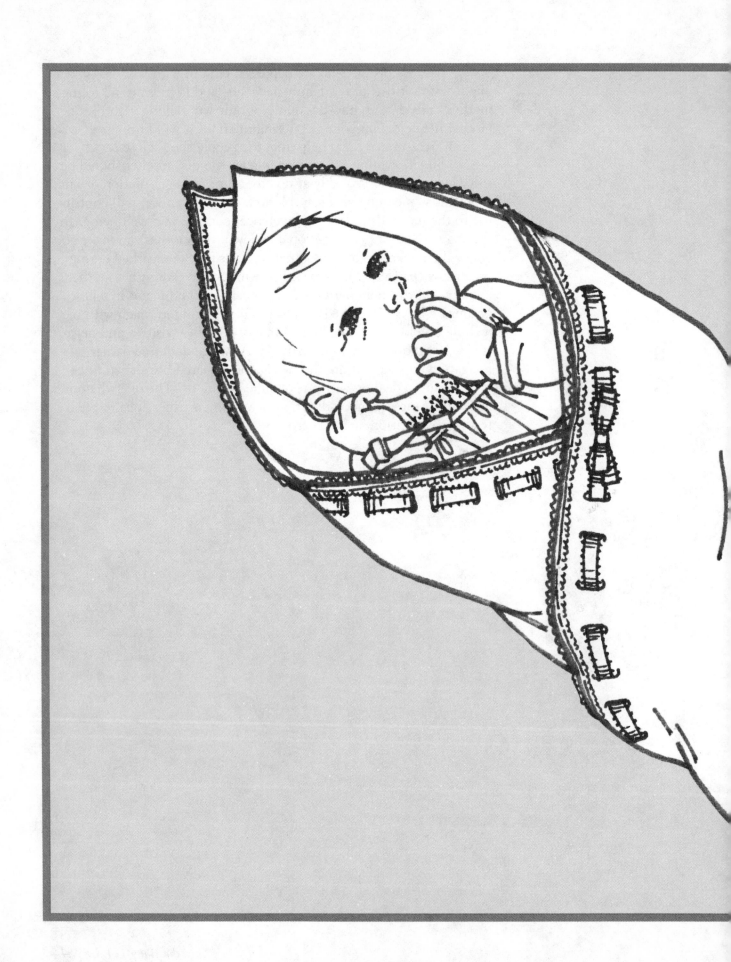

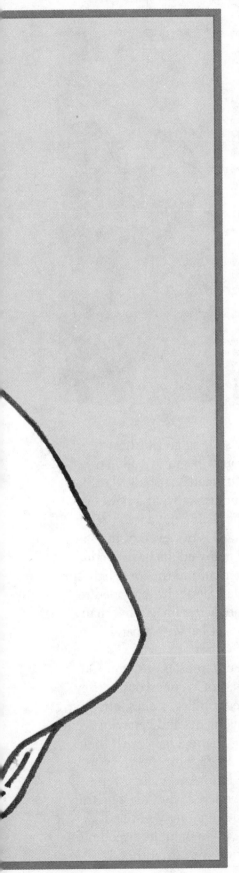

CHAPTER 20

The Newborn

The Newborn's Presence

The newborn is a magical and powerful creature who inevitably compels attention and elicits an intense emotional response. Parents are awed by the baby's perfection and by the realization of how little they did consciously to bring about such a miracle. A newborn brings everyone face to face with natural forces that have been at work for millions of years and that will persist long after we are gone. In this sense a baby represents a spiritual gift, a rebirth that profoundly reconnects us with the most fundamental issues of life. Paradoxically, the birth of a baby brings us in contact with dying as well as living, for we realize intuitively that beginnings imply endings and that all great undertakings involve risks. So there is an innate seriousness that deepens our sense of joy and our wonder.

The anticipation surrounding the baby's emergence and the awe inspired by the mother's efforts during delivery induce a heightened state of consciousness in all those who have participated in the experience. For the new parents, the baby's presence and this heightened awareness help sever the ties with pregnancy and enable them to become immersed in the concerns and activities of their new roles.

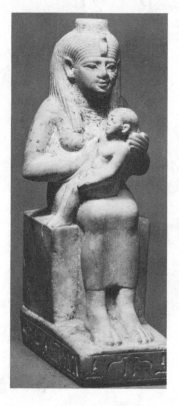 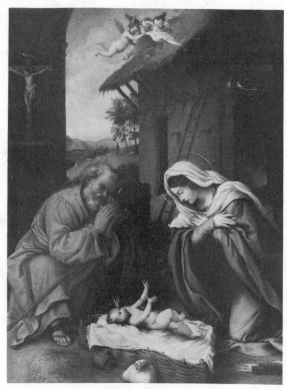 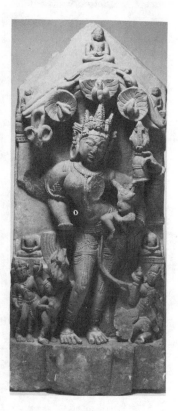

In all cultures and religions the newborn has inspired a sense of wonder and reverence because of its perfection and vulnerability.

Isis and Child Horus, Egyptian. The Metropolitan Museum of Art. Rogers Fund.

The Nativity, *Lorenzo Lotto, 1523. National Gallery of Art, Washington. Samuel H. Kress Collection.*

Ambika, The Universal Mother Goddess, Indian, 11th century. Asian Art Museum of San Francisco. Avery Brundage Collection.

Parents await their baby's arrival for so long and with such intensity that they consciously or unconsciously begin to build an image of what the baby will look like. Pediatrician Marshall Klaus believes that all parents have an idealized picture of what a newborn looks like, and that very often they find that their baby doesn't resemble the one they have visualized—and perhaps is not even of the same sex. One reason for this discrepancy is that many adults have spent little or no time with a newborn baby. In our culture the low birth rate and the geographic dispersion of the extended family have tended to isolate adults from newborns. As already noted, the image that many people have of newborns is based on pictures of babies who are actually several months old.

Real babies are very different from our fantasies of them. On one hand, they are shiny, smooth, and new, but incongruously, they are also ancient-looking creatures who have wrinkles, rashes, and hair in places we don't expect it. Even their movements and behavior seem strange at first. For some parents reconciling the real baby with their ideal takes several days. This process is aided by forming as clear an idea as possible of what newborns are really like. Also most parents have had moments of anxiety when they wondered whether something about their baby was normal, but such worries are rarely justified. A detailed description of the newborn can be very helpful in dispelling unnecessary concerns and easing the transition into parenthood.

In the newborn we see natural forces that have been at work for millions of years. Star Baby, *photo by Michael Samuels.*

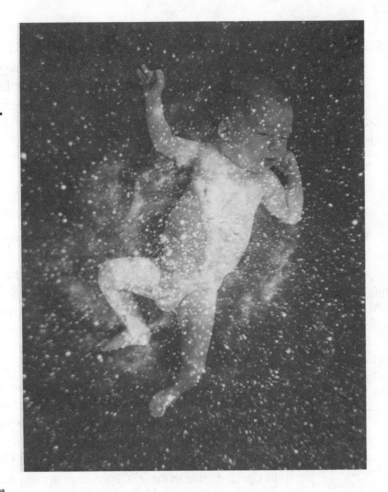

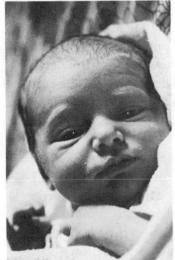

Real babies are different from our visualizations: they have wrinkles, rashes, and hair where we don't expect it. Photo by Michael Samuels.

Newborn Size and Proportions

On the average, newborns range from 18 to 22 inches in length (45 to 55 centimeters) and weigh between 5 pounds 8 ounces and 8 pounds 13 ounces. Babies who are above or below these standards are considered *small* or *large for their gestational age (SGA or LGA)*. Both the baby's length and weight are strongly influenced by its gestational age as well as by the genes it inherits, so the birth weight and height are not always reliable indicators of the baby's growth pattern or adult size.

The newborn's proportions are unique. In comparison with toddlers, adolescents, or adults, the newborn's head seems disproportionately large in relation to the rest of its body. At birth the baby's head averages 13 to 14 inches (33 to 35 centimeters) in circumference, which is slightly larger than its chest. In terms of height, the baby's head accounts for a quarter of its overall length, whereas in an adult this ratio drops to about a tenth. The midpoint of a baby's body is also very different from an adult's. Whereas the center of an adult's body lies at about the level of the pubic bone, the center of a baby's body is slightly above its navel.

During pregnancy human development focuses on the growth

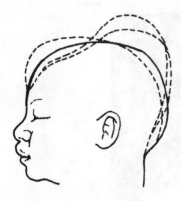

During a vaginal delivery the baby's head often becomes molded when the forces of labor and delivery cause the bones of the skull to override one another at the suture lines. Such molding can take several common shapes, as shown by the dotted lines. It normally disappears within several days after birth.

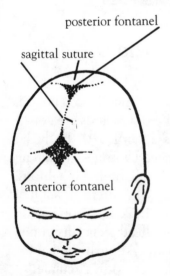

The two soft spots on the top of the newborn's head are called the anterior *and posterior fontanels.* At the soft spots the bony plates of the skull are connected with fibrous tissue.*

and refinement of the brain, as opposed to the muscles and bones of the trunk and limbs. The result of having such a well-developed brain is that humans are capable of incredibly complex behavior and thought. However, having such a relatively large head and small body means that a baby cannot get around by itself for many months and is much more dependent on its parents than are most other animals.

The Head

Just after delivery the newborn's head is often quite *molded,* that is, the pressure of the birth canal has caused the bones of the skull to override one another where they meet at the suture lines, making the baby's head appear quite pointed (see p. 294). Depending on the amount of molding, the suture lines may feel bumpy (overridden), flat, or slightly depressed (open between the plates). Such molding is quite normal, especially with first vaginal deliveries or with long labors in which the baby's head was engaged in the birth canal for some time. These effects disappear gradually over a period of several days.

The baby's *front* or *anterior fontanel* normally varies from 1 to 5 centimeters in diameter, while the *rear* or *posterior fontanel* is less than 1 centimeter. The fontanels are frequently referred to as *soft spots* because they are not hard like the rest of the skull. When the baby is held upright, the front soft spot may appear sunken or depressed, which is most noticeable in newborns with little hair. Often the front fontanel visibly pulses with the baby's heartbeat. There is no danger in touching or stroking the fontanels, although young children obviously have to be taught not to poke at this mysterious feature of the new baby. If the baby's head has been strongly molded, the front fontanel is likely to become slightly larger as the molding disappears. The rear fontanel closes by about 4 months, the front one sometime between 9 and 18 months.

In addition to molding, babies' heads sometimes show swelling of the soft tissues of the scalp after delivery. This condition, which is called *caput succedaneum,* from the Latin words for substitute or second head, tends to be more common after a long labor. It is due to pressure from the mother's cervix and is therefore greatest on the area of the baby's head that presented first. Generally it disappears within 48 hours.

A much less common kind of scalp swelling, called a *cephalohematoma,* is due to bleeding under the skin, like a bruise. It occurs when the presenting part of the head bumps against the bones of the mother's pelvis during labor. A cephalohematoma may not be apparent for several hours after birth and often doesn't reach a peak until the second or third day. No treatment is necessary, as the baby's body

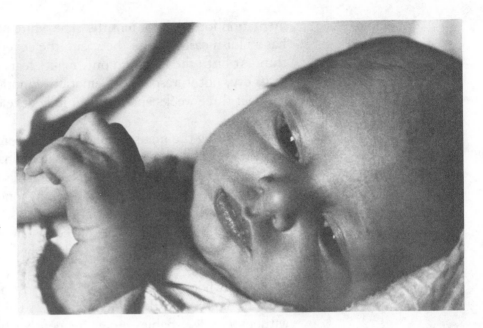

The shape and proportions of the newborn's face and eyes instinctively invite the care and attention of adults. Photo by Michael Samuels.

naturally reabsorbs the blood within 2 to 12 weeks, the average time being about 6 weeks. Finally, if a baby has had a fetal scalp monitor, it will have a red mark where the electrode was inserted and possibly some swelling around the site.

The shape and proportions of the newborn's face instinctively draw the attention of parents and other adults. A study in which adults were shown sketches of babies with varying facial proportions found that certain features commonly elicit the most nurturing responses. Interestingly, the features that drew the greatest response were those of the typical newborn: round face, chubby cheeks, large forehead, small mouth, and wide-set eyes.

Occasionally a baby's face will be swollen right after delivery, especially if it presented face-first. A newborn's face also may appear somewhat asymmetrical if the baby lay in utero with one shoulder pressed against its jaw. Since newborns often assume the same position that they spent the most time in before birth, the baby with facial asymmetry may choose to lie with its shoulder once again tucked under its jaw. Such asymmetry corrects itself in a matter of weeks or months.

For many people the most striking feature of the newborn is its eyes, probably because they are already three-quarters of their adult size. During the first hour or so after birth the baby's eyes will remain wide open and staring if the light in the room is dim. This alert quality, which is the result of the newborn's remarkable visual ability, plays an important part in the bonding process (see pp. 463 and 466–67).

Babies who have darker skins can show their true eye color within weeks, but fair-skinned babies may not develop their final pigmentation for weeks or months. The white part of all newborns' eyes has a bluish cast because the *sclera*, the covering of the eye, is still thin. At birth the newborn only makes tears in response to a particle in its eye, not in response to emotion. Emotional tearing first appears at about three weeks and does not fully develop until two or three months.

During the first several days of life some newborns develop swollen eyelids and tearing or a puslike discharge. This inflammation of the eyes, called *conjunctivitis,* is often a result of silver nitrate, a medicine used to prevent blindness from gonorrhea (see bonding chart, p. 472). It usually goes away within several days and does not need to be treated. Where permitted by law, erythromycin ointment is often substituted for silver nitrate drops because it is less irritating to the baby's eyes.

Newborns are nose-breathers by instinct, as they must be in order to nurse or bottle-feed. Their noses tend to be flat, broad, and without a bridge. Babies sneeze frequently when they need to clear their nose and become quite agitated if they have to resort to mouth breathing, especially during a feeding. If a newborn cannot clear its nose by sneezing, as occasionally happens, it will be more comfortable if the mucus is gently and carefully cleared away with a tissue, a cotton swab, or with gentle suction from a bulb syringe.

Babies' mouths are tiny but exquisitely formed and already reveal their adult shape. From birth, babies' mouths are highly mobile and can assume a number of different positions. Often in the first few days after birth babies develop sucking blisters, because their lips are not used to the pressures of nursing or bottle-feeding. The baby's gums and palate may also be dotted with tiny white nodules called *Epstein's pearls,* which disappear within a few weeks. On rare occasions babies are actually born with soft loose teeth, which will be removed so that the baby cannot choke on them. The newborn's tongue appears to be quite large and is more tightly attached at the base than an adult's. Extra fat pads stiffen the cheeks and upper lip and aid the baby in nursing. These fat pads disappear when the "suckling days" are over, as one of the major pediatric texts observes.

The baby's ears tend to be relatively large but, like those of adults, vary greatly in size and shape. The amount of cartilage in the newborn ear is one of the indicators used by doctors to establish gestational age. Newborns' necks are rather short and thick, which is a great help in holding up their ponderously heavy heads. For an adult it would be like having a head the size and weight of a large watermelon. Despite the sturdiness of their necks, most babies do not acquire really good head control for several months. Although newborns' heads tend to be wobbly in an upright position, their neck muscles are strong enough to turn their heads from side to side in order to breathe clearly when lying on their stomachs.

The Baby's First Breaths

Immediately after delivery the first and most critical task for the newborn is to begin breathing, to switch from passively receiving oxygen from the mother's blood to actively oxygenating its blood through its own lungs. At no other time in life will the baby make as profound a physiological transformation. By term the baby's body is remarkably prepared for the fundamental changes that take place in its respiratory and circulatory systems during and immediately after birth. But as parents touch and interact with their newborn in those first moments, few of them realize the extent of the baby's adjustments to its new environment. These sweeping changes are made with hardly any external indications.

During the last trimester two things happen that help to prepare the baby for breathing air (see p. 70). At around 25 weeks of gestation the tiny *air sacs* or *alveoli* in the lungs develop, and by 35 weeks the alveolar cells begin to produce a special wetting agent called *surface active material* or *surfactant*. Without this substance the walls of the alveoli tend to collapse and stick together whenever air is exhaled, and the baby must exert great force to reopen the alveoli with each breath. At term the baby produces enough surfactant to make breathing easy.

During pregnancy the air passages of the baby's lungs are filled with a special liquid called *fetal-lung fluid*. This fluid exerts great pressure on the alveoli and helps keep the tiny blood vessels in the lungs clamped down, so that very little blood flows through them. In fact, only 5 percent of the total blood volume goes to the lungs at this point, while 50 percent of the blood is in the placenta at any given time. After the baby is born these figures change radically. Late in pregnancy the baby actually makes tiny breathing motions, not inhaling the amniotic fluid as was previously thought, but shifting the fetal-lung fluid back and forth in a tidal movement. Doctors speculate that these movements are practice for the baby's first breaths of air.

In a vaginal delivery the baby's passage through the birth canal plays an important role in its first breath. Compared with an adult, the newborn's chest is barrel-shaped and very compressible, because the ribs are cartilage that has not yet calcified. This is a key factor in the events that occur right after the newborn emerges from the birth canal. The canal is so narrow that it constricts the rubbery bones of the baby's chest, squeezing out 5 to 10 milliliters of lung fluid and causing an elastic recoil as the baby's chest emerges from the vagina. The chest springs back out, sucking in enough air to fill the larger passages in the lungs, but not the alveoli.

The first half-breath is passive, but from that moment on the baby must use the muscles of its diaphragm and chest in order to breathe. Doctors are not yet certain what triggers active breathing, although there is evidence that cold, light, noise, and perhaps gravity serve to activate the brain center that controls breathing. Essentially it takes some kind of change or shock to make the baby start breathing on its own. That is why doctors and midwives used to hold newborn babies upside down and slap them on the bottom.

Another powerful stimulus to active breathing is the fact that after birth the placenta ceases to function, so the amount of oxygen in the baby's blood quickly drops and the amount of carbon dioxide rises. The change is registered in the baby's brain and signals the body to inhale. This response is greater when temperatures are cool and the baby is handled.

Once the newborn starts breathing a chain of events automatically takes place. Air forces the lungs to expand and quickly replaces most of the fetal-lung fluid. Although some fluid remains in the alveoli, the percentage of air in the lungs becomes much greater. Since air exerts far less pressure on the alveoli than did the fetal-lung fluid, the tiny blood vessels around the alveoli open and blood rushes into them in large amounts. All the baby's blood begins to pass through its lungs for the first time. The rush of blood is so sudden and so intense that it redirects much of the body's blood flow. The drop in lung pressure due to the fluid-air exchange also opens the nearby lymph vessels, and within six hours they drain virtually all the remaining fluid from the lungs.

As well as the newborn breathes, it does not breathe like an adult. Depending on whether it's crying, active, or sleeping, a healthy infant's respiratory rate fluctuates dramatically from 20 to 100 breaths per minute, the average being about 30 to 40, which is about three times the rate for an adult. Not only are a baby's lungs smaller than an adult's, initially they are less efficient. However, within an hour after birth the newborn is breathing efficiently, taking in the right amount of oxygen without any unnecessary breaths.

Babies breathe almost exclusively with the diaphragm rather than with the muscles of the chest. As a result, their stomach rises and falls much more with each breath than an adult's does. This movement is most noticeable when a baby is lying on its back. The newborn's rib cage is so soft, it sometimes drops lower than the stomach when the baby inhales. While this might be a sign of troubled breathing in an older baby, it is not abnormal for a newborn.

The Baby's Circulation

Paralleling the remarkable switch from placental oxygenation to air breathing, a series of equally incredible circulatory changes takes place after birth. While the baby is in the uterus, 50 percent of its blood is flowing throughout the vast network of blood vessels in the placenta.

After dropping off carbon dioxide and picking up fresh oxygen in the placenta, the blood returns to the baby's body through the umbilical cord. Half this incoming blood goes through the liver, and half of it bypasses the liver via a shunt called the *ductus venosus*. All the blood comes back together on the far side of the liver in the *inferior vena cava*, a large blood vessel that leads to the heart. Thus while the baby remains in the uterus, the blood coming to the heart is oxygen-rich.

Most of the blood entering the unborn baby's heart never even goes to the lungs, since the tiny capillaries are clamped down. Moreover, a large hole called the *foramen ovale* connects the two chambers at the top of the baby's heart and allows 90 percent of the entering blood to flow directly across to the left upper chamber of the heart. From there the blood passes into the bottom left chamber and is pumped out through the aorta. The 10 percent of the blood that does not go through the foramen ovale passes from the upper right chamber to the lower right chamber. From there a small amount of it goes to the lungs, but most is shunted through a vessel called the *ductus arteriosus*, which bypasses the lungs and empties into the aorta on the far side of the heart. Half of all the blood passing through the aorta goes out to the baby's body, while half goes directly back to the placenta to be reoxygenated.

Several of the structures just described are unique to the baby's circulatory system before birth: the artery and vein in the umbilical cord; the foramen ovale, the hole between the heart's upper chambers; and the two shunts, the ductus venosus that bypasses the liver and the ductus arteriosus that bypasses the lungs. These structures help complete the loop of the developing baby's utero-placental circulation. Once the baby is born and makes the shift to getting oxygen through its lungs, these structures are no longer needed and undergo radical changes in shape and function. Of all the miraculous changes that take place around the time of birth, these are the most profound.

Almost immediately after birth, as the newborn takes its first breaths, momentous changes start to occur within its circulatory system. As described earlier, the tiny capillaries in the baby's lungs suddenly open and large quantities of blood from the heart start flowing through them. At the same time the blood vessels in the umbilical cord clamp down quickly and vigorously due to a combination of increased oxygen from the lungs and the stretching of the cord. Interestingly, the umbilical artery that carries blood away from the baby to the placenta shuts down much more rapidly than the umbilical vein that carries blood from the placenta back to the baby. As a result, the placenta is efficiently drained and the blood passes into the baby's body, a process that is referred to as the *placental transfusion*. It is aided by uterine contractions, which simultaneously expel the placenta. Because of the transfusion effect, doctors and midwives wait several minutes after delivery until the umbilical cord stops pulsating before it

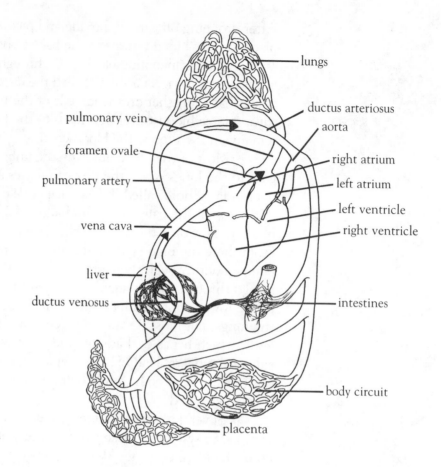

(a) While the baby is in the uterus it gets its oxygen and food through the placenta. The baby's blood flows from the placenta through the umbilical cord into the body. It reaches the heart either by going through the liver or the ductus venosus, a bypass around the liver. Instead of going to the lungs, the blood passes through the heart via a large hole called the fora-men ovale, *and then goes directly to the aorta or to the* ductus arteriosus, *a temporary shunt that connects to the aorta.*

a

lungs

pulmonary vein

foramen ovale

pulmonary artery

ductus arteriosus

aorta

right atrium

left atrium

left ventricle

right ventricle

vena cava

liver

ductus venosus

intestines

body circuit

placenta

is cut. This delay ensures that the newborn gets an average of 1½ cups of additional blood from the placenta.

With the placental circuit shut down, several other things happen to the baby's circulation. First, pressure rises in the arteries leading away from the heart, because the blood no longer travels the long distance through the placenta. Second, large quantities of blood returning from the lungs now pour into the upper left chamber, raising the pressure here as well. At the same time pressure drops in the upper right chamber, because large amounts of blood are no longer returning from the placenta. This combination of high pressure in the left upper chamber and low pressure in the right causes a large flap that is attached on the left side of the heart to slip across and cover the hole between the two chambers. This change takes place within minutes after the baby is born. Initially the pressure difference holds the flap or valve in place across the foramen ovale. Over a period of months or years, the valve actually becomes adhered to the middle wall of the heart, much as a cut heals, which is quite remarkable because this is not a cut and no other tissues in the heart stick together.

Once all the baby's blood is circulating through its lungs, the bypass called the ductus arteriosus is no longer necessary to shunt blood directly into the aorta. The force of blood pumping out of the

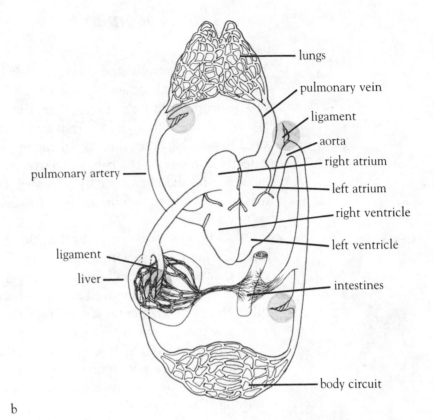

lungs

pulmonary vein

ligament

aorta

right atrium

left atrium

right ventricle

left ventricle

pulmonary artery

ligament

liver

intestines

body circuit

b

(b) Immediately after birth, blood vessels in the baby's lungs open, while those in the umbilical cord close down. At the same time a flap closes off the foramen ovale and the hole in the heart, and both shunts close off. Thus the newborn rapidly switches from being dependent on the placenta to oxygenating its own blood.

heart is now so great that some blood begins to flow backward through the shunt. At this point the ductus arteriosus starts to clamp down, much as the umbilical blood vessels did. This effect is due to the high oxygen content of the blood and to a special substance produced by the lungs. Closure starts within hours after delivery and is complete in about 24 hours. Within ten days or so after birth the ductus arteriosus shrivels and turns into a nonfunctional ligament, a tough fibrous band.

Meanwhile a clamping-down effect also takes place in the ductus venosus that was a bypass around the liver. With blood not circulating through the placenta, the ductus venosus is no longer needed. Unlike the ductus arteriosus, the liver bypass shuts down by itself. It too turns into a ligament, as do most of the umbilical blood vessels.

Thus within days of delivery the baby establishes a radically altered circulation system that is structurally like an adult's. But like the newborn's respiratory system, the circulatory system is much more labile than an adult's. The newborn's pulse varies widely, from 70 beats per minute when it is sleeping quietly to 180 when it is very active, but it averages around 120 to 160. Occasionally the heart may even skip a beat when the baby defecates or is startled, for instance. In the first hours after birth almost all babies have unusual heart sounds, called *murmurs*, due to the normal reversal of blood flow in the ductus arteriosus. These murmurs rarely indicate anything abnormal, and as the days and weeks go by the baby's heart begins to beat more and more steadily.

The Abdomen

Along with its barrel-shape chest, the newborn has an unusually large and protuberant abdomen because its abdominal muscles are not yet well developed. As we've said earlier, the baby breathes largely from its diaphragm, so its abdomen rises and falls with each breath. Compared to an adult, the rise and fall can appear quite dramatic, but it's perfectly normal. As the baby's digestive system fills with food and air, the size of its abdomen actually increases. Bowel sounds can be heard in as little as one to two hours after delivery, showing that digestion has already begun.

When the baby's umbilical cord is cut, it is clamped a short distance from the base with a plastic clip. The stub of cord beyond the clamp quickly dries up and turns leathery due to lack of blood flow. The clamp should be removed about 24 hours after birth. If the baby is still in the hospital, the nurses will take the clamp off; if the baby is at home, the parents can do it themselves.

After 5 to 10 days the remnant of the cord eventually falls off by itself. The process of separating is normally aided by bacterial action, which may give the cord a somewhat rotten odor shortly before it falls off. Parents should not tug at the cord or try to speed up its separation but should simply clean around the base of the cord daily with cotton applicators dipped in water, peroxide, or alcohol. Among some cultures the umbilical cord, like the placenta, is the object of tradition and an almost magical regard. The leathery remnant of the cord may be used to make medicines or may be buried with a special ceremony.

A slight bulge around the base of the cord, called an *umbilical hernia*, is not uncommon and is caused by a weakness in the connective tissue of the abdominal wall. The bulge appears most prominent when the baby is crying, coughing, or straining. Umbilical hernias normally heal themselves by the age of two or three years. In the past people used to tape a coin over an umbilical hernia, but most doctors today feel this remedy is ineffective. However, one study did support the idea that careful strapping with adhesive tape may help speed closure in hernias over 6 millimeters in diameter. Opposing sides of the abdomen are pulled together after the bulge has been pushed back in, and then tape is applied.

The newborn passes its first stool within a day or so. These early stools, called *meconium*, are dark greenish brown. They consist of bile and digested hair and skin cells that the baby has swallowed during the final weeks in utero, and contain no bacteria. About the third or fourth day, the meconium stools begin to be replaced with *transitional stools*, which contain milk curds. These stools are light greenish brown and loose.

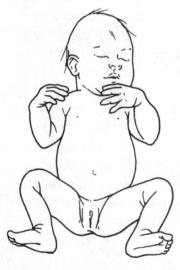

The newborn has a large abdomen, which tends to become even larger after a feeding. The abdomen normally rises and falls as the baby breathes.

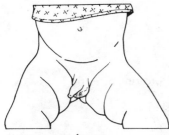

uncircumcised penis

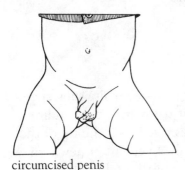

circumcised penis

The genitalia of newborn boys and girls appear quite swollen in the first few days after birth. This swelling is caused by female hormones that cross the placenta late in pregnancy.

The newborn has 2 to 7 stools per day, increasing toward the end of the first week. The amount of stool the baby passes depends upon the amount of milk it is getting. Breast-fed babies tend to have an average of 3 to 5 bowel movements per day. These stools have little or no odor and are soft, mushy, and golden in color. Bottle-fed babies have only 1 to 4 bowel movements per day. These movements have a fecal odor more like adult stool and are pasty, harder, and pale yellow.

The Genital and Urinary Systems

Apart from the baby's health, the most significant concern for the parents is probably the sex. Ironically, parents sometimes mistake the sex of the baby at first glance, because the genital organs tend to be quite swollen, due to female hormones that cross the placenta in the last part of pregnancy. In girls the labia can be so swollen that they appear like the two sides of the scrotal sac. In boys the scrotum appears large, red, and covered with folds. At birth the foreskin covering the end of the penis is not retractable.

In both sexes the breasts may also be enlarged and may even secrete a fluid like colostrum. This fluid, once referred to as witch's milk, is most likely to appear on about the third day after birth. As a result of maternal hormones that cross the placenta during pregnancy, newborn girls may also have a vaginal discharge. This discharge, which is grayish white and possibly tinged with blood, can last for up to two weeks.

Babies urinate for the first time soon after birth and at frequent intervals thereafter. The number of times a day they wet the diaper depends upon how much milk they are getting as well as on the temperature and humidity of the air. During the first several days after birth, babies lose excess body fluid that they have accumulated while in the uterus. The typical fluid loss amounts to 6 percent of the newborn's body weight. For the first week the baby's urine may have a pinkish tinge as a result of uric acid crystals made by the immature kidneys. This is normal and does not indicate a problem.

Circumcision

Parents of newborn boys face the decision of whether to circumcise their baby. *Circumcision* is a surgical procedure in which the foreskin of the penis is cut off with a scalpel or a metal or plastic bell. It is an ancient custom that is practiced by many religions. The foreskin is a double layer of skin, similar to a lined sleeve, that covers the tip of the penis. The top layer is continuous with the outer layer of the penis, while the inner layer is a mucous membrane similar to the lining of

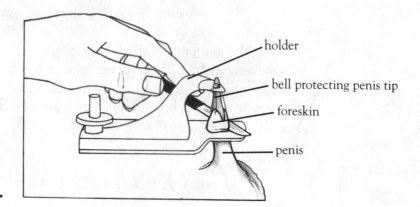

Circumcision is a surgical procedure in which the foreskin of the penis is cut off. Doctors often use a metal or plastic bell, as shown in the drawing, to protect the head of the penis. There is no medical reason for circumcision and it is no longer routinely done.

holder

bell protecting penis tip

foreskin

penis

the vagina. This mucous membrane secretes a cheesy white substance called *smegma* and is very sensitive because it has many nerve endings.

During gestation the foreskin becomes fused with the tip of the penis, and it is still largely fused at birth. Only 4 percent of newborn boys have a foreskin that is fully retractable at birth, and in almost 50 percent of boys the fusion is so great that the *urethra* or the urinary opening can barely be seen. Pediatricians used to think that such fusion represented abnormal adhesions that had to be forcibly separated, but it is now acknowledged that both the fusion and subsequent separation are normal processes. As the child grows, the foreskin generally separates gradually, so that by puberty it is fully retractable.

Circumcision is one of the few surgical procedures performed without anesthesia, probably because of an outdated idea that newborns do not really feel pain. If the newborn is only a few days old, it is simply strapped down or restrained during circumcision, but if it is more than a few weeks old it is admitted to the hospital and is given general anesthesia.

There are two types of reasons given for circumcision. The first is religious or cultural, which is a matter of the parents' personal value system and has inherent validity. The second is medical. Doctors used to think that problems could arise if the foreskin was too tight, and that circumcision would lower the incidence of cancer of the penis in men and cancer of the cervix in women. Both these medical arguments have been proved false. The foreskin is known to loosen naturally, and the rates of these two cancers are no higher among uncircumcised populations in which males practice reasonable cleanliness. These facts have led the American Academy of Pediatrics to state that "there is no absolute medical indication for routine circumcision of the newborn . . . a program of education leading to continuing good personal hygiene offers all the advantages of routine circumcision without the attendant surgical risk."[1]

In spite of the academy's sweeping recommendation, obstetricians, who perform the majority of circumcisions, sometimes do them with little or no discussion of the alternatives or explanation of the risks so that parents can make a thoughtful decision. Well over half of all newborn boys are still circumcised in the United States, as opposed to less than 1 percent in every other Western country besides Israel, but this number appears to be dropping. The most common reasons parents give for circumcising their newborn boys is cleanliness or social custom so that the boy resembles his father.

Like most procedures, circumcision is not without risk of complications: in studies various risks range from 4 percent to 28 percent. One study revealed that immediate problems arising from circumcision included excessive bleeding (2%), infection (1%), and faulty surgery (1.5%). Later complications included foreskin adhesions as a result of surgery (8%), irritation and infection (4%), and need for recircumcision (1%). In the same study no mother of an uncircumcised boy complained of problems of cleanliness or infection. However, some doctors claim that a definite percentage of uncircumcised boys will have to be circumcised at a later point to correct a tight foreskin or repeated infections. Their estimates range from .1 percent to 5 percent.

It only takes the doctor a few minutes to forcibly break the adhesions holding the foreskin and then cut it off, but the effects on the baby are significant. According to a recent study, all babies cried vigorously for a few minutes, then went into one of two different response patterns. Half of the babies became active, agitated, and fussy, while the other half became subdued, drowsy, or sleepy for a period of about 24 hours. Studies have also found that after being circumcised babies showed higher than normal levels of adrenal hormones (indicating stress) and that the babies' dream-state (REM) sleep cycles were disturbed. Both these findings indicate that the procedure is not without consequences for the baby.

The Limbs

The newborn's limbs are quite different from an adult's in shape and proportion. Babies have much longer arms than legs, and they often hold their arms and legs in a flexed position as a result of the crowded final weeks in the uterus. As we've mentioned, newborns tend to assume whatever position they were most commonly in before birth. Even when lying flat on their back, newborns rarely stretch out completely, preferring to keep at least one arm and leg drawn up.

The newborn's legs typically appear short and bowed. This is partly due to their position in the uterus and partly due to the fact that the outer muscles of the legs are more developed than the inner ones. The newborn's feet generally look chubby due to a special fat pad under the arch, and they appear to turn in due to the tucked-in position they assumed in the uterus. Babies also tend to hold their hands

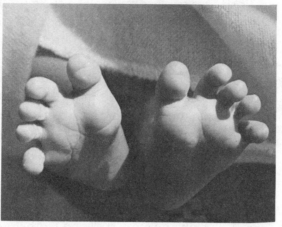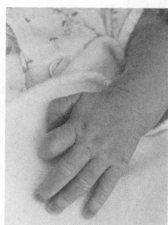

The newborn's feet and hands are astonishing in their miniature perfection. Photos by Michael Samuels.

in unusual positions. Frequently they curl their fingers in a fist with their thumb tucked inside the other fingers, or spread their fingers in a delicate C-shape arch formed by their thumb and index fingers.

The Skin

Parents notice almost immediately how remarkable the newborn's skin is. Like many other aspects of the newborn, it is quite different from that of the adult. At birth the newborn is covered with amniotic fluid and blood. This is perfectly normal, but it may be upsetting if parents are not expecting it. Once the baby is cleaned off, it can be seen that the skin is covered with a cheesy whitish substance called *vernix caseosa*, which protects the skin from the long immersion in amniotic fluid. Whereas preterm infants tend to be liberally covered with vernix caseosa, fulll-term infants show it only in the skin folds, and postterm infants show none at all.

Newborns are also covered with a very fine, downy hair called *lanugo*. As with vernix caseosa, the amount of lanugo varies according to the gestational age of the baby. Whereas preterm babies tend to be heavily covered with lanugo, full-term babies have it only on the backs of their shoulders, the tips of their ears, and on the forehead. Postterm babies have very little of it at all.

A baby's skin varies tremendously according to its gestational age, genetic background, and mood. Premature babies have a thin, tight, almost transparent appearance to their skin, while babies who are postdate have a thick, wrinkly, almost flaky look to theirs. Caucasian or light-skinned babies tend to be very pale at delivery, but their skin pigment immediately begins to darken in the presence of light. Just after birth light-skinned babies tend to be very pink except for their hands and feet, which have a blueish cast because their peripheral circulation is still sluggish. This blueishness is most pronounced when newborns are cool. When babies cry they can turn deep red or even purple. Newborns also show an effect called *mottling*, in which pink areas are interspersed with lighter ones. This is perfectly normal and disappears as the baby's circulatory system matures.

Approximately 60 percent of all newborns have a slight yellowish cast to the skin in the first week after birth. This condition, called *neonatal jaundice*, is usually mild and no cause for concern. It typically appears on the second or third day and peaks between the second and fourth days, decreasing thereafter. Neonatal jaundice results from the immature liver's inability to handle all the red blood cells that are normally being replaced by the baby's body. Within the liver the hemoglobin in the red blood cells is broken down to form *bilirubin*, a greenish yellow pigment that is an important part of the bile produced by the gall bladder. Before birth bilirubin crossed the placenta and was disposed of by the mother's liver, but following delivery the baby's body has to assume this task.

Feeding the baby shortly after delivery helps prevent neonatal jaundice because it keeps the baby's fluid levels high and stimulates digestion and elimination. Warmth tends to lessen the amount of bilirubin the newborn produces, and early exposure to sunlight accelerates the breakdown of bilirubin into products the baby can easily excrete. If jaundice appears earlier or later than the typical pattern or if the baby's bilirubin levels are very high, the pediatrician may want to watch the baby closely. Serious jaundice is more likely in preterm or low-birth-weight infants. In severe cases the baby may be treated with ultraviolet light or given an exchange transfusion, but this is uncommon.

The newborn's skin is soft, smooth and beautiful, and it is also

Normal newborn skin conditions

Milia—white dots on face in about 50 percent of newborns.

Acne—pimples on face, from 3 weeks to 6 months.

Mongolian spots—blue-black spots on back, buttocks, genital area in about 90 percent of black, Indian, and Asian babies.

Café-au-lait—light brown patches, a normal skin characteristic in 10 to 20 percent of babies.

Salmon patch—light red area on neck or eyelids in 50 percent of all babies; eyelid patches fade, neck patches may fade.

Strawberry birthmarks—red lumps; may appear at around 3 weeks of age, disappear as child grows.

fairly sensitive. Within a few days after birth the majority of babies experience some peeling, most commonly in the skin folds. Often the newborn also develops a variety of temporary skin rashes or eruptions that are pimplelike in nature and are caused by plugged skin ducts or by hormones. Many of the rashes, such as *newborn acne,* which appears in the second week, do not show the new baby at its best. But parents can be reassured that such skin conditions do not indicate any real medical problems, do not require treatment, and will quickly pass (see chart on p. 461).

The newborn may also have one of several birthmarks that are normal and that may or may not be transitory. Birthmarks are color changes that are due to slight differences in pigmentation (skin coloration) or to an overgrowth of blood vessels. Because parents often have an image of the baby's skin as flawless, they may be worried or upset by such birthmarks, but few require treatment.

Capabilities of the Newborn

As recently as fifty years ago doctors considered newborn babies to be "insensate," that is, unable to see, hear, or feel pain very acutely. At that time all the baby's reactions were believed to be reflexive rather than conscious or deliberate. The notion that a newborn could think or learn would have been flatly denied. The noted Harvard pediatrician T. Berry Brazelton suggests that this perspective allowed doctors to approach the baby from a depersonalized medical point of view, handling the delivery, performing medical procedures, and setting up nursery routines without really considering how they might affect the baby and its relationship with its mother. Essentially newborns were treated as if they were almost comatose, an attitude that resulted in what Marshall Klaus has called "bizarre policies of isolation and separation for the newborn."[2]

Parents, however, in their intuitive wisdom, have always realized that babies did not fit this insensate description. Indeed, scientists have now come to realize that newborns have remarkable capabilities at birth that are of great importance in their earliest and most profound social relationships. Babies react quite consciously, not reflexively, to the attention and caretaking they receive from their parents. A baby's responses reinforce the parents' nurturing and love and create a bond that is the beginning of a lifelong attachment. The infant's capabilities are essential to the creation of this bond, causing the parents to react with awe and appreciation.

According to Brazelton, parents' understanding of the importance of their earliest care gives them a sense of deep satisfaction that promotes earlier and more sensitive attachment between parent and infant. Thus newborn capabilities and bonding are inextricably inter-

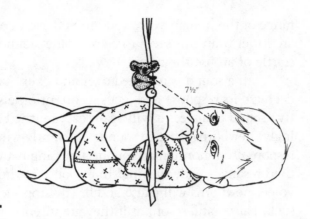

Initially the newborn has a fixed focal length of about 7½ inches, so it sees best at about that distance.

twined. Brazelton asserts that the newborn's capabilities are precisely the skills necessary for a reciprocal relationship. Babies are skillful at selectively focusing their attention, dismissing or shutting out extraneous sensory input. Not only do newborns have great ability to control their environment in terms of what they *let in*, but they also have tremendous control over the reactions they *put forth*, particularly in regard to their parents' attentions. As Brazelton points out, this makes the baby "a powerful force for stabilizing and influencing those around him."[3]

What are the newborn's capabilities? At birth all the newborn's senses work well, and it has the ability to react to the stimulation it receives. The newborn has 20/300 vision, so it sees rather well close up but not at far distances. Actually the baby has a *fixed focal length* of 19 centimeters, which means that it sees best at about 7½ inches; nearer or further away than that it sees less sharply, because its eye muscles are not yet used to adjusting their focus. Not surprisingly, 7½ inches is about the distance between the mother's face and her breast.

Visually, newborns prefer curved lines to straight lines, patterns to blanks, large patterns to those with tiny details, and outer contours to inner details. The newborn can follow horizontal and vertical motions with its eyes and is especially drawn to bright objects like lights. Some researchers think that this is why newborns so frequently become fixated on their parents' eyes, which are bright and shiny. Although the newborn is interested in faces and will tend to follow them with its eyes, it will look at but not follow a scrambled pattern of a face. Thus all the newborn's visual abilities seem well designed to foster social interaction with its mother and father.

Right from birth newborns respond to sounds, whether they are asleep or awake. A sleeping baby will become startled and blink in response to sound, but may or may not awaken. An awake baby will turn its head to follow a sound and will react to it with facial movements as well. Indeed, the baby's response to sound is at least as sophisticated as its response to visual stimuli. Studies have shown that newborns demonstrate the greatest responsiveness to sounds in the range of the human voice (500 to 900 cycles per second). Sounds that are lower than this seem to be soothing, sounds that are higher tend to startle or arouse the baby.

If a sound is repeated over and over, a newborn will tend to decrease its response and focus its attention elsewhere. But if a repetitive sound changes, it will again capture the baby's attention. Interestingly, newborns react to sounds differently when they are feeding. In response to a nonhuman sound, a nursing baby will pause to listen, then resume steady sucking. In response to the sound of the human voice, newborns will pause and briefly stop sucking, then suck, pause, suck, pause, and so on, as if they are intently waiting to hear more of an ongoing conversation. In an elaborate experiment in which newborns could activate a voice recording by a particular pattern of sucking, they were found to selectively modify their behavior in order to bring on the sound of the voice. Given a choice, newborns will choose a female (higher pitched) voice over a male (lower pitched) voice. Mothers and birth attendants seem instinctively to pitch their voices higher when talking to a newborn. Finally, there is some evidence to suggest that newborns learn to pick their mother's voices out of a group within a few days after delivery.

The newborn's senses of taste and smell are also highly developed. Within 1 to 3 days of birth, infants can already distinguish sweet from sour, less sweet from more sweet, and will also suck differently at a bottle of cow's milk formula and a bottle of breast milk. In terms of odor, the newborn can distinguish between milk and sugar water and shows a preference for milk. By 5 days a newborn can even smell the difference between its mother's breast milk pads and another woman's.

All of these abilities enable newborn babies to interact meaningfully with other people. Film research by Condon and Sander has shown that very young babies synchronize their movements to the speech and gestures of the person they are interacting with. In analyzing slow-motion footage, it was found that when the speaker paused to breathe, the baby would raise an eyebrow or reach out in response. This phenomenon, in which both the speaker *and* the listener move in time with the words of the speaker, is called *entrainment*. It is known to be characteristic of adult communication, but researchers were initially surprised that newborns were already capable of it. Only live speech elicited a high degree of entrainment from babies; neither tapping noises nor random vowel sounds drew forth the same degree of response. As Brazelton points out, the entrainment movements of newborns give such powerful feedback as to make them irresistible to their parents.

Newborns can respond to the environment in subtly different ways, depending on whether they are focused on an object or a person. Brazelton has done a number of film studies on infants, in which he found that this difference becomes apparent by about two weeks of

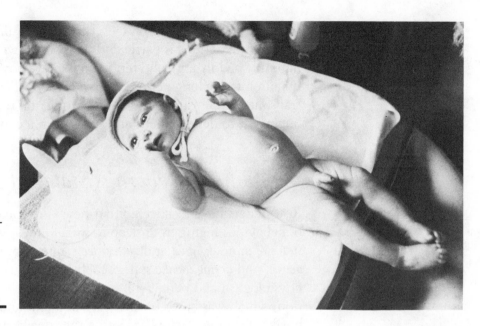

Newborns have good perception of nearby objects and often will reach out to touch them. Photo by Michael Samuels.

age. Faced with an attractive object, the newborn focused intently for a period of time and even tried to reach out with its fingers and toes before losing interest and turning away. Later the baby might renew its attention to the object and go through another episode with an abrupt beginning and ending. When the newborn focused on its mother, however, its attention was more sustained and its movements were much smoother. The baby showed an intent period in which it moved slightly toward its mother, then a somewhat less intent period in which it withdrew slightly. This cycle occurred at a rate of about four times per minute. The mother in such situations mirrored the baby's responses in a reciprocal way. Brazelton compares these complementary interactions to a swan's mating dance and notes that if the mother was not attentive to the baby's efforts at interchange, it shifted its attention away but kept the mother in its peripheral field of vision, ready to react should the mother become attentive again.

Brazelton believes that babies respond to external cues on the basis of innate abilities and that their responses are strongest in a cyclical, give-and-take situation. So characteristic are a baby's responses in these situations that it would seem they are important landmarks in its learning abilities and social development. Interestingly, Brazelton found that babies had very different patterns of interaction with their fathers. Whereas the mother-baby interaction was smooth, cyclical, and unhurried, the father-baby interaction was more playful and faster moving. In general, babies were more intense, wide-eyed, and exploratory in exchanges with their fathers.

For parents, the newborn's feedback is an important stimulus in developing their nurturing feelings; seeing the baby respond to their actions is very rewarding and tends to focus and deepen their attention toward the baby. Brazelton feels that parents' understanding of these mutual interactions is particularly important with babies who are not naturally cuddly and who tend to avoid eye contact. Brazelton sees the human infant's long period of physical dependency as the means of transmitting cultural mores and instrumental techniques that are important to development and survival in a complex world.

The Newborn's States of Attention

Researchers have discovered that newborns have six organized patterns of behavior ranging from sleep to wakefulness, which they refer to as *states of arousal: quiet* and *active sleep* states, *drowsiness,* and *quiet, active,* and *crying awake* states. Each state has its own recognizable physiological and behavioral characteristics (see chart). This information, which was based on the work of Wolff and Prechtl, was a major breakthrough in doctors accepting that newborns were capable of sensing things about their environment and responding appropriately.

In terms of the baby's capabilities, the quiet awake state is comparable to conscious attention in adults. In this state the baby

Newborn behavior states

STATE	BEHAVIOR	DURATION
Regular sleep	Baby's eyes are closed, eyes don't move, common household noises don't awaken the baby.	4–5 hours per day
Irregular sleep	Baby's eyes are closed, but eyes move under lids; breathing is irregular; slight muscle twitching. Corresponds to rapid eye movement (REM) sleep in adults.	12–15 hours per day
Drowsiness	Baby's eyes may be open and the baby reacts to noises.	Variable
Alert inactivity	Baby responds to noises with body movements and by focusing eyes.	2–3 hours per day
Waking activity	Baby's eyes are open, baby makes slight body movements and/or cries.	1–4 hours per day

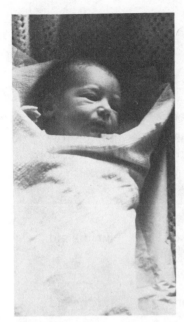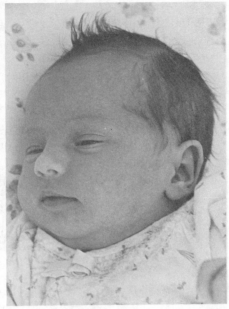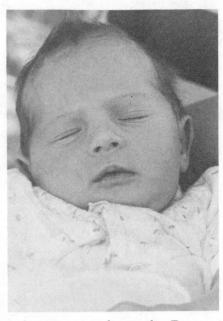

Newborns have distinct states of arousal, each one having its own characteristic behaviors. The quiet awake state corresponds to adult attention. Drowsiness precedes sleep, which separates into quiet and active segments. Photos by Michael Samuels.

focuses on objects, listens to sounds, and interacts with people. During the first week after birth the newborn spends only 8 to 16 percent of its time in this state, which may account for why doctors in the past so readily accepted the idea of newborns being insensate. But while infants are in a quiet awake state for only minutes at a time for the first week, during the first 45 to 60 minutes after birth they are *continuously* in a quiet awake state. This is one of the reasons that newborn experts feel that the first hour after birth is so important, and that if possible mother and baby not be separated during that time.

Parent-Infant Bonding

After the long months of preparing for the baby's arrival, parents' attitudes are generally totally transformed by the reality of delivery and the actual presence of the newborn. For the great majority of parents the time right after birth is filled with intense emotion. Until very recently Western doctors tended to deemphasize the fact that the drama and poignancy of these moments had any behavioral consequences for the mother and father. And they certainly never considered that the first hour might have far-reaching effects on the newborn as well. In the past psychiatrists have speculated on the results of birth trauma on the infant, but until recently no one had speculated on other than *medical* effects on the baby due to the period shortly after birth. Now it is recognized that the events of the first hour play a key role in the attachment that develops between parent and infant.

Two of the leaders in the emerging field of parent-infant attachment are neonatologists Marshall Klaus and John Kennell. Klaus

A partial list of the newborn's reflexes

NAME	TO ELICIT	BABY'S MOVEMENTS	POSSIBLE USE TO BABY
Moro, or startle	Suddenly change position, dropping baby's head backward; make a loud noise next to baby	Throws out arms and legs, then pulls them back convulsively	Attempt to grab mother for protection, comfort
Rooting	Touch baby's cheek or area around mouth	Turns head toward stimulus	Nursing aid
Sucking	Touch mucous membranes inside baby's mouth	Sucks on object	Nursing aid
Grasping	Touch palm of hand or sole of foot	Closes hand or curls foot	To hold mother while feeding, being carried
Babinski	Stroke outside of foot	Large toe curls up	Unknown
Hand to mouth	Stroke cheek or palm	Turns head toward stroke, bends arms up, and brings hand to mouth; mouth opens and sucks	Feeding aid; may help to clear baby's air passage

and Kennell's experience in caring for premature and/or high-risk infants led them to study the relationship between these babies and their parents. They found that parents whose newborns were hospitalized in intensive-care nurseries often had a difficult time relating to their baby once it was finally out of the hospital. They also found that newborns who had been hospitalized later showed higher than expected incidences of both physical abuse and *failure to thrive,* a condition in which an infant fails to grow normally without any apparent

NAME	TO ELICIT	BABY'S MOVEMENTS	POSSIBLE USE TO BABY
—	Bright light in eyes	Closes eyes	Protects eyes
Blink	Clap hands	Eyes close	Protects eyes
—	Cover mouth	Turns head away and flails arms	Prevents smothering
—	Stroke leg	Baby crosses other leg and pushes object away	Protection
Withdrawal	Give baby a pinch or painful stimulus	Baby withdraws	Protects body
—	Place baby on belly	Holds up head, and turns it	Prevents smothering
Tonic neck reflex (TNR)	Turn baby's head to side	Whole body arches away, arms and legs move to "fencing" position	Helps in birth
Step	Stand baby up	Baby walks	Practice walking movements

medical reason. Klaus and Kennell found these statistics perplexing in view of the extraordinary efforts that had been made to save these babies; and in an attempt to make sense of them, they began to study the factors affecting *attachment* between all newborns and their parents. The most obvious difference between hospitalized and healthy newborns was that the healthy ones did not undergo anywhere near the same degree of separation from their mothers (and fathers) as the sick babies did.

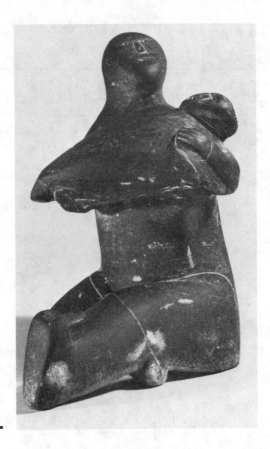

In 1972 Klaus, Kennell, and their associates did a landmark study comparing two groups of mothers who had different exposure patterns to their newborns. The control group followed the normal hospital routine, which included only a glimpse of the baby at birth, "contact for identification at 6 to 12 hours," and then 20 to 30 minutes for feeding every 4 hours until they left the hospital. By comparison, the experimental group was allowed 1 hour of contact with their unclothed newborn within the first 3 hours, and 5 hours of extra contact each day. Klaus and Kennell found that the behavior of mothers in the experimental group was very different from those in the control group and that this difference was sustained over a period of several years. Mothers who had greater early exposure to their infants showed more soothing, fondling, and eye-to-eye contact with their babies at one month still showed more soothing behaviors at one year. At two years they used more words and questions and fewer imperatives with their children. This study provided the earliest evidence for the existence of a *sensitive period* in human maternal-infant bonding. Klaus and Kennell define the sensitive period as the time "during which the parents' attachment to their infant blossoms . . . [and during which] complex interactions between the mother and infant help lock them together."[4]

Between 1972 and 1982 seventeen studies were done on the effects of separating babies from their mothers directly after birth.

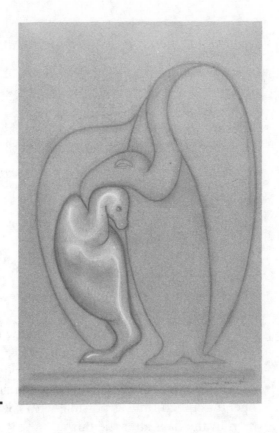

Skin-to-skin contact promotes a close bond between mother and baby. Maternity, *Max Ernst, 1942. Pencil and chalk on orange paper, 18⅞" x 12⅛". Collection, The Museum of Modern Art, New York. Gift in memory of William B. Jaffe.*

Thirteen of the studies dealt only with contact in the first hour of life. Of these, one Swedish study showed that mothers who were simply given an extra 15 minutes with their babies in the first half-hour of life spent significantly more time looking their infants in the face and kissing them at 3 months. Seven of the other studies showed that mothers who had longer initial contact with their infants tended to continue breast-feeding for significantly longer periods of time. One study of 301 mothers found that those women who had an extra 6 hours of contact with their babies on both the first and second day had one-fifth the rate of serious mothering problems. The remainder of the studies corroborated Klaus and Kennell's initial findings that extra

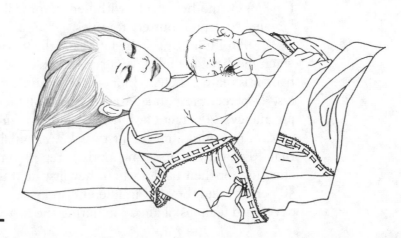

The events of the first hour after birth play a key role in the attachment that develops between parents and the newborn. This initial interaction is called bonding.

> ### Encouraging bonding between baby and mother
>
> - Prior to childbirth, evaluate the kind of birth you would ideally like to have, and then work to have those needs met as much as possible.
> - Educate yourself about the birth process in order to reduce anxiety about the unknown and enable you to participate fully in the experience.
> - Arrange for a supportive companion to stay with you throughout labor and delivery.
> - Spend at least twenty minutes with the baby, in privacy, after delivery is completed.
> - Hold the baby against your bare chest and allow the baby to nurse immediately after birth.
> - Delay eye medication until the baby becomes sleepy after the initial bonding experience.
> - Have continuous contact with the baby in the days after birth, and take primary responsibility for its care. Have nurses, family members, and other helpers take their direction from you.
> - Breast-feed the baby on demand if you are nursing.
> - Spend as much time as possible with the father and other children in the days after the birth.

contact in the first several days led to more physical contact and displays of affection between mothers and their infants.

Several other studies tend to broaden the definition of bonding and are of interest. A study by Siegel not only corroborated Klaus's findings but dealt with variables in addition to the first hour after birth. Siegel found that factors such as the mother's economic status, race, housing, education, number of previous children, and age also have significant effects on her relationship with her baby. It's important to note that these variables are all fixed, whereas the amount of time a new mother spends with her infant is flexible, determined largely by hospital nursery routines.

An interesting study by MacFarlane attempted to find out when mothers first felt love for their babies or when they first felt the baby was really "theirs." In a questionnaire given to 97 English mothers, 41 percent responded that they initially felt such feelings during pregnancy, 24 percent at birth, 27 percent during the first week, and 8 percent not until after the first week. A similar study by Robson found that 40 percent of first-time mothers reported they felt immediate affection for their babies when they first held them, whereas another 40 percent said they felt indifferent on first contact and gradually developed feelings of affection during the first week.

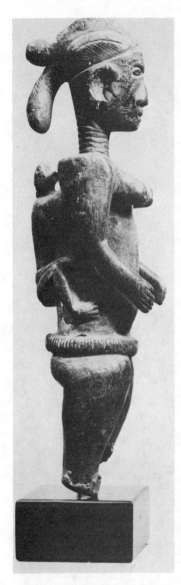

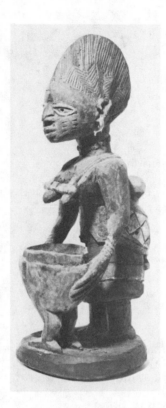

A bond is a unique relationship between two people that is specific and endures through time.

Mother and Child, Nigerian. The Metropolitan Museum of Art. The Michael C. Rockefeller Memorial Collection.

Mother and Child, Yoruba. Lowie Museum of Anthropology, University of California, Berkeley.

Studies such as these show that parent-infant attachment is a complicated, multifaceted phenomenon that is not determined purely by the interactions of the first hour after birth but by many factors that are operative over a long period of time. Marshall Klaus defines a *bond* as "a unique relationship between two people that is specific and endures through time."[5] He considers fondling, cuddling, kissing, and prolonged gazing to be behaviors that indicate parental-newborn attachment. Such a bond does not develop instantaneously; neither does it imply that the parties cannot be separated, as if joined by "epoxy glue." Klaus adds that humans are flexible creatures who have many "fail-safe" behaviors that enable them to bond even when conditions are not ideal.

Klaus divides the factors that produce a bond into two types: internal and external. *Internal factors* include how the mother and father were raised by their own parents and the cultural models available to them as they were growing up. The most obvious corroboration of this concept can be found in studies of battered children: a great number of parents who physically abuse their children were themselves abused as children. Likewise, women whose families had been disrupted by death or divorce as they were growing up showed that they interacted less with their 20-week-old babies than did a control group of mothers from undisrupted families. It's important to point out that parents are not necessarily bound to repeat the mistakes of their own parents, but that in times of stress people tend to revert to what was done to them.

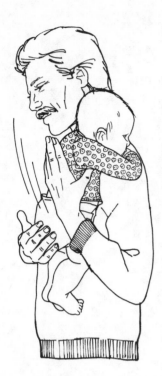

Often fathers can soothe crying babies by walking, rocking, or patting them.

Causes of crying and soothing techniques

REASONS BABIES CRY

Hunger

Need to suck

Pain—gas, indigestion, colic

Discomfort—too cold or too hot, diaper rash, straining to defecate

Wet diapers

Fear—sudden movement, loud noises, precarious (unsupported) position

Uncomfortable position

Overstimulation

Lack of body contact—the need to be held and touched

Boredom—lack of stimulation or attention

Tension—from self or others

Fatigue

TECHNIQUES FOR SOOTHING BABIES

Feed the baby

Burp the baby—put baby on its tummy or your shoulder, rub or pat its back

Change diapers

Pat baby while it lies on its stomach

Talk to baby

Give the baby a pacifier

Put baby where it can see activity

Distract baby from crying—engage baby's attention with a moving object or a music box or take the baby on a "tour" of the house

Walk the baby.

Rock the baby.

Give the baby a warm bath.

Pat the baby to sleep in a dark, quiet room.

The *external factors* affecting a new mother's reactions to her infant include the way in which a woman is cared for during pregnancy, labor, and delivery. Mothers who are subjected to a great deal of stress during pregnancy, a time when they themselves need tremendous support, may also be more likely to have problems with early caretaking. Hospital practices and the attitude of medical personnel profoundly influence how a woman experiences these stages in becoming a mother. A striking example of this is Klaus and Kennell's Guatemalan study on how mothers are affected by the constant presence of a supportive person during labor and delivery (see p. 200). As we have described, those women who had a *doula* with them were found to have shorter labors and significantly fewer complications during both labor and delivery. Moreover, those women who were attended by a doula tended to remain awake longer after the delivery and to stroke and touch their newborn babies more often. Klaus speculates that these women actually had lower epinephrine or stress levels. Both the mother's and the baby's medical condition play an incredibly important role in how they interact in the first hour after birth. If mother and baby have been heavily anesthetized or sedated, they will not benefit as much from the early sensitive period.

There are many reasons parent-infant attachment is strengthened during the first 30 to 60 minutes of life, and most of them have to do with the infant's capabilities. First, the healthy newborn is in a quiet awake state for the first 45 to 60 minutes, an unusually long period of time for a newborn, as we have said. In this state the newborn has reciprocal interactions with the mother in which their behaviors complement each other. Klaus believes that the most important behavior during the sensitive period is *touch*. Studies show that new mothers instinctively begin by touching their baby's hands and feet and progress to rubbing the baby's tummy and trunk within a few minutes. Almost simultaneously the mother and baby will lock eyes, staring intently at one another. Finally, the mother will begin crooning to the baby in a special high-pitched voice, often using both soothing sounds as well as intelligible words.

Awareness of these instinctive patterns combined with all that is known of the newborn's capabilities led Klaus and Kennell to recommend sweeping changes in delivery room and nursery routines. Although there are still major hospitals that do little or nothing to promote bonding between parents and their newborn, Klaus and Kennell's recommendations have been implemented on an unprecedented scale.

Klaus and Kennell's goal is to produce "conditions that are optimal for the development of parent-infant attachment in the first days of life."[6] They recommend that during pregnancy the mother and father learn about the birth process and engage in group discussions about the emotional and physical aspects of birth in order to allay the

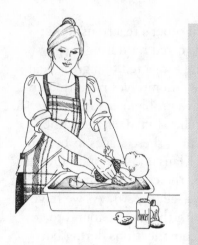

Bathing the baby is an enjoyable but challenging task for the new mother.

Layette for the first 6–8 weeks

CLOTHING

2–3 dozen diapers (cloth)

2–3 pair diaper pins or clips (for cloth diapers)

3–6 pair rubber pants and/or soaker pants

2–6 boxes of newborn disposable diapers

6–12 newborn undershirts

6–12 short-sleeved tops and/or long kimonos for warm weather

6–12 long drawstring nightgowns and/or newborn jump suits for cool weather and nighttime

2–6 warm buntings or sleep suits for daytime outings and nighttime sleeping in cold weather

1–2 sun hats (warm weather)

1–2 warm hats (cold weather)

2–3 pair washable booties

1–2 very small sweaters, preferably washable

BEDDING

6–12 receiving blankets

6–12 sets rubber pads and soaker mats to change baby on and protect laps and sheets (if cloth diapers are to be used)

3–6 crib sheets

2–3 baby towels, extra soft, absorbent, possibly with a hood

3–6 baby washcloths, for frequent change and laundering

2–4 medium-weight washable blankets

underlying anxieties that all prospective parents feel. Included in the parents' preparation should be a thoughtful evaluation of their own plans and wishes for the baby, as well as an examination of how their own mother and father functioned as parents.

Klaus and Kennell recommend that during labor the mother never be left alone and that she be attended constantly by a special person who acts as a *doula*, giving guidance and reassurance. This particular suggestion is perhaps least likely to be accepted or adopted by

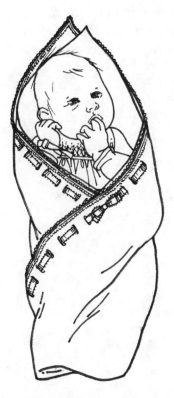

The newborn loses heat easily and needs to be bundled up unless the weather is quite warm.

most hospitals. Once all the medical procedures have been completed, Klaus and Kennell recommend that the mother and father be allowed at least 15 to 20 minutes alone with their baby in a comfortable room. At this time the mother should be encouraged to hold her baby naked against her bare chest. We would add that the mother should try this even if she has no plans to nurse her baby. Ideally even cesarean mothers should be able to hold their babies for a similar amount of time within the first hour (see p. 388).

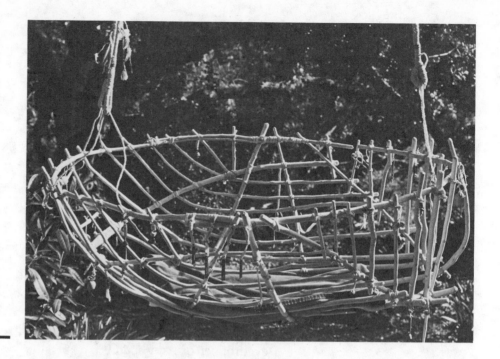

Cradle for Baby Roo, *James Surls, 1972. Collection of Michael and Nancy Samuels.*

Klaus and Kennell suggest that the baby be with the mother during the hospital stay either continuously or for long periods, with a minimum of 5 hours a day, and that the mother should be the major caregiver for her infant, even if the baby requires an incubator for extra warmth or is receiving ultraviolet treatments for neonatal jaun-

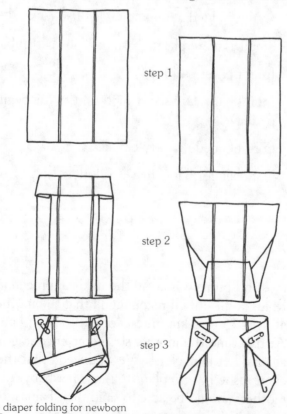

Because cloth diapers only come in one size, diapering the newborn can be a challenge and an art.

step 1

step 2

step 3

diaper folding for newborn

diaper folding tor older baby

dice. Such continuous care is particularly important if the mother has not been able to be with the baby in the first hour after delivery for medical reasons. If a newborn is quite ill and is in an intensive care nursery, Klaus and Kennell recommend that the parents be allowed to visit the baby at any time and be encouraged to touch and care for it.

By acting as the primary caregiver, the mother will acquire a good deal of competence and confidence in taking care of the baby and will have her own body rhythms tied in with those of the baby by the time she leaves the hospital. Such interaction will ensure that the mother is not left bewildered or anxious in the first days that she is alone with her baby. Klaus and Kennell also make several additional recommendations. With regard to breast-feeding, they, like the majority of pediatricians, recommend total on-demand feeding. They also suggest that siblings and fathers be encouraged to visit with mother and baby for long periods while they are in the hospital so as to strengthen intrafamily ties.

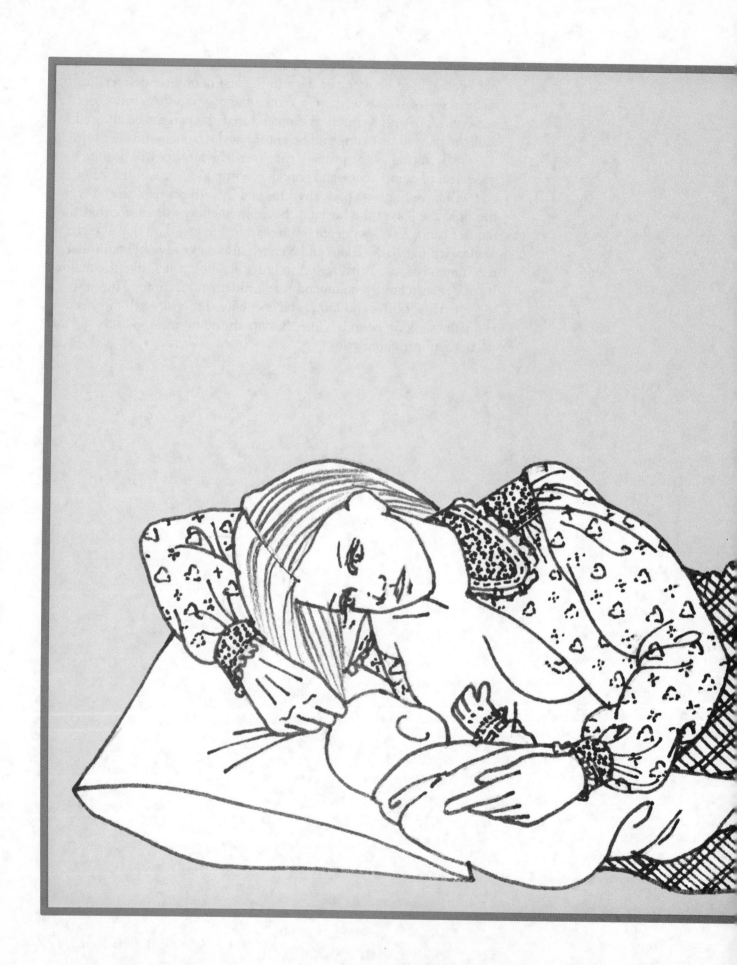

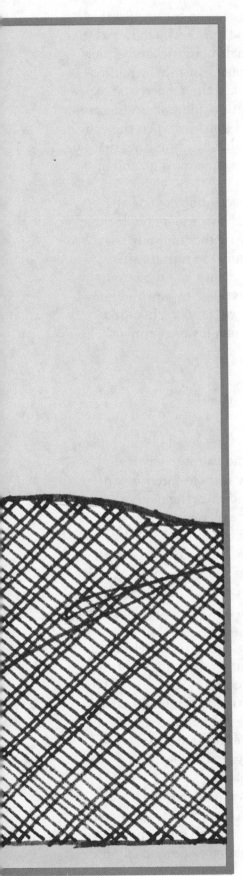

Breast-feeding

Breast-feeding—Learned and Instinctual

Most new mothers have an instinctive desire to touch and be touched by their newborn, and this naturally leads to the nursing act. Breast-feeding fulfills a mother's strong feelings of wanting to pour out her love and nurture her baby. As a result, in the first days after the birth, breast-feeding has tremendous emotional intensity.

The great majority of women ultimately find breast-feeding to be a deeply satisfying experience, both emotionally and physically, but this is not to say that there aren't a few moments in the first week when it all seems improbable and women may wonder if it will ever become second nature. As natural and instinctive as breast-feeding may be, there is much that mother and baby have to learn about this basic skill. Among primates this learning comes from observation of experienced females, which conveys information and allows the future mother to build up a climate of positive expectation. The importance of firsthand observation is dramatically demonstrated by chimpanzees raised in captivity. Females who have never observed another chimpanzee nurse and care for an infant find it difficult to nurse without the help and support of experienced caretakers.

Among humans, help and support has traditionally come from knowledgeable relatives, friends, or birth attendants. This practice worked effectively up until about fifty years ago, when a number of

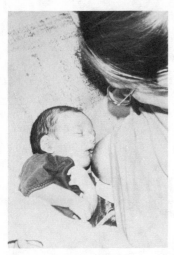

For the great majority of women, breast-feeding is a deeply satisfying experience that bonds them to their baby. Photo by Michael Samuels.

changes began to undermine it. First, bottle-feeding became feasible and popular, with the aid of both doctors and nurses who did much to promote it. Second, hospital deliveries by male obstetricians became popular at about this time, as opposed to home deliveries by midwives. This meant that the new nursing mother lacked the support and experience of the midwife and had to contend with rigid newborn nursery routines that generally had strictly scheduled times for when the baby was to nurse. This was such an unfavorable climate for nursing that by the 1950s, less than 25 percent of all mothers were nursing, and of those, most stopped within a month.

Today, due to a combination of new scientific data on the importance of breast-feeding (see p. 179) and lay pressure on doctors, nursing is again on the rise. The present-day mother not only has organizations like La Leche League International to turn to, she is much more likely to have the support of her doctor and the hospital, as well as experienced friends. The popular attitude toward and knowledge about breast-feeding is still not what it was fifty or a hundred years ago, but it is certainly more favorable than it was twenty or thirty years ago.

Beginning to Nurse

Currently most experts believe that breast-feeding should begin immediately after birth or as soon as the mother and baby are physically able. It appears that just being with the baby without interruption during the first several hours after delivery increases the mother's desire to nurse. Conversely, if a new mother experiences long separations from the baby right after birth, her interest in nursing is likely to wane. A number of studies show that mothers who breast-feed within an hour of delivery tend to have more success than those who wait for 2 to 16 hours. A Swedish study found that mothers who breast-feed immediately tend to nurse longer and more frequently, both at night and during the day.

Babies vary tremendously in their nursing patterns right from birth, but optimally a baby should nurse for at least 5 minutes at each breast shortly after birth, and thereafter as frequently as it wants. Until the mother's letdown reflex is well established, 3 to 5 minutes of strong, constant sucking is necessary to cause her brain to signal the release of oxytocin, the hormone that controls this reflex (see p. 414). Once the reflex becomes established, it is triggered immediately, sometimes even before the baby begins to nurse.

The amount a baby sucks during a session affects how much prolactin the mother produces, which in turn determines how much milk she will make. It is important for the mother to nurse the baby at both breasts from the first. If one breast is not emptied, residual milk or colostrum accumulates in the ducts, building up pressure, which tends to prevent blood and extracellular fluid from leaving the breasts. When this happens the breasts become swollen and hard, blocking the milk remaining in the ducts. Increased pressure in the ducts signals the mother's pituitary gland to decrease the production of prolactin. The result is a physiological process called *milk tension:* new milk is not produced, setting a pattern for low milk production. At the same time the breast becomes so hard that the baby has difficulty getting on the nipple effectively. Milk tension can occur at any time, but it is most common around the second or third day after delivery, when blood flow to the breasts suddenly rises and milk production begins in earnest. About 400 ounces of blood has to pass through the breasts for each ounce of milk. By the second day the *average* milk production is 180 milliliters or 6 ounces, which means that 2,400 ounces or 2½ quarts of blood will pass through the breasts.

Nursing Schedules

How often and how long to nurse in the first few days are questions of great concern to the new mother, and they have been the subject of great controversy over the last thirty or forty years. During the 1930s doctors advised an inflexible schedule of widely spaced feedings. In part, this schedule was based on bottle-feeding practices, but it also reflected the prevailing philosophy about babies, which recommended a rigid timetable for everything from bathing and changing to playing with the baby and putting it to sleep. It was felt that a baby would be spoiled by having its needs met immediately. The baby books of this era even advised letting the baby cry for long periods in order to build self-reliance and independence. Dr. Benjamin Spock was the first spokesperson for a more liberal approach to childrearing, but remnants of the old philosophy continued to affect breast-feeding instructions until fairly recently.

During the late 1970s physicians who had done research on breast-feeding radically altered their advice to new mothers, recommending total *on-demand nursing,* letting each baby and mother work out their own schedule. Currently there are no longer any rules to restrict the baby's sucking; rather, it is recommended that the baby be fed whenever it cries or fusses, for as long as it wishes. This is the "schedule" that has always been followed in virtually all cultures except Western industrial ones.

According to Dr. Niles Newton, a psychiatrist who specializes in childbirth, pregnancy, and newborn behavior, unrestricted breast-feeding has major psychophysiological effects on the mother. She believes that on-demand feeding provides the optimum psychological gratification for both mother and baby, which in turn tends to increase

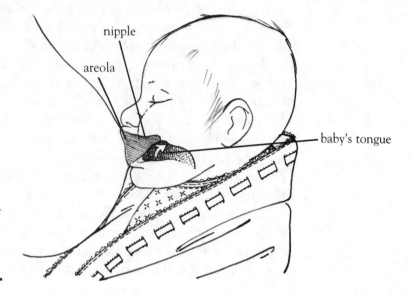

When a baby grasps the nipple correctly, most of the areola is in its mouth. In this position the baby uses its gums to squeeze milk from the sinuses behind the areola.

and enhance their interaction. Dr. Newton, like breast-feeding researchers, believes that unrestricted nursing is the optimum physiological means to ensure that the baby gets enough milk and that the mother does not become engorged. Unrestricted nursing stimulates milk production but empties the breasts so frequently that pressure never builds up in the ducts.

Unlike formula, breast milk is low in fat and low in protein and is therefore rapidly and easily digested (see p. 179), so a breast-fed baby, unlike one who is bottle-fed, is often hungry within 1½ to 2

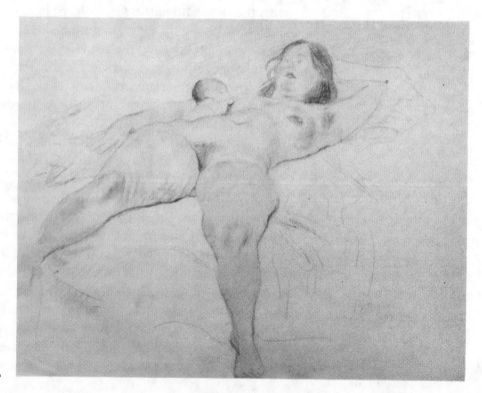

Doctors and midwives recommend that mothers nurse whenever the newborn is hungry. Mother and Infant, *Raphael Soyer, 1967. Collection of Whitney Museum of American Art, New York.*

hours after a feeding. The average breast-fed baby, particularly in the first several weeks, will need between 8 and 18 feedings a day, 10 being the average. Mothers who nursed 8 times a day during the first two weeks were found to have a larger milk output at the end of the first month and less nipple soreness than mothers who nursed less frequently.

Worries about the baby's weight gain and the adequacy of their milk supply are two of the most important concerns that new mothers have, especially if they have not nursed before. A recent study has shown that babies who nursed on demand, as opposed to ones that nursed on a 3- to 4-hour schedule, nursed more frequently (9.9 versus 7.3 feedings per day), got more milk (725 versus 502 milliliters per day), and gained more weight by the end of the second week (561 versus 347 grams). Interestingly, the on-demand babies spent no more time nursing in minutes per day, and in fact, during the second week they nursed less (130 minutes per day versus 170).[1]

The average number of feedings per day gradually drops from 10 to 5 after several months of regular nursing. At this point the mother's breasts replenish 75 percent of their supply within two hours. Thus if the mother nurses every 2 to 3 hours, she will empty her breasts completely with each feeding, preventing swelling and engorgement. At the same time she will satisfy the baby's hunger and most effectively build up her milk supply to meet the baby's nutritional needs.

If a mother delays feedings, her breasts are likely to become swollen with milk and the baby is likely to become fretful and uncomfortable with hunger. In this situation the baby finds it harder than usual to get on the breast but is less able to deal with the frustration. Typically, the baby will gnaw ineffectively at the nipple, become frantic, pull off to get air because the full breast blocks its nose, and finally cry out in hunger and exasperation. Understandably this sequence upsets the new mother, especially if she is inexperienced at nursing. Anxiety is likely to delay or block her letdown reflex, and the baby will repeat the sequence until it finally gets the milk or becomes exhausted and falls asleep. If such difficulties occur frequently, the baby's tugging at the nipple may cause the mother to develop sore or cracked nipples, which will make her very uncomfortable whenever the baby *initially* tries to get on, and thus further compounds the problem.

This sort of early nursing problem is somewhat analogous to the fear-tension syndrome in labor that Grantley Dick-Read wrote about (see p. 155). Ironically, what breaks the cycle is not feeding the baby less frequently but feeding it more often. A mother with sore nipples may be skeptical of this idea, but it's important she realize that frequent feedings promote good drainage, which prevents maternal

(text continues on page 488)

Information on nursing

Almost all women can nurse successfully.

Colostrum is secreted the first 1–4 days; milk comes in on the 3rd to 6th day.

Breast engorgement is possible in the first few weeks, especially when the milk first comes in.

Sore nipples are most likely on the 4th to 5th day of nursing.

Nursing is a learned skill that can take mother and baby a week or more to become adept at.

Worries and tension impair nursing; relaxation and positive visualization stimulate the mother's letdown reflex.

The more the baby nurses, the more the mother's milk supply builds up.

The baby nurses more frequently and for longer periods during growth spurts; the milk supply increases in 1–3 days of frequent, long feedings.

The baby grasps most of the areola in its mouth when nursing.

The baby gets most of the milk in the first 5–10 minutes of nursing.

A newborn with 5–6 wet diapers a day is getting enough milk.

A mother needs lots of fluids to produce milk. Milk and water are especially good for a mother. She needs high-protein, high-calcium diet (see table p. 88). *Note:* brewer's yeast supplies large amounts of protein and B vitamins, which are needed to fight fatigue and stress.

Avoid birth control pills. They reduce milk supply substantially; some pills actually alter the protein and fat composition of the milk.

HOW OFTEN AND HOW LONG?

Generally recommended the baby be fed entirely *on demand.* At first baby will want to nurse every 2–3 hours, sometimes hourly, and occasionally with one longer stretch. Frequent nursing in the first days probably helps bring in the milk more quickly.

Mothers who have fair or sensitive skin and who have not done nipple toughening exercises during pregnancy should be careful to avoid sore nipples from incorrect nursing techniques.

Initially try 7–10 minutes on the first breast, a little longer on the second. Gradually increase the time on each side until you and the baby are comfortable (10–15 minutes a side).

Mother can sit or lie down, hold baby in a variety of positions (see illustrations).

Pillows can be used to prop up mother and baby.

Mother should make sure baby's nose is clear and not turn baby's head forcibly while nursing.

Advice for getting the baby on the nipple in the early days

Both baby and mother can become frustrated if the baby has trouble getting on at the beginning of nursing. The mother should find a quiet place to nurse, get in a comfortable position, and try to relax so her letdown reflex will work.

Hold the nipple securely between two fingers.

Touch the baby at the corner of the mouth to stimulate its rooting reflex. (Newborns do not like something stuck in their mouths and may even try to spit out the nipple when it's inserted directly.)

Keep the baby's nose away from the breast by holding the nipple between two fingers or by depressing the areola.

Don't put the baby on the nipple when it is very excited. The best time to begin nursing is when the baby is just waking up or has been soothed. This prevents the baby from "chewing" at the nipples and making them sore.

Bundle the baby if its hands get in the way or scratch the breast.

Try different positions for nursing.

Shift to the other breast if one is sore.

Hand-express some milk if nipples are engorged.

Actively wake baby when breasts are full.

Encourage the baby to take most of the areola in its mouth.

Get the baby sucking vigorously on an orthodontically shaped pacifier first, then gently remove the pacifier and put the baby on the nipple.

engorgement and keeps the baby from becoming a fretful, anxious learner. Just as nursing is a half-instinctive, half-learned act for the mother, so it is for the baby. And a new baby tends to forget much of what it knows when it is ravenous or frustrated.

Factors That Affect Nursing

In addition to frequency of feedings, there are several other factors that affect early nursing sessions. First, mothers who have had general anesthesia or pain medication during labor and delivery may find that their babies don't seem very alert (see chart on page 503), and therefore may have a harder time with their part in the dual experience of learning to nurse. This drowsiness and lack of alertness has very general effects that can persist to up to five days. Dr. T. Berry Brazelton has found that these babies suck at lower rates and pressures and drink less milk than those whose mothers did not have any anesthetics. It is also important that new mothers avoid pain relievers or sleeping medication if possible after the delivery. Not only do these drugs pass on to the baby through the breast milk, they slow down the mother's basal metabolism or metabolic rate and decrease her milk production. Mothers whose babies are affected by drugs may find it helpful to arouse the baby intentionally (see pp. 504–05) and to manually express some milk before attempting to nurse.

Another factor that affects nursing, especially in the early days, is any kind of supplemental feeding. Although this sounds rigid, there are very good reasons for it. Extra formula or glucose water fills up the baby, so that it is not able to eat as much at the next nursing session, which tends to cut back on the mother's elaborate and complex milk production cycle. In the relatively uncommon situation that supplemental feeding is indicated for *medical* reasons, a mother needs to be aware of what effects it will have. But otherwise mothers are advised not to use supplemental feeding to solve relatively minor problems in the early days. In particular, a mother should not give a baby bottles because she is worried that she does not have enough milk (see p. 505).

A second and more subtle problem with supplemental feeding is that bottles alter the baby's feeding patterns. Drinking from a bottle, even one with a "naturally shaped nipple," requires a different technique than nursing. Breast-feeding requires strong and steady pressure from the baby's gums, tongue, and cheeks to squeeze the milk out. To bottle-feed, the baby needs to exert only slight pressure to get out a great gulp of milk, and then must squeeze the nipple shut to keep from choking. With bottle-feeding the gums are open in an O shape, the muscles of the cheeks and mouth are relaxed, and the tongue is thrust straight out. In breast-feeding, the baby's mouth is drawn back into a

C shape, the tongue moves back and up to press the nipple against the roof of its mouth, and the muscles of the jaw and cheek contract strongly to make the gums press together. Thus for the newborn supplemental feedings involve a whole new, complex learning task.

Studies show that alternating bottle and breast-feeding is very confusing for new babies and that they tend to mix up the two techniques. When they suck on the bottle like a breast, they choke; when they suck on the nipple like a bottle, tonguing it rather than pulling it fully into their mouth, the milk does not come down as readily and the mother's nipples often become sore. Since getting milk from a bottle is somewhat easier at first, a very young baby who is exposed to both kinds of feeding is likely to lose interest in the task of breast-feeding. Thus La Leche League International now advises that any supplemental liquid necessary in the first weeks be given with a teaspoon or even an eyedropper. Later, when a baby is older and has mastered nursing, it can easily handle the two types of feeding.

Breast-feeding Techniques

For a nursing session to be successful and easy in the first few days, it is important that both mother and baby be physically comfortable, relaxed, and undistracted. The baby should be relatively clean, dry, and warm, although it doesn't necessarily need to be washed or changed before every feeding. A baby may be fretful or distracted if it's wet, and changing its diaper may help to wake up a sleepy baby. If a

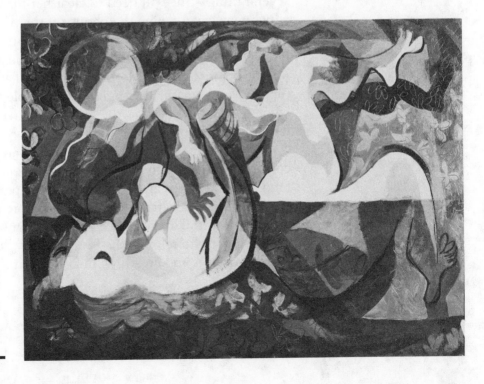

For nursing to be successful, it's important that mother and baby be comfortable, relaxed, and undistracted. Mother and Child, *Abraham Rattner, 1938. Oil on canvas, 28¾" x 39⅜". Collection, The Museum of Modern Art, New York.*

baby has been awake for some time and is likely to fall asleep at the breast, rediapering it first also makes sense. A mother who is a novice at diapering won't want to chance changing a well-fed baby who has contentedly gone to sleep at the breast.

With an on-demand schedule, nursing will generally be initiated by the baby's hunger signs, although in some instances a mother may occasionally start a feeding if the baby has not nursed in several hours and her breasts are beginning to feel uncomfortable. In this situation it is especially important that the baby be alert and focused.

Just as the mother needs to concentrate on the task at hand in the early days of nursing, so does the baby. And some babies are very outwardly oriented, their concentration easily interrupted by voices, faces, or nearby moving objects or light. Conversation and company can be equally distracting for both the new mother and the baby. In fact, the mother may find it's best if *she* doesn't even talk when the baby is cranky or easily interrupted when it's first getting on. Often it's best for mother and baby to go into a room by themselves, or to send all but one or two people out of the room.

Another reason for mother and baby to go off by themselves is that mothers sometimes find themselves a little embarrassed or uncomfortable at baring their breasts in front of even their oldest friends, especially if those friends are male. Or they may feel slightly tense about being watched by relatives or friends who are "experts" on breast-feeding or who believe the mother would be better off to bottle-feed anyway.

For the new mother preparing for a nursing session involves several things. She will need to clear her time for a half-hour or so, which may mean taking the phone off the hook if she's at home or closing her door if she's in the hospital. If she's experiencing any after-birth pains (see p. 419) or episiotomy discomfort, she should be sure to urinate before nursing. Mothers who have flaccid or nonprotruding nipples should manually stimulate the nipple they plan to start on before putting the baby to the breast. An erect nipple is much easier for an unskilled baby to get hold of.

The initial moments at each breast are usually a time for quiet concentration for both mother and baby. Especially for mothers who tend to feel tense or anxious, it may be helpful to spend a few minutes doing relaxation exercises (see p. 163) before picking up the baby. If the baby is fretful and can't be soothed by anyone else, a mother can consciously try to relax at the beginning of the nursing session by closing her eyes and breathing in and out in a slow, even rhythm.

POSITIONS FOR NURSING

Lying down or sitting up are the two basic positions for nursing. Which position a mother chooses will depend upon several factors—

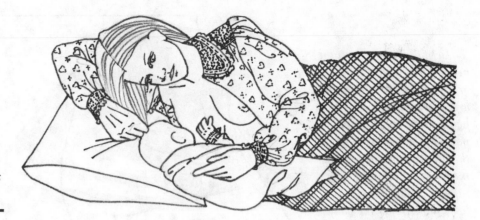

Often during early nursing sessions the mother prefers to lie down. When she lies on her side, the starting breast is the lower one.

where she is, what time of day it is, how skillful she and the baby are, and whether or not her nipples are sore. For the first few sessions the mother is usually lying in bed. Generally she turns on her side with the starting breast the lower one and places the baby on its back across her lower arm, perhaps with a pillow or two to hold the baby steady and to raise it to the height of her nipple.

Nursing experts refer to the arm supporting the baby as the *holding arm,* and call the opposite hand the *steering hand.* With the thumb and index finger (or the index and third finger) of her steering hand, the mother should grasp her nipple *behind* the areola, using the remaining fingers to support her breast. This position allows the mother to stroke her nipple against the baby's cheek or the side of its mouth, which will elicit the baby's *rooting reflex,* causing it to turn toward the nipple (see p. 468). If the mother simultaneously expresses a few drops of milk for the baby to smell and taste, it will be a powerful inducement for even the sleepiest baby.

As the baby roots toward the nipple, the mother should press her fingers back slightly so that her nipple protrudes more, making it easier for the baby. When the baby grasps the nipple, it is also helpful if the mother leans back slightly and lifts the baby, which will enable

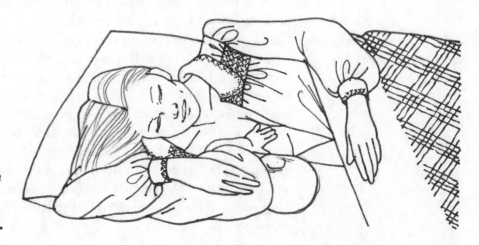

As an alternative, the baby can be turned backward when the mother nurses lying down.

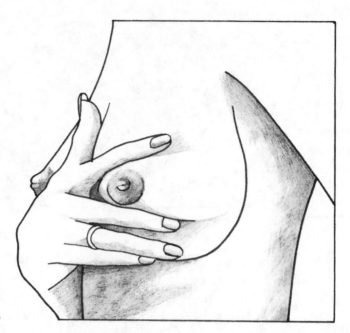

To help the baby get on the nipple, the mother should grasp her breast behind the areola with two fingers from her steering hand. In this position the mother can make the nipple protrude, stroke the baby's cheek with the nipple, and even express a little milk. After the baby has gotten on, the mother can also use her steering hand to depress her breast so the baby's nose is clear and it can breathe comfortably.

it to get the nipple way back in its mouth and the areola between its gums. This is the correct position for nursing. It prevents the baby from "hanging on" the nipple itself, which makes sucking ineffective and may cause the mother to have sore nipples (see p. 499).

Once the baby has firmly grasped on to the nipple, the mother can use her steering hand to depress the area of her breast near the baby's nose so that the baby is able to breathe comfortably. If a baby senses that its air space is blocked, it will tend to tug at the nipple or pull off repeatedly. A clear air space is especially important with new babies or when the mother's breasts are engorged. It is less important for a baby who is an experienced nurser, unless it has a stuffy nose. Getting the baby properly on the nipple is at least half the work for the new nursing pair.

Sitting up is the other basic position for nursing. When a mother sits to nurse, it's important that she be in a comfortable chair, such as a rocker, or be well-supported with pillows when she's in bed. If she is in bed, a mother will find it helpful to raise the baby by drawing up her legs; if she is in a chair, she can raise the baby by crossing her legs or putting them on a stool. By placing pillows in her lap, the mother can get the baby exactly equal to the level of her breast. This relieves her of having to support the baby with her arms for the entire nursing session, a tiring job that some doctors feel can result in enough neck and back strain to cause a tension headache. Whether sitting or reclining, the mother's holding arm positions and supports the baby, while the steering hand maneuvers her nipple to help the baby. In either position, the mother is advised to lean back and elevate the baby slightly to ensure that it gets a good hold on the nipple and areola, and to prevent the baby's gums from sliding down onto the nipple.

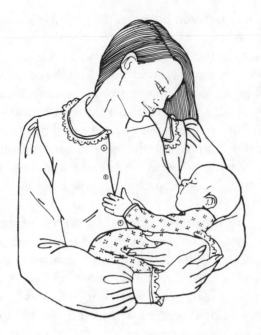

In the most common position for nursing the mother sits upright in a comfortable chair and holds the baby in her arms. In the first days after delivery the mother may find it helps to prop the baby on pillows.

The mother can tell that the baby has not gotten the nipple in its mouth properly if much of the areola shows or if the baby makes slurping noises. When this happens the mother should remove the nipple from the baby's mouth and start over again. This is more of a challenge than it sounds, because even the tiniest baby exerts powerful suction on the mother's nipple. If the mother simply attempts to pull away, the baby is likely to suck even harder and may bruise her nipple. Instead the mother should slide one finger of her steering hand into the corner of the baby's mouth until the baby lets go. This technique is also useful if the mother has to interrupt nursing for some other reason, or if the baby falls asleep with the nipple firmly grasped in its mouth. No matter how idyllic a new baby asleep on the breast may look, the mother should not let it continue, because once the baby falls asleep, it no longer squeezes and lets up on the nipple in an alternating rhythm. Instead it maintains a steady suction that can result in bruises if capillaries in the top layer of the nipple break. Such bruises are small but can become quite uncomfortable in subsequent nursing sessions.

WHEN THE MILK COMES IN

The mother's regular milk, as opposed to the colostrum, generally comes in sometime between the second and fourth day after the baby's birth. When the milk first comes in, the mother is likely to experience some degree of engorgement and possibly nipple soreness. Also she will probably be aware of warmth, tingling, or tightening in her breasts when the letdown reflex occurs.

During the first month or so mothers may notice milk leaking

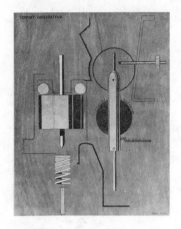

Babies are not machines—they do not behave the same throughout a single feeding or in successive feedings. The Child Carburetor, Francis Picabia, 1919. Solomon R. Guggenheim Museum, New York.

from the unsucked breast as they begin to nurse. This happens because the letdown reflex is stimulated chemically, not mechanically, and oxytocin in the blood reaches both breasts at the same time. After 6 to 8 weeks the ducts around the areola have enlarged sufficiently to hold the milk without dripping from the second breast. Leaking can be annoying, but it does not continue indefinitely and it tends to be less common in mothers who have nursed before. If a mother is bothered by it, she can put a cloth under the second nipple or a pad in that side of her nursing bra when she begins a feeding. Leaks are less likely to show on light-colored clothes, and some mothers choose them for this reason.

It's important for mothers to realize that babies will not behave in the same manner throughout a given feeding or at successive feedings. Just as adults do not eat at a constant rate of speed, neither do babies. They suck, rest, suck more actively, swallow, and look around. Generally a baby gets 75 percent of its total feeding within the first 5 minutes, and 90 percent within the first 10. But babies like sucking and many will continue to suck for 20 or 30 minutes, or until they fall asleep.

How energetically a baby begins a feeding depends on how hungry and how alert it is. An alert, hungry baby will usually suck quite actively at first in order to get the mother's letdown reflex to take place. Then once the milk begins to come down, the baby will slow to swallow. If a great gush of milk comes down, the baby, especially one who's just learning to nurse, may even choke or splutter and pull off the nipple to catch its breath. The baby soon becomes proficient in these skills, although the problem tends to solve itself because the mother's letdown reflex eventually becomes better conditioned.

The more frequently a mother nurses in the first few days, the more quickly her letdown reflex tends to become conditioned. By nursing as soon as she can after she feels the letdown reflex, the mother will help coordinate the reflex with the act of nursing. Within several weeks the mother's letdown reflex will become so attuned to the baby's schedule that she will find herself letting down when the baby cries or even when she thinks of an upcoming feeding. Occasionally a mother may let down at "inappropriate" times—when the baby is sleeping or being bathed. Such occurrences are perfectly normal and will stop when the reflex becomes well conditioned.

During a feeding it's important that the baby nurse at each breast, especially in the early weeks. If the baby only nurses at one breast, the second breast will have high pressure in its ducts for twice as long as the other breast, and the mother is more likely to become engorged. Her letdown reflex will also take longer to condition, and she will tend to build up her milk supply more slowly, as we've mentioned.

Even though a mother nurses at both breasts, often the second one is not emptied completely, since the baby gets approximately 75 percent of its feeding after 5 minutes on the first breast. Thus most doctors and midwives suggest that the mother switch to the second breast after 5 to 10 minutes of good nursing at the first, or about halfway through the entire feeding if the baby consistently nurses for longer than 10 to 20 minutes a feeding.

Sometimes a mother is disturbed at the idea of shifting the baby when it seems to be doing well at the first breast, but she should realize that the important thing is to see that the second breast is largely emptied. A mother who has ample milk or finds her breasts even slightly engorged should make a special point of switching promptly. If a baby is allowed to nurse for 15 minutes at the first breast, it is likely to fall asleep and never even nurse at the second breast during that feeding.

Until nursing is well established it may be useful for the mother to use a watch or clock to keep track of how long the baby has nursed on the first side. As the baby grows, it will need more milk and it will nurse longer and longer at each breast until the mother's milk supply catches up. The mother will come to recognize her baby's own patterns, and she will be able to adjust the amount of time at each breast accordingly. In general, by the end of the first month babies nurse for 10 to 15 minutes at the first breast and up to 20 minutes at the second breast.

Another important reason for nursing at both breasts during each feeding is that the milk from the second breast is generally richer because it contains high-calorie, high-fat hindmilk (see p. 415) left over from the previous feeding because the starting breast is often not emptied completely. Nursing expert Dr. R. M. Applebaum has coined the adage, "Infants grow best at the second breast."[2] He goes so far as to suggest that a mother can manually express extra hindmilk into the baby's mouth at the end of the feeding. Obviously this would be of most benefit to babies who were slow to gain weight, but it would tend to build up any mother's milk supply.

A corollary to the rule of nursing at both breasts is that a mother should begin each feeding on the side she *ended* the last feeding on. The reason for this, once again, is that often the second breast is not emptied. Following this pattern ensures that each breast is fully emptied at least at every other feeding, so it is encouraged by almost all breast-feeding authorities. Surprisingly, it may be difficult for new mothers to keep track. They nurse so often in the first days that they are likely to forget which side the baby last nursed on. The old trick of pinning a diaper pin on the second side doesn't always work, either, because a mother may forget to move the pin or be uncertain if she did. Eventually most mothers can tell by the fullness of their breasts, but for the first week or so they may find it useful to write down the time of each feeding and which breast they started on. This also gives

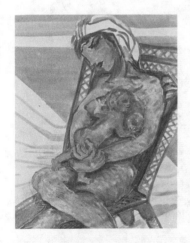

Especially during the first weeks, it's important that the baby nurse at both breasts during each feeding. Mother and Child, *Schuyler Harrison, 1970. Courtesy of the artist.*

mothers some idea of how long and how often the baby nurses if it is on a totally on-demand schedule.

Nursing Problems

Although breast-feeding is a natural act, many nursing mothers experience some concerns or troubles, especially in the early days. Problems include difficulty getting the baby on, engorgement, nipple soreness, delay with the letdown reflex, inadequate milk supply, and sleepiness or poor weight gain in the baby. It's reassuring for mothers, particularly those who are nursing for the first time, to realize that most of these problems are resolved by the second or third week. In addition, a new mother should remember that her emotions tend to be very labile in the first few weeks, so she is likely to react more strongly than usual to any stress. Thus, as with other problems of the early days, breast-feeding difficulties that initially loom large will seem much smaller when looked back upon later.

Despite the growing approval of breast-feeding among obstetricians and pediatricians, the general attitude toward nursing is not as supportive as it might be, especially when it comes to problems. Thus a mother may find that friends, relatives, or even her obstetrician or

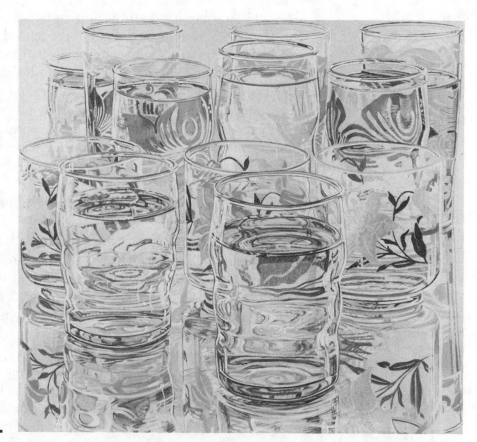

Nursing mothers need to drink lots of liquids, especially water. Painted Water Glasses, *Janet Fish, 1974. Collection of Whitney Museum of American Art, New York. Gift of Sue and David Workman.*

pediatrician are all too ready to advise her to give up nursing if she or the baby encounters anything more than the slightest difficulty. Unfortunately this is the time when a mother most needs encouragement. If she cannot get sufficient information or support from friends who are experienced at nursing or from her medical personnel, she should contact La Leche League International (see p. 207). Often her difficulties may stem from friends' or even doctors' well-meaning but misguided advice, or from inappropriate hospital routines. If a problem should arise, the sooner a mother recognizes it and takes steps to deal with it, the sooner it will be solved and the less likely it is to become a major problem. A mother should realize that such problems are not her fault, that they can be remedied, and that in all likelihood she can enjoy a successful nursing relationship with her baby.

Dealing with Engorgement

Engorgement is one of the most common breast-feeding problems that new mothers experience. As we described, *engorgement* is swelling in the breasts that results from a normal increase in blood flow to the area combined with insufficient emptying of the breasts (see pp. 482–83). It occurs most often when the milk comes in, between the second and fourth day after the baby is born, and it happens to mothers who don't breast-feed as well as to those who do. If taken care of promptly, engorgement lasts only a day or two.

The day before a mother becomes engorged she is likely to be aware of unusual sensations of heaviness and fullness in her breasts. Once the breasts become engorged, she may experience noticeable swelling, tautness, increased warmth, and tenderness. If the engorgement is significant, the breasts can become hard and painful, the skin may become shiny and red, and veins may be clearly visible under the skin. These symptoms were once thought to be signs of "breast milk fever" or an infection, but now they are considered the natural result of abundant milk production and lack of drainage.

In general, engorgement can be prevented by the promotion of good milk drainage. This begins with prenatal breast exercises (see p. 189) and is aided by putting the baby to the breast immediately after delivery and feeding frequently thereafter. It is important that a mother not skip or delay feedings or give the baby supplemental bottles at the beginning. Finally, it is helpful if the mother nurses the baby at both breasts during each feeding.

The treatment for engorgement is very similar to the method of prevention. The mother is advised to feed the baby often and always at each breast. Those babies who are sleepy, "lazy," or affected by anesthesia or pain medication should be encouraged to nurse frequently even if it means waking them up (see pp. 504–05). If the

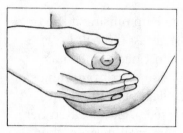

Manual expression can be very helpful if the mother's breasts become engorged. Not only does it start the milk flowing and relieve pressure, it makes it easier for the baby to grasp the nipple.

mother's areola and breast are so swollen that the baby has difficulty grasping the nipple, the mother should manually express enough milk to soften the areola before the baby begins to nurse at that breast. This will prevent the baby from hurting her nipple and will help keep the baby from becoming frustrated in its attempts to get the nipple far enough into its mouth.

Mothers who are painfully engorged often become anxious about getting the baby on, especially if their nipples are sore. While tension tends to block the letdown reflex, manual expression helps to physically stimulate it. If the baby does not nurse long enough to relieve the mother's engorgement, she should manually express milk (see illustration) at the end of the feeding until the flow ceases or her breasts feel comfortable. Manual expression is a relatively easy task, but it does require a little dexterity and practice. Also, some women may be emotionally uncomfortable about manually expressing milk in quantity. For them, and for women who plan to express and store their milk regularly, a breast pump offers a convenient solution.

There are two types of breast pumps for home use: manual and battery-powered. Both are small, relatively inexpensive devices that suction while the mother holds her areola. A manual style has to be pumped by hand; a battery-powered style is somewhat easier to use because it provides suction automatically. In addition to relieving immediate engorgement, expressing milk will give a mother practice for those times when she wishes to leave the baby for longer than the period between two feedings because she has to go out or she returns to work (see p. 504).

If a mother is experiencing problems with engorgement she will probably find it helpful to apply heat to her breasts, especially right

There are two types of breast pumps for home use: manual (left) and battery powered (right). Both can be used to express milk to relieve engorgement or for breast-feeding while the mother is away. Photo by Michael Samuels.

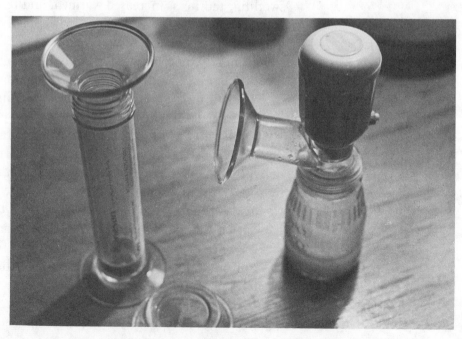

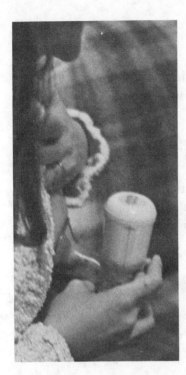

A battery-powered breast pump is a convenient way for the mother to express and store milk. Photo by Michael Samuels.

before she nurses. Taking a warm shower or applying hot, wet compresses will serve the purpose and make the mother more comfortable. Heat stimulates blood flow, thereby increasing circulation and encouraging milk flow as well. Between feedings, if a mother is very uncomfortable, ice packs or cool compresses may help relieve discomfort but shouldn't be used just before feedings because they do not promote milk flow.

Many women find that engorgement discomfort can also be alleviated by wearing a well-fitting nursing bra. Care should be taken to make sure the bra does not fit too snugly, as this can aggravate the problem and cause blocked ducts. Pain medication is to be avoided if possible because it passes in the milk, but if a mother is uncomfortable enough to require it, she should realize that the slight doses that come through won't harm the baby. The drugs most commonly prescribed for engorgement pain are aspirin, phenacetin (Tylenol), or codeine.

Occasionally a nursing mother will develop an infection called *mastitis.* It occurs most commonly with first-time mothers in the second week. Generally the bacteria causing the infection is *staphylococcus aureus,* which has been transmitted from the mother's hands or the baby to the breast. Signs that precede mastitis are severe engorgement combined with slight fever and increased tenderness in one area of the breast. These symptoms should be treated promptly. The symptoms of an actual infection are a fever of 103 to 104 degrees Fahrenheit, chills, and a red, very tender area in the breast. It is important that a mother with symptoms of mastitis call her doctor or midwife. Most practitioners will prescribe heat, a bra for support, and an antibiotic. They will also advise the mother to continue nursing and to pump the breast if necessary to drain it completely. If mastitis is not treated, the mother can develop an abscess with pus, in which case she may have to give up breast-feeding temporarily. If the symptoms are treated promptly, the condition can be cleared up within several days.

Dealing with Sore Nipples

Nipple soreness is another common problem in the early days of nursing. All nursing mothers are likely to experience some degree of nipple tenderness because of the sudden amount of manipulation, rubbing, and pulling they receive from the baby's mouth and gums, and because of the constant moistening the nipples get from the baby's saliva and the milk itself. Nipple soreness is the most common reason for giving up breast-feeding in the first weeks after birth. Even the most dedicated nurser may wonder if it is worth it when her nipples become very painful. Once her nipples hurt, a mother is likely to become anxious about nursing, which tends to weaken or interfere with her letdown reflex. All too often this leads to further problems with getting on and

Encouraging the letdown reflex

- Begin breast-feeding immediately after birth.
- Avoid medication before and after birth if possible.
- Feed the baby on demand.
- Do relaxation exercises before nursing.
- Use a comfortable chair with arm support for nursing.
- Drink warm herb tea before nursing.
- Take a warm shower shortly before nursing.
- Nurse in a quiet, private area with subdued lighting.
- Send people out of the room or go into a separate room if it helps you and the baby focus on the task at hand.
- Avoid supplementary bottles for the baby.

TIPS FOR RELIEVING DISCOMFORT FROM ENGORGEMENT IN THE EARLY DAYS OF NURSING

Use nursing bra for support.

Nurse frequently enough at both breasts to prevent engorgement.

Limit the amount of nursing on the first side, so the baby doesn't fall asleep without nursing on the second side.

Manually express milk if necessary or use a breast pump.

Apply heat or take a warm shower.

TIPS FOR RELIEVING SORE NIPPLES DURING EARLY NURSING DAYS

Give baby a pacifier between nursings.

Apply lanolin and mild creams to protect nipples.

Don't let baby chew on nipple.

Allow nipples to air-dry after nursing.

Sunbathe nipples.

Apply dry heat briefly to nipples—a heater or even a light bulb will do.

Limit nursing to short times and try not to nurse more frequently than every couple of hours.

Avoid engorgement by not going long stretches between nursings—if necessary wake the baby.

Avoid nursing on only one side at a feeding—shift to second breast after 5–7 minutes.

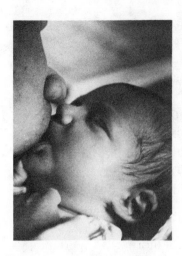

Frequent nursing in the early days helps to avoid engorgement.

Change baby's nursing position to alter pressure on sore areas of nipple. Lean forward so baby doesn't hang on nipple.

Manually stimulate nipple so it's erect before putting baby to breast.

Sore nipples generally are most tender about 4–5 days after delivery if the baby feeds on demand; they may be tender later if the baby is kept to a schedule.

If one nipple is especially sore, briefly start baby on other side, then switch back to sore nipple when milk has let down.

engorgement. What results is an upsetting cycle that can be hard to break.

Much can be done to prevent such problems, including nipple-toughening exercises during pregnancy and good nursing techniques after the baby is born. When the new mother nurses the baby she should take great care to see that the baby gets enough of the nipple in its mouth (see p. 493). Any problem of nipple soreness should be treated promptly if it arises. And the new mother should continue to be careful not to get soaps, perfumes, or drying agents such as alcohol near her nipples. Not only are they unnecessary in terms of cleanliness, they can aggravate the problem.

There are actually two different kinds of nipple soreness. The first type, which ranges from burning to a very uncomfortable searing sensation, takes place for several minutes at the beginning of a feeding *before* the letdown reflex has occurred. At this point there is little milk in the ducts around the areola and the baby is sucking vigorously at the breast. As the ducts fill with milk after the letdown reflex starts, the baby eases its powerful suction and the mother experiences relief and even pleasure in the baby's nursing. This kind of soreness is generally fairly transient and tapers off as the mother's letdown reflex becomes better conditioned, unless her nipples become bruised.

The second type of nipple soreness, which is a more serious problem, involves a variety of injuries to the thin, sensitive skin over the nipple. Occasionally blood blisters and cracks or fissures form in the area right around the nipple itself. They can cause pain and discomfort throughout the feeding. Such symptoms are less common than ordinary nipple soreness, and they require treatment (see below).

Some experts feel that the major cause of nipple soreness is the baby not getting on completely and then mouthing the nipple. Several factors can hinder the baby's attempts to get on. If the mother's nipple is not erect, the baby can have difficulty getting the nipple far enough into its mouth. Engorgement can add to the baby's difficulties. The baby can also have trouble problems on if the mother leans forward to nurse rather than back. When she leans forward, the tendency will be for the baby to dangle at the end of the nipple, putting all the pressure on this sensitive area rather than on the areola.

Often mothers wonder how long the baby should stay on the breast. Until recently many breast-feeding authorities suggested letting the baby nurse for only short periods at each breast during the first several days. But new studies indicate that unrestricted or on-demand feeding actually produces less nipple soreness. Babies who are limited to short feedings may not be getting all the milk they need and at the next feeding may initially tug at the nipple in hunger and frustration, then nurse longer in order to catch up.

Nipple care becomes very important if a mother is experiencing sore nipples or has injured nipples. Following a feeding, a mother may be more comfortable if she gently washes her nipples with plain water, then leaves her breasts exposed to air for the next 15 to 20 minutes. If she is wearing a nursing bra, she can simply lower the flaps. This allows the nipples to dry completely after the constant moisture of the nursing session. After washing, the nipples can be patted with a towel, but should never be rubbed.

Dry warmth, such as sunshine or a 40-watt light bulb placed about 18 inches from the breast, will further the drying, speed healing, and soothe and toughen the nipples. This procedure should be repeated after each feeding if a mother is having problems. Some mid-wives go so far as to suggest that *all* new nursing mothers apply heat several times a day to prevent sore nipples. Care should be taken to see that the nipples are not burned, and the heat should be applied for 15 to 20 minutes at a time. Afterward, a cream such as A and D ointment, hydrous lanolin, or Massé cream may be applied. These creams do not need to be removed before the baby begins its next feeding.

Special nursing techniques can be very helpful to a mother with sore nipples. First, if a mother's nipples do not tend to be erect, she may find it helpful to stimulate the areola until her nipple stands out. If her breasts are engorged or her letdown reflex tends to be slow, she should not only stimulate the area around the nipples, she should manually express some milk so that the baby has to do a minimum of sucking to bring the milk down. Another way to deal with a slow letdown reflex is to start the baby on the less sore breast, regardless of which side was last nursed, then as soon as the milk lets down switch the baby to the breast last nursed, returning to the other breast for the end of the feeding.

To help deal with nipple soreness it's good for the mother to vary her nursing position from feeding to feeding (see p. 490). This keeps the baby from repeatedly exerting pressure on the same tender spot. Also, instead of cradling the baby across her stomach when she's

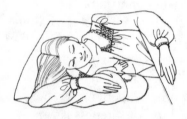

One way the new mother can help relieve or prevent sore nipples is to vary the position in which she nurses. This tends to keep the baby from repeatedly exerting pressure on the same sore spot. When the mother lies down, the baby can be placed upside down in relation to her; when she is sitting, the baby can be held under her arm instead of across her lap.

sitting up to nurse, the mother can adopt the "football position," tucking the baby under one arm with its feet pointing toward her back. When the mother nurses lying down, she can try leaning way over the baby so that it nurses from the higher breast rather than the lower one. Both this and the football position tend to be a little more awkward than the standard sitting or lying positions, but they will be worth the extra effort if a woman's nipples are truly uncomfortable. In both cases pillows can be used to help prop the baby at the proper height and angle. Finally, the mother can gently turn the baby as it nurses or can gradually rotate her nipple in the baby's mouth with the fingers of her steering hand.

Whenever the mother is taking the baby off the breast, she should carefully break the baby's suction by putting her finger in its mouth; she should not pull the baby off. A mother with sore nipples should never let the baby fall asleep with the nipple in its mouth or suck for long periods of time after both breasts have been emptied. Babies who seem to need to suck all the time can be given an orthodontically shaped pacifier or allowed to suck on someone's finger rather than the mother's nipple. Paradoxically, if a mother has been delaying feedings because of discomfort, she is likely to find she's more comfortable if she switches to more frequent short feedings. Most experts now advise mothers to use nipple shields only as a last resort, because they interfere with the baby's normal sucking patterns and are confusing to the baby in much the same way that a bottle is. Some doctors will recommend that mothers with sore nipples wear shields *in between* nursings, because they allow air to circulate around the nipples and promote drying.

Getting the Baby on the Nipple

For many mothers the hardest part of early breast-feeding is getting the baby on the nipple. Difficulty at the beginning of a feeding can be frustrating and upsetting for baby and mother. Probably the most common cause of this problem is some degree of engorgement. This is best dealt with by expressing some milk from each breast until the areola becomes soft. Another cause of difficulty in getting on is due to nipples that do not protrude. In this case the mother is advised to stimulate the nipple manually before the baby begins to feed.

Problems in getting the baby on can also arise from incorrect nursing techniques. These include holding the baby's head and neck too firmly; leaning too far forward, which causes the baby to slide off the nipple; and not depressing the breast under the baby's nose, which makes the baby less secure about its breathing. Also, mothers sometimes interfere with the baby's natural rooting reflex, either by attempting to put the nipple directly into the baby's mouth or by acci-

Nursing and returning to work

- Practice manual expression of milk, especially when the baby sleeps through a feeding.
- Clean hands and bottle carefully before expressing milk. Freeze or refrigerate milk immediately. Transport the milk in a small ice chest.
- If you are using a breast pump, practice and become familiar with its use several weeks prior to returning to work.
- If you are planning to supplement, teach the baby to drink from a bottle a week or two before returning to work. If you do not plan to express and store milk, introduce the baby to formula in advance of returning to work.
- Have the person who will care for the baby feed it a bottle several times in the weeks before you return to work. Warm the milk before serving.
- Before returning to work, arrange for breaks to express your milk, or arrange to go home or to have the baby brought to you if you live nearby.
- The baby will need one bottle if you are working a part-time job, two bottles if you are working longer.

dentally touching the baby's cheek while it is trying to grasp the nipple (see p. 468). The mother needs to remember that the baby automatically turns its head toward anything that touches its cheek; when the baby is touched by two things at the same time, it tends to become confused.

Occasionally problems getting on have to do with the baby's mood or character. Babies have very different personalities, which is readily seen in their nursing styles. When they are excited, some babies alternately grasp the nipple and then let go and scream. If possible, these babies should be quieted or soothed with walking or rocking before being put back on the breast. In general with this type of baby, nursing is easiest if the mother responds promptly to cries of hunger and if she seeks out a quiet, undistracting place to nurse.

Other babies tend to show only mild interest in nursing, especially for the first few days. They may spend most of their time licking the mother's nipple, or they may nurse a little and then lose interest. Such reactions can be caused by drugs in the baby's system as well as by the baby's personality. In either case, most of these babies become hungrier and more attentive by the fourth or fifth day. Until then holding the baby upright, rubbing its back, and talking to it before a feeding may help to stimulate the baby. A special maneuver called *jackknifing* will actually make the baby physiologically more alert. The mother bends the baby's head and feet toward each other 15 to 30

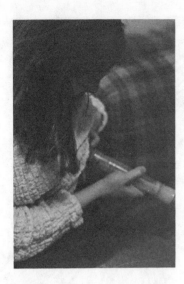

Breast pumps are very useful when a mother returns to work, but still wishes to breastfeed. Photo by Michael Samuels.

times fairly rapidly in succession. This increases blood flow to the heart from the vena cava, the major vein returning blood from the lower body. Increased blood flow, in turn, causes the heart to pump more freshly oxygenated blood to the brain, making the baby more alert. Some doctors advise doing this procedure right before a feeding if a baby is consistently sleepy or disinterested in eating.

Many mothers and sometimes even their pediatricians wonder if the baby is getting sufficient milk. According to most nursing experts, there are very few babies who fail to get enough milk because their mother has an inadequate supply. A woman who nurses on demand and who drinks a reasonable amount of liquids virtually always has enough milk for her baby. Problems with insufficiency are most often due to not nursing enough or to difficulties with nursing technique.

In addition to the nursing problems we have already discussed, concern over adequacy of milk may be due to difficulties with the letdown reflex. Other than engorgement or nipple soreness, the most common reasons for letdown problems are tension, anxiety, fatigue, fear, and worry. The letdown reflex is profoundly influenced by the mother's feelings and her environment (see p. 414). This is because the muscle cells in the breast that control the letdown reflex are regulated by the *autonomic nervous system,* which is not under as direct control as are voluntary movements. Often a new mother's worries and concerns can be put to rest by talking with a knowledgeable, sympathetic person—a doctor, midwife, relative, or friend. Fatigue can be combatted with frequent naps, since a full night's sleep is unlikely in the first few weeks after delivery. And immediate easing of tension can often be achieved by relaxation techniques or by engaging in physically relaxing activities (see p. 163).

According to pediatricians, it's not difficult at all to tell if a baby is getting enough milk. If a baby appears satisfied at the end of feedings and sleeps contentedly for an hour or so afterward, its milk intake is probably ample. Wakefulness by itself indicates a restless baby, but not necessarily one who is hungry. Babies who are getting enough to eat can be soothed between feedings by rocking or body contact, and they appear full after nursing. If, in addition, the baby has frequent wet diapers and every day or so has the characteristic loose stools of a breast-fed baby (see p. 457), the mother can be assured that the baby is getting sufficient food. Over a period of time weight gain is a good indicator of adequate milk supply. But most doctors feel it is not useful to weigh babies more than once a week, because their weight fluctuates enough so that frequent weighing can be misleading and can make the mother unnecessarily anxious rather than reassured.

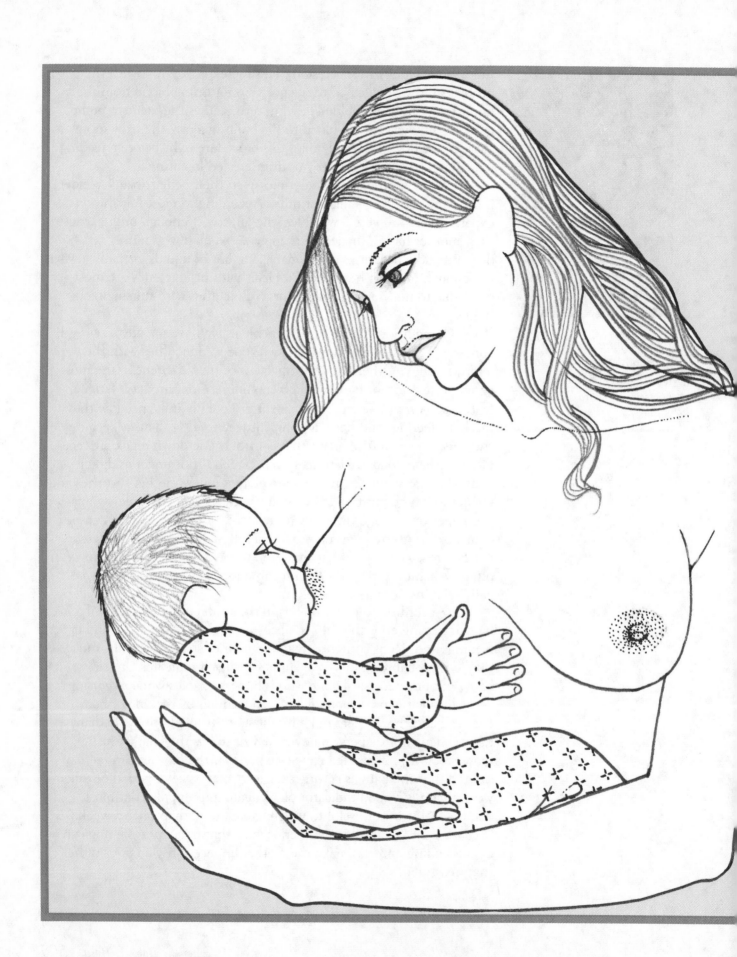

Epilogue

Final Thoughts

Writing *The Well Pregnancy Book* has been a fascinating and intense experience. Having written *The Well Baby Book*, which included chapters on prenatal development and delivery, we felt we knew a great deal about pregnancy and childbirth. But in doing in-depth research for this book, we learned much more. As we described the complex anatomy and physiology of pregnancy and delivery, we came to have a profound respect for what we call *the three-million-year-old mother* within every woman. The extraordinary mystery and capability of the human body is never more clearly demonstrated than in the process of conception, prenatal development, and birth. By the end of the book we felt more than ever that the basic lesson of childbirth is to help a woman trust in her own body.

At the same time, we are increasingly impressed by the value of good prenatal care—both by the mother herself and by her doctor or midwife. All the research we did pointed to the overwhelming importance of getting good nutrition, exercising regularly, avoiding substances that can harm the baby, and achieving support and relaxation throughout the whole of pregnancy. We feel that one of the most valuable aspects of this book is its emphasis on *preventive* medicine and

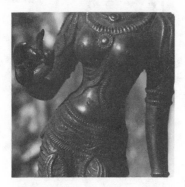

The basic lesson of childbirth is to help a woman trust in her own body. The Three-Million-Year-Old Mother. Photo by Michael Samuels.

the way prenatal care can avoid complications in pregnancy and delivery and improve the health of the baby as well as the mother.

Although we have always been advocates of prepared childbirth, we have developed increased respect for the value of relaxation and visualization in coping with the demands of labor and delivery. Putting together all the pieces of information on how the mind affects the uterus through the autonomic nervous system impressed upon us the great power of relaxation and prepared childbirth techniques. At the same time we became even more concerned with the tremendous, often overlooked, effect that the caregiver and the delivery environment have on the mother's frame of mind and thereby on her labor and delivery. More than ever, in the face of increasing technology, the field of obstetrics must humanize the birth process so that the mother is confident and unafraid, and is able to participate in this primeval experience with joy and enthusiasm. We believe that such humanization is not only necessary for the mother's comfort, but is essential to optimize the physiology of labor and delivery, reduce complications, and maximize the health of the newborn.

Future Trends

In this regard, we see trends in obstetrics that please us and others that disturb us. Trends that concern us are the increased technicalization of obstetrics without sufficient studies demonstrating the value of some procedures, and the implementation of new techniques without suffi-

This book is our way of sharing what we have learned with pregnant women everywhere. Nancy Pregnant. Photo by Michael Samuels.

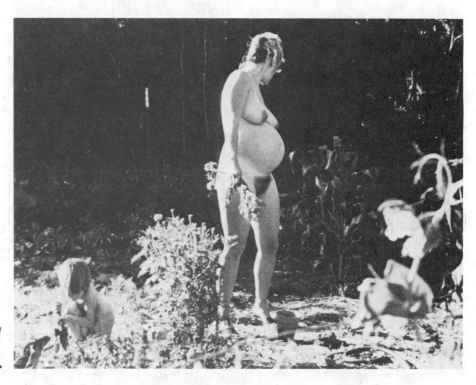

cient regard to how they can be used without distracting from the human character of the mother's birth experience. These trends are most apparent in the spiraling cesarean section rates.

There are several trends in obstetrics that we find heartening and that we believe point to the future. The widespread changes in nursery routines brought about by Klaus and Kennell's studies on bonding is an example of implementing humanistic concerns without sacrificing the quality of technical care. We feel that Klaus and Kennell's research on the value of a continuous caregiver during labor and delivery are of equal importance. We strongly believe that if undertaken widely, this concept could lead to a reduction in complication rates, as well as improving women's experiences. We hope that there will be more careful studies on the role of the autonomic nervous system and how stress and relaxation affect labor and delivery. The ultimate goal would be for science to work hand-in-hand with the three-million-year-old mother and the miraculous process humans have evolved for having babies.

We have tremendous empathy for pregnant women and new mothers and their babies. Having a baby is an act of commitment, courage, and optimism about life. We want to support these feelings. This book is our way of sharing what we have learned with pregnant women everywhere.

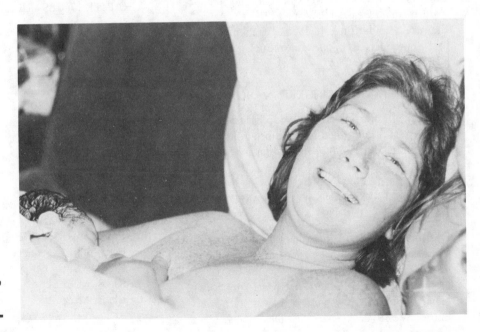

When a mother is confident and unafraid and able to participate in the birth experience with joy and enthusiasm, she optimizes her physiology for labor and delivery, reduces complications, and maximizes the health of her newborn. Photo by Linda O'Neil.

Notes

CHAPTER 5: NUTRITION DURING PREGNANCY

1. Worthington, B., Vermeersch, J., and Williams, S. 1977. *Nutrition in Pregnancy and Lactation.* C. V. Mosby, p. 55.
2. Ibid.

CHAPTER 6: EXERCISE AND SEX DURING PREGNANCY

1. Noble, E. 1984. "Pre-natal Exercise," in Sagov, S. *Home Birth.* Aspen Systems, p. 137.
2. *Op. Cit.,* p. 149.
3. Naeye, R. 1979. "Coitus and Associated Amniotic Fluid Infections." *New England Journal of Medicine* 301: 1198.
4. Herbst, A. 1979. "Coitus and the Fetus." *New England Journal of Medicine* 301: 1235.

CHAPTER 7: ENVIRONMENTAL AGENTS THAT AFFECT THE BABY DURING PREGNANCY

1. Catz, Charlotte. 1976. *Prevention of Embryonic, Fetal, and Perinatal Disease.* HEW, p. 123.
2. Stein, Z., and Kline, J. 1983. "Smoking, Alcohol, and Reproduction." *American Journal of Public Health* 73: 1154.

CHAPTER 8: STRESS DURING PREGNANCY

1. Norbeck, J., and Tilden, V. 1983. "Life Stress, Social Support, and Emotional Disequilibrium in Complications of Pregnancy." *Journal of Health and Social Behavior* 24: 33.

CHAPTER 9: RELAXATION AND PREPARED CHILDBIRTH TECHNIQUES

1. Heardman, H. 1959. *Physiotherapy in Obstetrics And Gynecology.* Livingstone, p. 90.
2. Ibid.
3. Noble, E. 1984. "Prenatal Exercise," in Sagov, S. *Home Birth.* Aspen Systems, p. 150.
4. Luthe, W. 1970. *Autogenic Therapy, Vol 4.* Grune & Stratton, p. 4.
5. Dick-Read, G. 1959. *Childbirth Without Fear.* Harper & Brothers, p. 13.

CHAPTER 10: PREPARING TO BREAST-FEED

1. Barnes, L., et al. 1978. "Breastfeeding." *Pediatrics* 62: 591.

CHAPTER 11: CHOICES FOR CHILDBIRTH

1. Sagov, S. 1984. *Home Birth.* Aspen Systems, p. 33
2. Kitzinger, S. 1981. *The Experience of Childbirth.* Penguin, p. 61.
3. Klaus, M. 1982. *Parent-Infant Bonding.* C. V. Mosby, p. 33.

CHAPTER 16: FETAL MONITORING

1. Varney, H. 1980. *Nurse-Midwifery.* Blackwell Scientific Publications, p. 180.
2. Lauersen, N. 1983. *Modern Management of High-Risk Pregnancy.* Plenum, p. 217.
3. National Institute of Child Health and Human Development. *Antenatal Diagnosis.* U.S. Department of Health, Education, and Welfare, p. 161.
4. Ibid., p. 165.
5. Ibid., p. 165.
6. Ibid., p. 168.

CHAPTER 17: CESAREAN BIRTH

1. National Institute of Child Health and Human Development. 1981. *Cesarean Childbirth.* U.S. Department of Health, Education, and Welfare.
2. Klaus, M. 1982. *Parent-Infant Bonding.* C. V. Mosby, p. 3.

CHAPTER 20: THE NEWBORN

1. Committee on Fetus and Newborn. 1975. "Report of The Ad Hoc Task Force On Circumcision." *Pediatrics* 56: 610.
2. Klaus, M. 1982. *Parent-Infant Bonding.* C. V. Mosby, p. 5.
3. Brazelton, T. B. "Behavioral Competence of the Newborn Infant." *Seminars in Perinatology* 3: 36.
4. Klaus, M., p. 39.
5. Klaus, M., p. 2.
6. Klaus, M., p. 98.

CHAPTER 21: BREAST-FEEDING

1. DeCarvalho, M. 1983. "The Effect of Frequent Breastfeeding on Early Milk Production and Infant Weight Gain." *Pediatrics* 72: 309.
2. Applebaum, R. 1975. "The Obstetrician's Approach To The Breasts and Breastfeeding." *The Journal of Reproductive Medicine* 14: 109.

Bibliography

CHAPTER 1: INTRODUCTION

Samuels, M., and Bennett, H. 1972. *The Well Body Book.* Random House/Bookworks.

Samuels, M., and Samuels, N. 1979. *The Well Baby Book.* Summit Books.

Samuels, M., and Samuels, N. 1982. *The Well Child Book.* Summit Books.

CHAPTER 2: BIRTH IN DIFFERENT CULTURES

Berndt, R. 1974. *Australian Aboriginal Religion.* E. J. Brill.

Berndt, R., and Berndt, C. 1951. *Sexual Behavior in Western Arnheim Land.* Viking Fund Publications in Anthropology.

Eliade, M. 1963. *Patterns in Comparative Religion.* Meridian Books.

Elkin, A. P. 1977. *Aboriginal Men of High Degree.* St. Martin's Press.

Engelmann, G. 1882. *Labor Among Primitive Peoples.* H. Chambers & Company.

Evans-Wentz, W. Y. 1960. *The Tibetan Book of the Dead.* Oxford University Press.

Ford, C. 1964. *A Comparative Study of Human Reproduction.* Human Area Relations File.

Hanks, J. 1963. *Maternity and Its Rituals in Bang Chan.* Cornell University.

Hart, D. 1965. *Southeast Asian Birth Customs.* Human Relations Area File.

Jordan, B. 1980. *Birth in Four Cultures.* Eden Press.

Mead, M., and Newton, N. 1967. "Cultural Patterning of Perinatal Behavior," in Richardson, S., and Guttmacher, A. 1967. *Childbearing—Its Social and Psychological Aspects.* Williams & Wilkins Co.

Montagu, A. 1937. *Coming Into Being Among the Australian Aborigines.* George Rutledge and Sons.

Stevenson, I. 1974. *Twenty Cases Suggestive of Reincarnation.* University Press of Virginia.

CHAPTER 3: ANATOMY AND PHYSIOLOGY OF THE MOTHER

Benson, R. 1982. *Current Obstetric and Gynecological Diagnosis and Treatment.* Lang Medical Publications.

Danforth, D. 1971. *Textbook of Obstetrics and Gynecology.* Harper & Row.

Jensen, M. 1981. *Maternity Care.* C. V. Mosby.

Pritchard, J., and MacDonald, P. 1980. *Williams Obstetrics.* Appleton-Century-Crofts.

Varney, H. 1980. *Nurse Midwifery.* Blackwell Scientific Publications Inc.

CHAPTER 4: DEVELOPMENT OF THE BABY

Balinsky, B. I. 1975. *An Introduction to Embryology.* W. B. Saunders.

Hamilton, W. J., and Mossman, H. W. 1972. *Human Embryology.* Williams & Wilkins Co.

Moore, K. 1982. *The Developing Human.* W. B. Saunders Co.

Nielsen, L. 1977. *A Child Is Born.* Dell.

Rugh, R., and Shettles, L. 1971. *From Conception to Birth.* Harper & Row.

CHAPTER 5: NUTRITION DURING PREGNANCY

Anderson, G. 1979. "Nutrition in Pregnancy." *Southern Medical Journal* 72: 1304.

Brewer, G. 1977. *What Every Pregnant Woman Should Know: The Truth About Diets And Drugs in Pregnancy.* Random House.

Burke, B. S., et al. 1943. "The Influence of Nutrition Upon the Condition of the Infant at Birth." *Journal of Nutrition* 26: 569.

California Department of Health. 1975. *Nutrition During Pregnancy and Lactation.* California Department of Health.

Hart, D. 1965. *Southeast Asian Birth Customs.* Human Relations Area File.

Higgins, A. 1976. "Nutritional Status and the Outcome of Pregnancy." *Journal of the Canadian Dietary Association* 37: 17.

Leader, A., Wong, K., and Deitel, M. "Maternal Nutrition in Pregnancy." *California Medical Journal* 125: 545.

Varney, H. 1980. *Nurse Midwifery.* Blackwell Scientific Publications, Inc.

Williams, S. 1974. *Essentials of Nutrition and Diet Therapy*. C. V. Mosby.

Winick, M. 1968. "Nutrition and Cell Growth." *Nutritional Review* 26: 195.

Worthington, B., Vermeersch, J., and Williams, S. 1977. *Nutrition In Pregnancy And Lactation*. C. V. Mosby.

CHAPTER 6: EXERCISE AND SEX DURING PREGNANCY

Bing, E., and Coleman, L. 1977. *Making Love During Pregnancy*. Bantam Books.

Collings, C., et al. 1983. "Maternal and Fetal Responses to a Maternal Aerobic Exercise Program." *American Journal of Obstetrics and Gynecology* 145: 702.

Edwards, P., et. al. 1983. "Fitness and Pregnancy." *Canadian Journal of Public Health* 74: 86.

Eichner, E. 1983. "Exercise and Heart Disease." *The American Journal of Medicine* 75: 1008.

Goodlin, R. 1971. "Orgasm During Late Pregnancy: Possible Deleterious Effects." *Obstetrics and Gynecology* 38: 916.

Herbst, A. 1979. "Coitus and the Fetus." *New England Journal of Medicine* 301: 1235.

Mills, J., et al. 1981. "Should Coitus Late in Pregnancy Be Discouraged?" *Lancet*, July 18, 1981: 136.

Naeye, R. 1979. "Coitus And Associated Amniotic-Fluid Infections." *The New England Journal of Medicine* 301: 1198.

Naeye, R. 1981. "Coitus and Antepartum Haemorrhage." *British Journal of Obstetrics and Gynecology* 88: 765.

Noble, E. 1982. *Essential Exercises for the Childbearing Year*. Houghton Mifflin.

Noble, E. 1984. "Prenatal Exercise," in Sagov, S. *Home Birth*. Aspen Systems Corporation.

Paffenbarger, R., et al. 1978. "Physical Activity as an Index of Heart Attack Risk in College Alumni." *American Journal of Epidemiology* 108: 161.

Pomerance, J., et al. 1974. "Physical Fitness and Pregnancy: Its Effect on Pregnancy Outcome." *American Journal of Obstetrics and Gynecology* 119: 867.

CHAPTER 7: ENVIRONMENTAL AGENTS THAT AFFECT THE BABY DURING PREGNANCY

Bracken, M., and Holford, T. 1981. "Exposure to Prescribed Drugs in Pregnancy and Association With Congenital Malformations." *Obstetrics & Gynecology* 58: 336.

Catz, C. 1976. *Prevention of Embryonic, Fetal, and Perinatal Disease*. DHEW Publication 76-853.

Cordero, J., and Oakley, G. 1983. "Drug Exposure During Pregnancy." *Clinical Obstetrics and Gynecology* 26.

Cushner, I. M. 1981. "Maternal Behavior and Perinatal Risks: Alcohol, Smoking, And Drugs." *Annual Review of Public Health* 2: 201.

Dunn, G. 1977. "Maternal Cigarette Smoking During Pregnancy and the Child's Subsequent Development: Neurological and Intellectual Maturation at the Age of 6½ Years." *Canadian Journal of Public Health* 68: 43.

Greenland, S., et al. 1982. "The Effects of Marijuana Use During Pregnancy." *American Journal of Obstetrics and Gynecology* 143: 408.

Heinonen, O., et al. 1977. *Birth Effects and Drugs in Pregnancy*. Publishing Sciences Group.

Hemminki, K., et al. 1983. "Assessment of Methods and Results of Reproductive Occupational Epidemiology: Spontaneous Abortions and Malformations in the Offspring of Working Women." *American Journal of Industrial Medicine* 4: 293.

Jensen, M. 1981. *Maternity Care*. C. V. Mosby.

Jones, K., and Smith, D. 1973. "Recognition of the Fetal-Alcohol Syndrome in Early Infancy." *Lancet* 2: 999.

Kirkinen, P., et al. 1983. "The Effect of Caffeine on Placental and Fetal Blood Flow in Human Pregnancy." *American Journal of Obstetrics and Gynecology* 147: 939.

Kline, J., et al. 1981. "Epidemiological Detection of Low Dose Effects on the Developing Fetus." *Environmental Health Perspectives* 42: 119.

Lemoine, P., et al. 1968. "Les Enfants de Parents Alcooliques." *Ouest Med* 21: 46.

Picone, T., et al. 1982. "Pregnancy Outcome in North American Women: Effects of Diet, Cigarette Smoking, and Psychological Stress on Maternal Weight Gain." *American Journal of Clinical Nutrition* 36: 1205.

Saxton, D. 1978. "The Behavior of Infants Whose Mothers Smoke in Pregnancy." *Early Human Development* 2: 363.

Shepard, T. H. 1980. *Catalogue of Teratogenic Agents*. The Johns Hopkins University Press.

Stein, Z., and Kline, J. 1983. "Smoking, Alcohol, and Reproduction." *American Journal of Public Health* 73: 1154.

Surgeon General's Report. 1979. *Healthy People*. U.S. Department of Health, Education, and Welfare.

U.S. Department of Health, Education, and Welfare. 1982. *Prevention of Embryonic, Fetal, and Perinatal Disease*. U.S. Government Printing Office.

Zacharias, J. 1983. "A Rational Approach to Drug Use in Pregnancy." *JOGN Nursing*, May 1983: 184.

CHAPTER 8: STRESS DURING PREGNANCY

Barnett, B., et al. 1983. "Life Events Scales for Obstetric Groups." *Journal of Psychosomatic Research* 27: 313.

Cramden, A. 1978. "Maternal Anxiety and Obstetric Complications." *Journal of Psychosomatic Research* 23: 109.

Gorsuch, R., and Key, M. 1974. "Abnormalities of Pregnancy as a Function of Anxiety and Life Stress." *Psychosomatic Medicine* 36: 353.

Gottschalk, L. 1983. "Vulnerability to Stress." *American Journal of Psychotherapy* 37: 5.

Holmes, T. H., and Rahe, R. H. 1967. "The Social Readjustment Rating Scale." *Journal of Psychosomatic Research* 11: 213.

Lederman, R. P., et al. 1978. "The Relationship of Maternal Anxiety, Plasma Catecholamines and Plasma Cortisol to Progress in Labor." *American Journal of Obstetrics and Gynecology* 132: 495.

McDonald, R. 1968. "The Role of Emotional Factors in Obstetric Complications: A Review." *Psychosomatic Medicine* 30: 224.

Norbeck, J., and Tilden, V. 1983. "Life Stress, Social Support, and Emotional Disequilibrium in Complications of Pregnancy." *Journal of Health and Social Behavior* 24: 30.

Nuckolls, K., et al. 1972. "Psychosocial Assets, Life Crisis and the Prognosis of Pregnancy." *American Journal of Epidemiology* 95: 431.

Pelletier, K. 1978. *Toward a Science of Consciousness*. Dell.

Picone, T., et al. 1982. "Pregnancy Outcome in North American Women. I. Effects of Diet, Cigarette Smoking, and Psychological Stress on Maternal Weight Gain." *American Journal of Clinical Nutrition* 36: 1205.

Smilkstein, G., et al. 1984. "Predictions of Pregnancy Complications: An Application of the Biopsychosocial Model." *Social Sciences in Medicine* 18: 315.

CHAPTER 9: RELAXATION AND PREPARED CHILDBIRTH TECHNIQUES

Bradley, R. 1974. *Husband-Coached Childbirth*. Harper & Row.

Buxton, C. 1962. *A Study of Psychophysical Methods for Relief of Childbirth Pain*. W. B. Saunders.

Chertok, L. 1959. *Psychosomatic Methods in Painless Childbirth*. Pergamon Press.

Dick-Read, G. 1959. *Childbirth Without Fear*. Harper & Brothers.

Heardman, H. 1959. *Physiotherapy in Obstetrics and Gynecology*. Livingston.

Jacobson, E. 1965. *How to Relax and Have Your Baby*. McGraw-Hill.

Kitzinger, S. 1974. *The Experience of Childbirth*. Penguin.

Lamaze, F. 1970. *Painless Childbirth: Psychoprophylactic Method*. Henry Regnery.

LeBoyer, F. 1977. *Inner Beauty, Inner Light*. Knopf.

Luthe, W. 1970. *Autogenic Therapy*. Grune & Stratton.

Noble, E. 1984. "Prenatal Exercise," from Sagov, S. *Home Birth*. Aspen Systems Corporation.

Odent, M. 1984. *Birth Reborn*. Pantheon.

Samuels, M., and Samuels, N. 1975. *Seeing With the Mind's Eye*. Random House/Bookworks.

CHAPTER 10: PREPARING TO BREAST-FEED

Barnes, L., et al. 1978. "Breast-Feeding." *Pediatrics* 62: 591.

Klaus, M., et al. 1981. "Child Health and Breast Feeding: The Effect of a Supportive Woman During Labor and the Effect of Early Suckling." *Pediatric Research* 15: 450.

Mata, L. 1978. "Breastfeeding and Infant Health." *American Journal of Clinical Nutrition* 31: 2058.

Ogra, P. L., and Greene, H. 1982. "Human Milk and Breastfeeding: An Update on the State of the Art." *Pediatric Research* 16: 266.

Ogra, S. S., and Ogra, P. L. 1978. "Immunological Aspects of Human Colostrum and Milk." *The Journal of Pediatrics* 92: 546.

Waletzky, L. 1976. *Symposium on Human Lactation*. U.S. Department of Health, Education, and Welfare.

CHAPTER 11: CHOICES FOR CHILDBIRTH

Cohen, N., and Estner, L. 1983. *Silent Knife*. Bergin and Garvey.

Kitzinger, S. 1978. *The Place of Birth*. Oxford University Press.

Kitzinger, S. 1979. *Birth at Home*. Oxford University Press.

Klaus, M., and Kennell, J. 1982. *Parent-Infant Bonding*. C. V. Mosby.

Lumley, J. 1983. "Preschool Siblings at Birth: Short-Term Effects." *Birth* 10: 11

McRae, M. 1983, "Alternatives in Childbirth," from Cohen, W., and Friedman, E. *Management Of Labor*. University Park Press.

Odent, M. 1984. *Birth Reborn*. Pantheon.

Sagov, S. 1984. *Home Birth*. Aspen Systems Corporation.

Sosa, R., et al. 1980. "The Effect of a Supportive Companion on Perinatal Problems, Length of Labor, and Mother-Infant Interaction." *New England Journal of Medicine* 303: 597.

CHAPTER 12: PRENATAL CARE AND MEDICAL CONCERNS

Baker, D. 1983. "Herpes Genitalis." *Clinics in Obstetrics and Gynecology* 10: 3.

Benson, R. 1982. *Current Obstetric and Gynecologic Diagnosis and Treatment*. Lang Medical Publications.

Bishop, E. 1982. *Perinatal Medicine: Practical Diagnosis And Management*. Addison-Wesley.

Blum, M. 1979. "Is the Elderly Primipara Really at Risk?" *Journal of Perinatal Medicine* 7: 108.

Bolognese, R., et al. 1981. "Prenatal Care and the Prevention of Infection." *Clinics In Perinatology* 8: 617.

Brann, A. 1980. "Perinatal Herpes Simplex Virus Infections." *Pediatrics* 66: 147.

Cohen, W., et al. 1980. "Risk of Labor Abnormalities With Advancing Maternal Age." *Obstetrics and Gynecology* 55: 1980.

Fadel, H. 1982. *Diagnosis and Management of Obstetric Emergencies*. Addison-Wesley.

Frenkel, J. 1981. "Congenital Toxoplasmosis: Prevention or Palliation?" *American Journal of Obstetrics and Gynecology* 141: 359.

Grimes, D., and Gross, G. 1981. "Pregnancy Outcomes in Black Women Aged 35 and Older." *Obstetrics and Gynecology* 58: 614.

Jensen, M. 1981. *Maternity Care*. C. V. Mosby.

Lauersen, N. 1983. *Modern Management of High-Risk Pregnancy*. Plenum Medical Book Company.

Nahmias, A., and Roizman, B. 1973. "Infections With Herpes Simplex Viruses 1 and 2." *New England Journal of Medicine* 289: 667.

National Institute of Child Health and Human Development. 1979. *Antenatal Diagnosis*. U.S. Department of Health, Education, and Welfare.

National Institute of Child Health and Human Development. 1976. "Mid-Trimester Amniocentesis for Prenatal Diagnosis: Safety and Accuracy." *Journal of the American Medical Association* 236: 1471.

Pritchard, J., and MacDonald, P. 1980. *Williams Obstetrics*. Appleton-Century-Crofts.

Sabbagha, R., et al. 1982. "The Use of Ultrasound in Obstetrics." *Clinical Obstetrics and Gynecology* 25: 735.

Simpson, H., et al. 1976. "Perinatal Diagnosis of Genetic Disease in Canada." *Canadian Medical Association Journal* 115: 739.

Simpson, J., and Verp, M. 1982. "The Prenatal Diagnosis of Genetic Disorders." *Clinical Obstetrics and Gynecology* 25: 635.

Stein, A. 1983. "Pregnancy in Gravidas Over Age 35 Years." *Journal of Nurse-Midwifery* 28: 17.

Stratmeyer, M. 1980. "Research in Ultrasound Bioeffects: A Public Health View." *Birth and the Family Journal* 7: 92.

Wilson, C., and Remington, J. 1980. "What Can Be Done to Prevent Congenital Toxoplasmosis?" *American Journal of Obstetrics and Gynecology* 138: 357.

Working Party on Amniocentesis. 1978. "An Assessment of the Hazards of Amniocentesis." *British Journal of Obstetrics and Gynecology* 85: 2.

CHAPTER 13: THE PHYSIOLOGY OF LABOR

Caldeyro-Barcia, R. 1979. "The Influence of Maternal Position on Time of Spontaneous Rupture of the Membranes, Progress of Labor, and Fetal Heal Compression." *Birth and the Family Journal* 6: 10.

Danforth, D. 1971. *Textbook of Obstetrics and Gynecology*. Harper & Row.

Dick-Read, G. 1959. *Childbirth Without Fear.* Harper & Brothers.

Friedman, E. 1978. *Labor: Clinical Evaluation and Management.* Appleton-Century-Crofts.

Oxorn, H., and Foote, W. 1975. *Human Labor and Birth.* Appleton-Century-Crofts.

Pajntar, M. 1982. "Psychosomatic Disturbances in the Course of Labor." In Prill, H. *Advances In Psychosomatic Obstetrics and Gynecology.* Springer-Verlag.

Pritchard, J., and MacDonald, P. 1980. *Williams Obstetrics.* Appleton-Century-Crofts.

CHAPTER 14: THE MOTHER'S EXPERIENCE OF LABOR AND HOW IT IS MANAGED

Barnett, M. 1982. "Infant Outcome in Relation to Second Stage Labor Pushing Method." *Birth* 9: 221.

Beynon, C. 1957. "The Normal Second Stage of Labor: A Plea for Reform in Its Conduct." *Journal of Obstetrics and Gynecology* 64: 815.

Caldeyro-Barcia, R. 1979. "The Influence of Maternal Bearing-Down Efforts During Second Stage on Fetal Well-Being." *Birth and the Family Journal* 6: 19.

Cohen, W., and Friedman, E. 1983. *Management of Labor.* University Park Press.

Friedman, E. 1978. *Labor: Clinical Evaluation And Management.* Appleton-Century-Crofts.

Hassid, P. 1978. *Textbook for Childbirth Educators.* Harper & Row.

Kitzinger, S. 1981. *The Experience of Childbirth.* Penguin Books.

LeBoyer, F. 1976. *Birth Without Violence.* Knopf.

Noble, E. 1982. *Essential Exercises for the Childbearing Year.* Houghton Mifflin.

Varney, H. 1980. *Nurse-Midwifery.* Blackwell Scientific Publications.

CHAPTER 15: THE MOTHER'S EXPERIENCE OF DELIVERY

Banta, D. 1982. "The Risks and Benefits of Episiotomy: A Review." *Birth* 9: 25.

Caldeyro-Barcia, R. 1960. "The Effect of Position Changes on the Intensity and Frequency of Uterine Contractions During Labor." *American Journal of Obstetrics and Gynecology* 80: 284.

Caldeyro-Barcia, R. 1975. "Some Consequences of Obstetrical Interference." *Birth and the Family Journal* 2: 34.

Cohen, W., and Friedman, E. 1983. *Management of Labor.* University Park Press.

Friedman, E. 1978. *Labor: Clinical Evaluation and Management.* Appleton-Century-Crofts.

Kitzinger, S. 1981. *The Experience of Childbirth.* Penguin Books.

LeBoyer, F. 1976. *Birth Without Violence.* Knopf.

Newton, N. "Interrelationships Between Sexual Responsiveness, Birth, and Breastfeeding," in *Maternalism and Woman's Sexuality.* p. 77–98.

Oxorn, H., and Foote, W. 1975. *Human Labor and Birth.* Appleton-Century-Crofts.

Pritchard, J., and MacDonald, P. 1980. *Williams Obstetrics.* Appleton-Century-Crofts.

Varney, H. 1980. *Nurse-Midwifery.* Blackwell Scientific Publications.

CHAPTER 16: FETAL MONITORING

Haverkamp, A., et al. 1976. "The Evaluation of Continuous Fetal Heartrate Monitoring in High-Risk Pregnancy." *American Journal of Obstetrics and Gynecology* 125: 310.

Kelso, H., et al. 1978. "An Assessment of Continuous Fetal Heartrate Monitoring in Labor." *American Journal of Obstetrics and Gynecology* 131: 526.

Lauersen, N. 1983. *Modern Management of High-Risk Pregnancy.* Plenum.

National Institute of Child Health and Human Development. 1979. *Antenatal Diagnosis.* U.S. Department of Health, Education, and Welfare.

Neutra, R., et al. 1978. "The Effect of Fetal Monitoring on Neonatal Death Rates." *New England Journal of Medicine* 299: 324.

Paul, R., and Hon, E. 1974. "Clinical Fetal Monitoring." *American Journal of Obstetrics and Gynecology* 118: 529.

Schifrin, B. 1982. "The Fetal Monitoring Polemic." *Clinics in Perinatology* 9: 399.

Varney, H. 1980. *Nurse-Midwifery.* Blackwell Scientific Publications.

Wood, C., et al. 1981. "A Controlled Trial of Fetal Heartrate Monitoring in a Low Risk Obstetric Population." *American Journal of Obstetrics and Gynecology* 141: 527.

CHAPTER 17: CESAREAN BIRTH

Cohen, N., and Estner, L. 1983. *Silent Knife*. Bergin and Garvey.

Dewhurst, C. 1968. "The Ruptured Cesarean Scar." *Journal of Obstetrics and Gynecology* 75: 1296.

Donovan, B. 1977. *The Cesarean Birth Experience*. Beacon Press.

Haverkamp, A., et al. 1979. "A Controlled Trial of the Differential Effects of Intrapartum Fetal Monitoring." *American Journal of Obstetrics and Gynecology* 134: 399.

Kehoe, C. 1981. *The Cesarean Experience*. Appleton-Century-Crofts.

Klaus, M., and Kennell, J. 1982. *Parent-Infant Bonding*. C. V. Mosby.

Levin, J. 1983. "Vaginal Delivery After Cesarean Birth: Frequently Asked Questions." *Clinics In Perinatology* 10: 439.

Monheit, A., and Resnik, R. 1981. "Cesarean Section: Current Trends and Perspectives." *Clinics In Perinatology* 8: 101.

National Institute of Child Health and Human Development. 1979. *Antenatal Diagnosis*. U.S. Department of Health, Education, and Welfare.

National Institute of Child Health and Human Development. 1981. *Cesarean Childbirth*. U.S. Department of Health, Education, and Welfare.

O'Sullivan, M., et al. 1981. "Vaginal Delivery After Cesarean Section." *Clinics In Perinatology* 8: 131.

Shy, K., et al. 1981. "Evaluation of Elective Repeat Cesarean Section as a Standard of Care." *American Journal of Obstetrics and Gynecology* 139: 123.

Sosa, R., et al. 1980. "The Effect of a Supportive Companion on Perinatal Problems, Length of Labor, and Mother-Infant Interaction." *New England Journal of Medicine* 303: 597.

CHAPTER 18: THE MOTHER'S PHYSIOLOGY AFTER CHILDBIRTH

Benson, R. 1982. *Current Obstetric and Gynecologic Treatment*. Lang Medical Publications.

Pritchard, J., and MacDonald, P. 1980. *Williams Obstetrics*. Appleton-Century-Crofts.

Varney, H. 1980. *Nurse-Midwifery*. Blackwell Scientific Publications.

CHAPTER 19: CONCERNS OF THE FIRST FEW WEEKS AFTER DELIVERY

Benson, R. 1982. *Current Obstetric and Gynecologic Treatment*. Lang Medical Publications.

Bing, E. 1982. *Making Love During Pregnancy*. Bantam Books.

Kitzinger, S. 1981. *The Experience of Childbirth*. Penguin Books.

Noble, E. 1982. *Essential Exercises for the Childbearing Year*. Houghton Mifflin.

Pritchard, J., and MacDonald, P. 1980. *Williams Obstetrics*. Appleton-Century-Crofts.

Varney, H. 1980. *Nurse-Midwifery*. Blackwell Scientific Publications.

CHAPTER 20: THE NEWBORN

Brazelton, T. B. 1979. "Behavioral Competence of the Newborn Infant." *Seminars In Perinatology* 3: 35.

Brazelton, T. B. 1983. "Developmental Framework of Infants and Children: A Future for Pediatric Responsibility." *The Journal of Pediatrics* 102: 967.

Committee on Fetus and Newborn. 1975. "Report of the Ad Hoc Task Force on Circumcision." *Pediatrics* 56: 610.

Condon, W., and Sander, L. 1974. "Neonate Movement Is Synchronized With Adult Speech." *Science* 183: 99.

Kempe, C., et al. 1982. *Current Pediatric Diagnosis and Treatment*. Lang Medical Publications.

Klaus, M., et al. 1982. "Maternal-Infant Bonding: A Joint Rebuttal." *Pediatrics* 72: 569.

Klaus, M., and Kennell, J. *Parent-Infant Bonding*. C. V. Mosby.

Lamb, M. 1982. "Early Contact and Maternal-Infant Bonding: One Decade Later." *Pediatrics* 70: 763.

Lester, B., et al. 1982. "Regional Obstetric Anesthesia and Newborn Behavior." *Child Development* 53: 687.

Lubchenco, L. 1980. "Routine Neonatal Circumcision: A Surgical Anachronism." *Clinical Obstetrics and Gynecology* 23: 1135.

MacFarlane, J., et al. 1978. "The Relationship Between Mother and Neonate," in Kitzinger, S. *The Place of Birth*. Oxford University Press.

Marshall, R., et al. 1982. "Circumcision: Effects Upon Mother-Infant Interaction." *Early Human Development* 7: 367.

Metcalf, T., et al. 1983. "Circumcision." *Clinical Pediatrics* 22: 575.

Samuels, M., and Samuels, N. 1984. "All About Circumcision." *Medical Self-Care* 20: 20

Siegel, E. 1982. "Early and Extended Maternal-Infant Contact." *American Journal of Diseases of Children* 136: 251.

Sosa, R., et al. 1980. "The Effect of a Supportive Companion on Perinatal Problems, Length of Labor, and Mother-Infant Interaction." *New England Journal of Medicine* 303: 597.

Vaughan, V., et al. 1979. *Nelson Textbook of Pediatrics.* W. B. Saunders.

Wallerstein, E. 1980. *Circumcision: An American Health Fallacy.* Springer.

Wolff, P. and Ferber, R. 1979. "The Development of Behavior in Human Infants, Premature and Newborn." *Annual Review of Neurosciences* 2: 291.

CHAPTER 21: BREAST-FEEDING

Applebaum, R. 1975. "The Obstetrician's Approach to the Breasts and Breastfeeding." *The Journal of Reproductive Medicine* 14: 98.

DeCarvalho, M., et al. 1983. "The Effect of Frequent Breast-feeding on Early Milk Production and Infant Weight Gain." *Pediatrics* 72: 307.

Esterly, N., et al. 1975. "The Obstetrician and Breast-feeding: Some Views of Women Physicians." *Journal of Reproductive Medicine* 14: 89.

Shepherd, S., and Yarrow, R. 1982. "Breastfeeding and the Working Mother." *Journal of Nurse-Midwifery* 27: 16.

Slaven, S., and Harvey, D. 1981. "Unlimited Suckling Time Improves Breast Feeding." *Lancet* (1981) 1: 392.

Index

A and D ointment, 502
abdominal muscles:
  exercise of, 38, 102–4, 105, 232, 410, 434–35
  of newborn, 456
  after pregnancy, 410, 434–35
abdominal pain, 260, 261, 263
  in active phase of labor, 316
  as early symptom, 228, 229
  in postdelivery period, 408
  spontaneous abortion and, 258–59
abdominal rubs, in labor, 318
aborigines, Australian, 12, 13
abortion, induced, 244–45
abortion, spontaneous, 119, 133, 258–60
  alcohol consumption and, 126, 127
  amniocentesis and, 244
  caffeine consumption and, 129
  cigarette smoking and, 123, 124
  cocaine and, 130
  sexual intercourse and, 111
  stress and, 145
abruptio placenta, 213, 261–62, 372
abusive parents, 473
acceleration phase of labor, 287–88, 307
acetone, 81
acne, 37, 461, 462
acrosome, 55
active phase of labor, 286, 287–88, 313–322
  prolonged, 315
active segment, 281–82
adrenal glands:
  fetal, 34
  in onset of labor, 274
  stress and, 138, 159
adrenaline (epinephrine), 139, 415
  caffeine and, 127–29
  exercise and, 99
  labor slowed by, 278–79
aerobic exercise, 98, 108–9, 232
aerosol propellants, 134
Africa:
  birthing practices in, 12, 14
  spiritual views of births in, 12–13, 15
after-baby blues, 440–43
afterbirth pains, 409, 419–21, 424
AFV (amniotic fluid volume test), 245

age:
  gestational, 224–25, 237, 381–82
  maternal, 250–52, 253
alcohol consumption:
  as controllable environmental agent, 121, 232
  fetal breathing movements affected by, 249
  male reproduction affected by, 135
  pregnancy affected by, 125–27, 133, 232
allergens, 183
allergies, 179, 182–83, 189
all-fours position, 313, 316
Alor tribe, 19
alpha fetoprotein, 241–42
alpha receptors, 278
alpha waves, 72
alternative birth centers, see birth centers
alveoli:
  breast, 30, 40, 43, 188, 412, 413
  pulmonary, 70, 451
American Academy of Husband Coached Childbirth, 206
American Academy of Pediatrics, 154, 177–78, 206, 381
American College of Home Obstetrics, 206
American College of Nurse Midwives, 206
American College of Obstetricians and Gynecologists, 206, 210, 212, 381
American Foundation for Maternal and Child Health, 206
American Journal of Public Health, 124
American Society for Psychoprophylaxis in Obstetrics, 206
amino acids, 179, 180
Aminopterin, 122, 133
amniocentesis, 197, 213, 237, 238–44
  indications for, 239–42
  procedure for, 242–43
  safety of, 243–44
amniotic cavity, 60
amniotic fluid, 69
  infection of, 114
  meconium staining of, 129, 213
amniotic fluid volume test (AFV), 245

amphetamines, 122, 131
ampicillin, 131
ampulla, 57
anacephaly, 241
android pelvic shape, 29
anemia, 228, 235
anesthesia:
  breast-feeding and, 488, 497
  for cesarean sections, 380, 381, 383–385, 386, 387, 390, 391
  for episiotomies, 339–40, 352
  fetal heart rate and, 359
  general, as childbirth hazard, 153–54
  hypnosis as, 154–55
  as occupational hazard, 133, 134, 135
  spontaneous abortion and, 133
  topical, 424
ankles, swollen, 37, 230
anovulatory state, postpartum, 435
anoxic infants, 153–54
anterior-posterior (A-P) distance, 28–29
anthropoid pelvic shape, 29
anti-amoeba drugs, 135
antibodies, 181–82, 183
  Rh, 48, 228
antibody titers, 255, 256
anticonvulsants, 135
antimetabolites, 503
anxiety, see stress
Apgar scores, 213, 349, 388
Applebaum, R. M., 495
Arabian Nights, The, 102
Arapesh tribe, 19
areola:
  changes of, during pregnancy, 43
  engorgement and, 498
  nursing and, 233, 486, 487, 492
  soreness in nursing and, 501
asbestos, 134
asexual reproduction, 52
aspiration, 383
aspirin, 131, 254, 255
Association for Childbirth at Home, International, 206
atenolol, 503
auricular hillocks, 62, 64
Australian aborigines, 12, 13
Autogenic training, 160–61

pituitary gland, 32, 64
  in beginning labor, 274, 409
  in menstrual cycle, 33, 34
  in nursing, 188
PKU (phenylketonuria), 120
placenta:
  abnormal placement of, 213, 261–62
  appearance of, 351
  blood flow to, 122–23
  chemicals affecting function of, 133
  disposal of, 17–18
  eating of, 19
  expulsion of, 298–301, 350–51
  genesis of, 34, 61
  hormones produced by, 31, 34, 35, 40,
    274–75, 412–13
  locating of, with ultrasound, 237
  maternal nutrition and, 78, 79, 80–81
  removal of, in cesarean section, 387
  retained, 213
  separation of, normal, 299–300, 351
  separation of, premature, 213, 261–62
placental barrier theory, 117
placental lactogen, 40
placental transfusion, 453–54
placenta previa:
  cesarean delivery and, 371, 372
  home delivery and, 213
  in third trimester bleeding, 261–62
platypelloid pelvic shape, 30
pleural fluid, 343
pneumonia, 182
polio, 181, 233
polychlorinated biphenyls (PCBs), 133
position, in uterus, 292, 293
postpartum period, 417–43
  afterbirth pains in, 409, 419–21, 424
  caring for new mother in, 418–19
  constipation in, 421–22
  emotions in, 437–43
  estrogen in, 409, 411
  exercise in, 100, 410, 432–35
  outside help and support in, 428–31
  perineal care in, 422–25
  rest and recuperation in, 425–28
  sexual activity in, 435–37
postural hypotension, 394
posture:
  exercises for, 38, 42, 104
  tips for, 39, 106, 232
poverty, maternal nutrition and, 79, 83
preeclampsia, 228, 265
pregnancy testing, 40, 61, 224
premature delivery:
  by cesarean section, 370
  cigarette smoking and, 124
  gestational age and, 225
  low birth weight and, 77
  marijuana and, 129–30
  orgasm and, 114
premature labor, 262–64
prenatal care, 223–67, 507–8
  diagnostic tests in, 235–50
  for high-risk pregnancies, 252–66
  hygiene in, 233

laboratory tests in, 228
physical exams in, 225–35, 309
  see also exercise; nutrition and diet,
    maternal
prep, for delivery, 197, 309
preparatory division of labor, 291
prepared childbirth techniques, 153–75,
    202–3
  Autogenic training, 160
  Bradley, 158, 159, 197, 206
  episiotomies and, 338
  historical roots of, 154–57
  hypnosis in, 154–55
  Lamaze, 158–59, 197, 206, 318
  natural childbirth, 155
  Progressive Relaxation, 155, 161
  psychoprophylaxis, 157–58
  psychosexual, 158
  rationale for, 153–54
  relaxation in, 159–64, 174
  visualization in, 165–75, 196
presentation, 291–93
  breech, 198, 213, 224, 292, 293, 371
prezepam, 503
primitive streak, 60
Prochownick, Ludwig, 76
progesterone, 31, 44, 275
  after delivery, 411
  immune responses and, 48–49
  in menstrual cycle, 33, 34
  pregnancy affected by, 35–40
programmed visualization, 165, 168–69,
    170–71
Progressive Relaxation, 161–62
prolactin, 411, 435
  milk production and, 188, 412, 413–
    414, 482
prolactin-inhibiting factor, 413
prolapsed cord, 371, 372
propylthiouracil, 122
prostoglandins, 275
protein metabolism, 47
protein requirements, calculation of, 86,
    87, 88, 93
proteinuria, 228, 265–67
psychoprophylaxis, 157–58
puberty, 55
pubic bone, 28, 29
pubic symphysis, 28
Public Health Service, U.S., alcohol
    consumption guidelines of, 127
pudendal block, 339–40
puerperium, 405
pulse-echo sonography, see ultrasound
Punjab:
  birthing practices in, 16
  postpartum care in, 18
pupillary light reflex, 72

quickening, 13

rabies immunization, 233
radiation, 134

birth defects and, 117–18, 119, 120–
  121
  critical periods for fetus and, 119
  ultrasound sonograms and, 236
radiopharmaceuticals, 503
Rahe, Richard, 142–43
raised skin areas, 256
rapid eye movement (REM) sleep, 72,
  426, 459
rashes, 256
receptive visualization, 165, 168, 171–72
rectal pain, 256
rectal sphincter, 101
rectus abdominus, 103, 105, 410, 434–35
reddened palms, 37
reddened skin, 256
reduction division, 55
reflexes:
  conditioned, in prepared childbirth,
    155, 157
  fetal, 67, 72
  letdown, 191, 391, 413, 414–15, 486,
    494, 500, 505
  in newborn, 468–69, 487, 491, 503–4
reincarnation, 14
relaxation response, 276
relaxation techniques, 159–64, 174, 233
  autosuggestion as, 162–64
  common elements of, 162
  during labor, 159–60, 277–78, 331
  after pregnancy, 169–71, 399, 427,
    429
  when to perform, 161, 164
  see also visualization techniques
REM (rapid eye movement) sleep, 72,
  426, 459
respiratory distress syndrome, 355
respiratory system:
  embryonic, 64
  fetal, 69, 70, 451
  maternal, effect of pregnancy on, 38,
    45
  of newborn, 153–54, 342, 343, 346–
    347, 358–59, 360, 450, 451–52
restitution, in delivery, 295, 334, 342
Rh incompatibility, 48, 228, 372
RhoGam shots, 228
rickets, 76
ripening, 273
rooting reflex, 468, 487, 491, 503–4
rotation:
  external, 295–98, 342
  internal, 295, 296
rubella, see German measles

sacral promontory, 227
sacred places, 12
sacroiliac joints, 28
sacrum, 28, 227
saline abortions, 244
salmon patches, 461
salt, in maternal diet, 76, 92
Sanpoil Indians, 15
Santa Maria Indians, 16
Sarason, Irwin, 144

About
the Authors

Mike Samuels is a physician and author. He attended Brown University and New York University College of Medicine. He has been interested in public health and preventive medicine since medical school. After internship he worked on the Hopi Indian Reservation for the U.S. Public Health Service and then worked for the Marin County Health Department. During the early 1970s he helped set up one of the first holistic medicine clinics in northern California and wrote a pioneering self-help medical book, *The Well Body Book*, with Hal Z. Bennett. Recently they have written an environmental health sourcebook, *Well Body, Well Earth*.

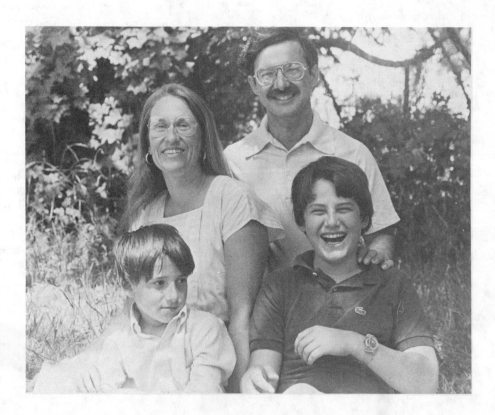

Nancy Harrison Samuels is an author and former nursery school teacher. She attended Brown University and Bank Street College of Education. After several years of teaching she did editorial work on *The Well Body Book*, and began to write with Mike. Together they have written *Seeing with the Mind's Eye*, a book on relaxation and mental imagery, and three books in a self-help series, *The Well Baby Book*, *The Well Child Book*, and *The Well Child Coloring Book*.

The Well Pregnancy Book is a natural addition to the Samuelses' work on child care. Its goal is to optimize pregnant women's health and their experience of having a baby. The Samuelses believe that self-help medical books are preventive medical tools for learning that provide valuable information and relieve natural concerns. Although they are unable to answer all letters individually, they appreciate hearing about readers' experiences and suggestions.

Mike and Nancy Samuels live in a small seacoast town in northern California, in a house they built themselves and continue to work on, much like their series of self-help books. They have a close family life and spend much of their free time doing projects with their sons, Rudy and Lewis. Together the family enjoys building, gardening, traveling, and camping.

About the Illustrator

Wendy Frost left Australia in 1965 to live in London where she worked for *The Observer* and various magazines and publishers. Since 1969 she has lived mainly in New York, with sojourns in Italy and Australia. She has also had numerous exhibitions of her paintings in Europe, the U.S.A., and Australia. Mike and Nancy Samuels have worked with her on three previous books. She now lives in New York with her eight-year-old son, Darcy Darwin.

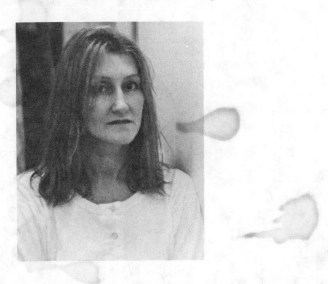